Adolescents with Down Syndrome

This book is printed on recycled paper. ♲

Adolescents with Down Syndrome
Toward a More Fulfilling Life

edited by

Siegfried M. Pueschel, M.D., Ph.D., J.D., M.P.H.
Child Development Center
Rhode Island Hospital
Providence
and
Mária Šustrová, M.D., Ph.D.
The Institute of Preventive and Clinical Medicine
Bratislava, Slovakia

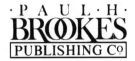

·P·A·U·L·H·
BROOKES
PUBLISHING CO.

Baltimore • London • Toronto • Sydney

Paul H. Brookes Publishing Co.
Post Office Box 10624
Baltimore, Maryland 21285-0624

Typeset by PRO-Image Corp., York, Pennsylvania.
Manufactured in the United States of America by
The Maple Press Company, York, Pennsylvania.

Some of the case studies described in this book are completely fictional, some are composites, and some are taken from actual experiences of real people. In the case of the fictional and composite case studies, any similarity to actual individuals or circumstances is coincidental and no resemblance to actual people or events should be inferred.

Library of Congress Cataloging-in-Publication Data
Adolescents with Down syndrome: toward a more fulfilling life / [edited by]
    Siegfried M. Pueschel, Mária Šustrová.
       p.   cm.
    Includes bibliographical references and index.
    ISBN 1-55766-281-9
    1. Down syndrome.   2. Handicapped teenagers—Rehabilitation.
  I. Pueschel, Siegfried M. II. Šustrová, Mária.
  RJ506.D68A34   1997
  616.85'8842'00835—dc21   96-52748
                                               CIP

British Cataloguing in Publication data are available from the British Library.

Contents

About the Editors

Siegfried M. Pueschel, M.D., Ph.D., J.D., M.P.H., Child Development Center, Rhode Island Hospital, 593 Eddy Street, Providence, Rhode Island 02903.

Dr. Pueschel studied medicine in Germany and graduated from the Medical Academy of Düsseldorf magna cum laude. He then pursued his pediatric residency training and subsequently was a fellow in biochemical genetics and metabolism. In 1967, he earned a master's degree in public health from the Harvard School of Public Health; in 1985, he was awarded a doctoral degree in developmental psychology from the University of Rhode Island; and, in 1996, he was granted a law degree from the Southern New England School of Law.

From 1967 to 1975, Dr. Pueschel worked at the Developmental Evaluation Clinic of Children's Hospital in Boston. There he became Director of the first Down Syndrome Program and also provided leadership to the PKU and Inborn Errors of Metabolism Program. In 1975, Dr. Pueschel was appointed Director of the Child Development Center at Rhode Island Hospital in Providence. He has continued to pursue his interest in clinical activities, research, and teaching in the fields of developmental disabilities, biochemical genetics, and chromosome abnormalities. Dr. Pueschel has lectured extensively, both nationally and internationally. He has authored or coauthored 15 books and has written more than 200 scientific articles. Dr. Pueschel is certified by both the American Board of Pediatrics and the American Board of Medical Genetics. His academic appointments include Lecturer in Pediatrics, Harvard Medical School; and Professor of Pediatrics, Brown University School of Medicine.

Mária Šustrová, M.D., Ph.D., The Institute of Preventive and Clinical Medicine, Limbová 14, SK-83301 Bratislava, SLOVAKIA.

Dr. Šustrová graduated from the Medical School of Comenius University in Bratislava, Slovakia, with an M.D. degree in 1972. She also earned a Ph.D. degree in immunology from Comenius University in 1992. In 1987, Dr. Šustrová was appointed Director of the Department of Clinical Immunology at the Children's Hospital in Bratislava. Since 1994, she has worked in The Institute of Preventive and Clinical Medicine in Bratislava as Head of the first Down Syndrome Program in Slovakia. Dr. Šustrová is active in research involving the immune system and antioxidants in people with Down syndrome. Her clinical activities include evaluation and follow-up of children with Down syndrome, primary immune disorders, and allergic diseases. She teaches in the field of developmental disabilities and mental retardation at Trnava's University. Dr. Šustrová has lectured on the national and international levels. She is the author of 6 chapters in monographs and more than 50 scientific articles. She is certified by the Slovak Board of Clinical Biochemistry and Clinical Immunology. Dr. Šustrová has been involved in many nongovernmental organizations such as the Down Syndrome Society in Slovakia, the European Down Syndrome Association, and the Association for Help to Persons with Mental Handicap in Slovakia.

The Contributors

David Behen, M.P.A.
Intern
Special Olympics International
1325 G Street, N.W., Suite 500
Washington, D.C. 20005

Robin S. Chapman, Ph.D.
Professor of Communicative Disorders
University of Wisconsin–Madison
Waisman Center
1500 Highland Avenue
Madison, Wisconsin 53705

Christine E. Cronk, Sc.D.
Adjunct Associate Professor
College of Nursing
Marquette University
Emory Clark Hall
530 North 16th Street
Milwaukee, Wisconsin 53201-1881

Nick Crowley
13 King George Drive
Londonderry, New Hampshire 03053

Theresa Crowley
13 King George Drive
Londonderry, New Hampshire 03053

Monica Cuskelly, Ph.D.
Fred and Eleanor Schonell Special
  Education Research Centre
The University of Queensland
Brisbane, Queensland Q-4072
AUSTRALIA

Jeanie P. Edwards, D.S.W.
Professor
Department of Special Education
Portland State University
Post Office Box 751 SPED
Portland, Oregon 97207

Thomas E. Elkins, M.D.
Professor
Department of Obstetrics and
  Gynecology
Louisiana State University Medical
  Center
1542 Tulane Avenue
New Orleans, Louisiana 70112-2822

Michelle Evans, B.A.
Database Manager
Special Olympics International
1325 G Street, N.W., Suite 500
Washington, D.C. 20005

Ellen S. Fabian, Ph.D.
Research Associate Professor
Department of Counseling and
  Personnel Services
University of Maryland
J.M. Patterson Building, Room 3229
College Park, Maryland 20742

Eileen M. Falvey, A.A.
Case Manager
Westside Regional Center
5901 Green Valley Circle
Culver City, California 90230

Mary A. Falvey, Ph.D.
Professor
Department of Special Education
California State University–Los
   Angeles
5151 State University Drive
Los Angeles, California 90032

Karen F. Flippo, M.R.A.
Training Associate
Rehabilitation Research and Training
   Center on Supported Employment
Virginia Commonwealth University
1314 West Main Street
Richmond, Virginia 23284-2011

H.D. Bud Fredericks, Ph.D.
Professor Emeritus
3420 Southwest Cascade
Corvallis, Oregon 97333

Elizabeth Evans Getzel, M.A.
Collateral Faculty
School of Education
Rehabilitation Research and Training
   Center on Supported Employment
Virginia Commonwealth University
1314 West Main Street
Richmond, Virginia 23284-2011

Karen E. Gibson, M.S.
Vocational Employment Counselor
Rehabilitation Research and Training
   Center on Supported Employment
Virginia Commonwealth University
1314 West Main Street
Richmond, Virginia 23284-2011

Patricia Gunn, Ph.D.
Fred and Eleanor Schonell Special
   Education Research Centre
The University of Queensland
Brisbane, Queensland Q-4072
AUSTRALIA

David T. Helm, Ph.D.
Director of Interdisciplinary and
   Preservice Training
Institute for Community Inclusion
University Affiliated Program
Children's Hospital
300 Longwood Avenue
Boston, Massachusetts 02115

Linda A. Heyne, Ph.D., C.T.R.S.
Research Associate
Rehabilitation Research and Training
   Center
University of Minnesota
109 Norris Hall
172 Pillsbury Drive, S.E.
Minneapolis, Minnesota 55455

Salome M. Heyward, J.D.
Attorney
100 Memorial Drive, Apartment 2-7A
Cambridge, Massachusetts 02142

Robert M. Hodapp, Ph.D.
Associate Professor
Graduate School of Education and
   Information Studies
University of California at Los
   Angeles
405 Hilgard Avenue
Los Angeles, California 90095-1521

William E. Kiernan, Ph.D.
Director
Institute for Community Inclusion
University Affiliated Program
Children's Hospital
300 Longwood Avenue
Boston, Massachusetts 02115

Charles R. Kingsley
Contractor
226 South Greeley Avenue
Chappaqua, New York 10514

Emily Perl Kingsley
Television Writer, *Sesame Street*
226 South Greeley Avenue
Chappaqua, New York 10514

Debra R. Langseth, M.S.
Chief Operating Officer
R&D Instructional Services, Inc.
2605 Rolling Road, Suite 408
Baltimore, Maryland 21244

Janet D. Lawson, M.D.
Director
Division of Women's Health
Texas Department of Health
1100 West 49th Street
Austin, Texas 78756-3199

Richard G. Luecking, M.Ed.
President
TransCen, Inc.
451 Hungerford Drive, Suite 700
Rockville, Maryland 20850

Sara Miranda, L.C.S.W.
Director of Social Work
Institute for Community Inclusion
University Affiliated Program
Children's Hospital
300 Longwood Avenue
Boston, Massachusetts 02115

Dawn Munson, B.A.
Research Manager
Special Olympics International
1325 G Street, N.W., Suite 500
Washington, D.C. 20005

Beverly A. Myers, M.D.
Clinical Associate Professor of
    Psychiatry
Brown University School of Medicine
Consultant in Child Psychiatry
Child Development Center
Rhode Island Hospital
593 Eddy Street
Providence, Rhode Island 02903

Jan A. Nisbet, Ph.D.
Associate Professor
Department of Education
Director, Institute on Disability
University Affiliated Program
University of New Hampshire
7 Leavitt Lane, Suite 101
Durham, New Hampshire 03824

Wendy S. Parent, Ph.D.
Assistant Professor
Department of Counseling and Human
    Development Services
College of Education
University of Georgia
402 Aderhold Hall
Athens, Georgia 30602-7142

Laurie E. Powers, Ph.D.
Associate Professor of Medical
    Psychology
Child Development and Rehabilitation
    Center
Oregon Health Sciences University
707 Southwest Gaines Avenue
Portland, Oregon 97207

Julie Ann Racino, M.A.P.A.
President and Director
Community and Policy Studies
208 Henry Street
Rome, New York 13440

Richard L. Rosenberg, Ph.D.
Program Specialist
Whittier Union High School District
9401 South Painter Avenue
Whittier, California 90605

Douglas L. Russell, M.Ed.
Regional Transition Specialist
Virginia Departments of Education and
    Rehabilitative Services
8004 Franklin Farms Drive
Richmond, Virginia 23288-0300

John E. Rynders, Ph.D.
Professor
Department of Educational Psychology
University of Minnesota
255 Burton Hall
178 Pillsbury Drive, S.E.
Minneapolis, Minnesota 55455

Stuart J. Schleien, Ph.D.
Professor and Division Head
Recreation, Park, and Leisure Studies
University of Minnesota
1900 University Avenue, S.E.
Minneapolis, Minnesota 55455

Darryn M. Sikora, Ph.D.
Assistant Professor
Department of Pediatrics
Oregon Health Sciences University
707 Southwest Gaines Avenue
Portland, Oregon 97207

George Smith, M.A.
Vice President of Sports Training
Special Olympics International
1325 G Street, N.W., Suite 500
Washington, D.C. 20005

Thomas B. Songster, Ph.D.
Senior Vice President of Sports Policy
    and Research
Special Olympics International
1325 G Street, N.W., Suite 500
Washington, D.C. 20005

Joan Tanenhaus, M.A., CCC
Speech-Language Pathologist
Assistive Technology Specialist
5 Tameling Road
East Rockaway, New York 11518

Darlene D. Unger, M.Ed.
Instructor
Rehabilitation Research and Training
    Center on Supported Employment
Virginia Commonwealth University
1314 West Main Street
Richmond, Virginia 23284-2011

Paul Wehman, Ph.D.
Director
Rehabilitation Research and Training
    Center on Supported Employment
Virginia Commonwealth University
1314 West Main Street
Richmond, Virginia 23284-2011

Katherine Mullaney Wittig, M.Ed.
Work/Transition Coordinator
Henrico County Public Schools
2206 Mountain Road
Glen Allen, Virginia 23060

Foreword

President John F. Kennedy in the early 1960s said, "We as a nation have for too long postponed an intense search for solutions to the problems of the mentally retarded," and, when subsequent legislative initiatives gave birth to innovative programs for people with developmental disabilities, including those with Down syndrome, a new era had begun. During the ensuing years, not only did biomedical issues start to be studied but also new directions were developed in education, vocational, sport competition, and recreational programs. Thus, we have witnessed significant advances in both the medical and the behavioral sciences since the mid-1960s, and this book captures the progress that has been made. The scientific progress relating to adolescents with Down syndrome is presented here in a comprehensible fashion so that parents of children with Down syndrome will be able to understand and gain from the information provided.

This book focuses on the total person with Down syndrome, with all his or her biomedical, maturational, sexual, behavioral, cognitive, educational, and vocational functions and needs. Of significance also is that issues such as leisure-time activities, participation in Special Olympics sports, community involvement, as well as self-determination, self-esteem, and the gaining of independence during the adolescent years are emphasized.

Also important are the attitudinal changes that have taken place in society toward people with Down syndrome. Whereas previously institutionalization of young people with Down syndrome had been recommended, today we champion integration, independence, community involvement, full citizenship, and empowerment of these youngsters. The latter message is illuminated in this book with the primary goal of improving the quality of all aspects of life of adolescents with Down syndrome. Instead of being given lip service, youngsters with Down syndrome should be offered a status that observes their rights and privileges as citizens in a democratic society and, in a real sense, preserves their human dignity.

Eunice Kennedy Shriver
Founder
Special Olympics International
Washington, D.C.

Preface

This book concerns the issues that young people with Down syndrome confront as they emerge from childhood and make the transition through adolescence into adulthood.

Adolescence is a challenging time in every person's life, and perhaps more so for individuals with special needs including those with Down syndrome. It is a stage when young people with Down syndrome are attempting to free themselves from the role of a child, while still not yet fully equipped to assume the responsibilities of a mature adult. Although many adolescents with Down syndrome have the physical attributes of youngsters without this chromosome abnormality, they frequently lack the intellectual or behavioral capabilities to cope with either the demands of the environment or their own desire for independence. They are faced with preparing for vocational pursuits as well as developing an array of social skills needed to function optimally in society.

This volume provides vital information on many aspects in the life of an adolescent with Down syndrome. By featuring the *total* young person with Down syndrome and exploring his or her major life patterns, this volume aims to provide a more holistic perspective on the adolescent's life. This book's contributing authors, who have worked extensively in the field, discuss innovative programs and trends, appropriate strategies for management and support, and underlying philosophies, all within the context of a host of issues and concerns that emerge during adolescence. Readers of this volume, whether parents of a son or daughter with Down syndrome or professionals, will appreciate the comprehensive perspectives that are brought to bear on the complex issues of adolescence that are presented here.

Section I of this book focuses on biomedical concerns, emphasizing the importance of a healthy lifestyle that includes appropriate nutrition, physical exercise, and various preventive measures in health care. The physical growth and sexual maturational processes of young men and women with Down syndrome are highlighted. Discussion of gynecologic concerns is also included. Various medical conditions that are known to occur at a higher frequency in young people with Down syndrome are also discussed.

Section II examines behavioral, cognitive, and psychiatric issues. Self-competence, self-esteem, and self-empowerment are stressed. The manifold roles of parents and other family members are crucial as the adolescent forces issues to the forefront at home, at school, and in the community. Theoretical and practical issues relating to cognitive functions of young-sters with Down syndrome are also described, in addition to the development of communicative skills. The chapter on behavior concerns disposes of the stereotype of people with Down syndrome as placid and amiable people; research reveals that no one pattern of temperament portrays all children with Down syndrome and that each person has his or her own unique personality. This section ends with a discussion of psychiatric disorders, emphasizing that the majority of adolescents with Down syndrome do not have psychiatric illnesses. Yet, certain psychiatric disorders may be encountered, and depressive disorders, which require prompt and appropriate treatment, may be observed during late adolescence more frequently than in those without the disorder.

Section III delves into educational pursuits. Academic considerations and curricula planning for secondary education are highlighted, with emphasis on inclusive education. Legal issues as they relate to the adolescent with Down syndrome are reviewed. The importance of computer learning during the adolescent years is outlined. Moreover, postsecondary education issues as transition outcomes for adolescents with Down syndrome are discussed.

The transition process from school to the world of work is illuminated in Section IV. This section emphasizes that appropriate transition planning improves employment outcomes and increases the adolescent's quality of life. Prevocational skill training and career preparation are detailed. Supported employment issues and creative job options and how they affect the adolescent with Down syndrome are also reviewed. In particular, active involvement in the planning and implementation of supported employment among all parties is paramount to achieve the adolescent's career goals. All of the authors in this section make the point that many adolescents with Down syndrome will be successful on the job if appropriate support is provided.

Section V underscores the importance of recreational activities in the daily lives of young people with Down syndrome as well as the pivotal role of communities in supporting inclusive lifestyles and individuals' self-determination. The chapters in this section stress that through developing various leisure repertoires, new skills can be mastered, physical and mental well-being can be strengthened, and the adolescent's self-esteem can be enhanced. Special Olympics represents a good example of the way in which involvement in community-supported sports and recreational activities not only improves health, fitness, and sport skills but also promotes self-confidence and fosters acceptance of young people into society. This section concludes with a discussion of public policy frameworks in regard to community support and services.

Thus, from many angles, this volume imparts important new knowledge relating to issues and concerns of adolescents with Down syndrome. The emergence of unforeseen progress in both the biomedical and behavioral sciences, as well as scholarly pursuits in medical and psychoeducational arenas, has brought about a better understanding of the total person with Down syndrome. Ultimately, it is hoped that the information provided here will lead to lives of greater fulfillment for these adolescents.

To Chris and Jurko

Introduction

Emily Perl Kingsley
Charles R. Kingsley

Adolescence! The very word strikes terror into the hearts of most parents!

A friend of ours once said, "Wouldn't it be nice if we could just go to sleep when our kids are about 13 and wake up when they are 21 and skip the whole thing?" That parent happened to be referring to the adolescence of his "normal," "ordinary," "typical" child, that is, his child without any disability. Needless to say, the adolescence of a child with Down syndrome brings with it its own special set of complications, challenges, and, yes, even rewards.

Some of the unique challenges we parents must face result from a relatively new philosophy about our youngsters with Down syndrome. Today's young people with Down syndrome are achieving more than was ever thought possible in previous generations. It is now taken for granted that our children will be raised at home and educated in community schools, alongside siblings and neighbors. It is now assumed that most children with Down syndrome are capable of academic learning, and, because these children have so many more opportunities, they can achieve more independence than was thought possible before.

Kids with Down syndrome are no longer considered "eternal children" who will spend the rest of their lives within our protective embrace or the safety of a sheltered workshop. As a result, we must help them to prepare to take their place out in the "real world" . . . where they will live, work, and have relationships with other people with and without disabilities.

We now recognize that *all* young people strive, need, and, in fact, have a right to separate from their parents. Smoothly accomplishing this separation is a hard enough job with our children who do *not* face special challenges, and the road to independence is often a rocky one under the best of circumstances. Adolescents with Down syndrome have the same needs to separate from their parents as their peers without disabilities and to achieve whatever level of independence they can accomplish.

And that's not easy.

It is right around the start of adolescence that all young people begin to wrestle with the complicated issues of identity. For adolescents with Down syndrome, this often includes becoming aware of their disability and struggling to come to grips with their "differentness." They see their schoolmates and often their own siblings doing things that they are not doing, such as driving and going on dates independently, and enjoying a lifestyle that may not be available to them. This can be extremely frustrating for the adolescent with Down syndrome, and parents need to be aware that ordinary sibling and peer relationships may intensify around these issues. It is important to understand what is really going on so that you can be there to support *all* the kids in the family during this challenging time.

Parents need to help by clarifying the issues, offering support and understanding, and, if necessary, providing their child with professional counseling to help with the difficult adjustment process. Some parents, because of their own pain and discomfort with these issues, try to pretend that their child is blissfully unaware of any difference or disability. As a result, parents may not be available to be the very important resource they need to be when the child is confused or upset by these topics. It is important to try to be tuned in to your child's real feelings and to encourage him or her to express those feelings.

We may find our children with Down syndrome start to exhibit some of the typical adolescent rebelliousness that we expect and take for granted from their siblings who do not have Down syndrome. When you add that to the tendency toward stubbornness that seems to "come with" Down syndrome, it can seem like you suddenly have an entirely different child! At times, we have let ourselves be lulled into a false sense of complacency, expecting our children with Down syndrome to be pleasant, cheerful, and compliant forever. Their sweetness is still there, but when they display the same kinds of adolescent moodiness or oppositionalism that "ordinary" kids manifest every day, somehow we are surprised and bewildered. At these times, we should remember that our children with Down syndrome have the same rights as their brothers and sisters—even if it means the right to be totally obnoxious now and then.

It is not entirely unreasonable for parents to perceive the outside world as a perilous place, especially for our youngsters with Down syndrome, who tend, for the most part, to be trusting, unsophisticated, and susceptible to suggestion and exploitation. Because of this added vulnerability, we often tend to overprotect them and not give them all the opportunities they need to experience the world, take risks, become problem solvers, and develop coping strategies. Our children without disabilities have such opportunities in abundance in school, among their friends, in after-school activities, on weekends, and in myriad situations where they are constantly testing, trying, succeeding, failing, learning, and growing, much of the time without our protective supervision.

For our children with Down syndrome, however, there is a strange contradiction. Especially at this time in their lives, we parents want to give our adolescent children with Down syndrome *more* freedom, *more* latitude, and *more* opportunities to be off on their own. Sadly, this is precisely when their peers without disabilities are often pulling away into their own groups and becoming *less* available as friends, cohorts, and peer-teachers.

Our good intentions notwithstanding, our children with Down syndrome generally do not have very much freedom or enough of the opportunities they need to experiment, evaluate, try, test, and learn from their own mistakes. In addition, they do not have much significant interaction with and input from their peers without disabilities that would enable them to learn what is appropriate and what is not, what is acceptable, and what is expected.

As a result, parents may need to be creative and actually structure opportunities to learn and grow because these opportunities may not occur spontaneously. Opportunities to learn and grow include specific independent living and learning experiences (e.g., shopping; cooking; grooming; learning about teenage or adult styles in dress, makeup, and hairstyling; learning to navigate public transportation). Learning to use public transportation, where available, is particularly important. It is very difficult for young people to feel grown up and independent when they must continue to rely on other people to get them wherever they want to go.

Structuring age-appropriate social experiences is also important. In our area, for example, we established regular monthly teen parties held at a different young person's home each month. The teens love having the experience of a "grownup" Saturday night party with music, dancing, and food. Each family brings something to the party. The parents scrupulously stay in a separate part of the house so as not to interfere with the young people's fun and sense of being on their own. Often a sibling or two or some local high school students volunteer to be on hand in case any subtle supervision or assistance is required. The parents enjoy getting together separately to socialize and discuss their own concerns about their kids' adolescence, and the young people have a chance, on a regular basis, to form relationships, practice social interaction, and have a good time. Telephone lists are made up to encourage the teens to be in touch with each other and possibly to get together in between the monthly parties.

So, the quandary is, must *we,* their parents, step in, *yet again,* and be the ones to provide the intense step-by-step training and preparation for independence, just as our children are trying to disconnect from us?

Well . . . (sigh) . . . yes, I suppose we must.

The schools are doing a better job of preparing our kids academically and vocationally, providing more inclusion and transitional programs; but they still are not fully, directly addressing the specific problems of emerging adulthood, sexuality, and needs for personal independence as well as interpersonal relationships. Some specific programs are emerging that do deal directly with these issues. They are wonderful and tremendously helpful, but they are not universally available yet. Other teens—well, in our experience, other teens are happy to be friendly, cordial, and pleasant to our kids with Down syndrome, especially in school—but they are absorbed with their own lives, loves, cars, colleges, and growing-up problems. Sadly, they rarely reach out to our youngsters in a really meaningful way on a regular basis in their free time. No, we cannot really expect that our kids with Down syndrome will "learn a lot from their friends" as our other kids without Down syndrome do.

We must take advantage of any and all programs, support groups, seminars, and resources that are available to help, but, basically, it seems again that it's mostly up to us.

There can be real confusion when parents start thinking ahead and begin coming to grips with realistic future adult goals for their children, just as the children are starting to develop goals of their own. It's very delicate because the dreams of adolescents with Down syndrome should be encouraged and supported, but, at the same time, kids often need guidance to help them define which goals are reasonable and something to work toward and which are not. Moreover, much flexibility is needed because, as growth and change occur and the youngster develops more skills, goals that were unreal yesterday may become more feasible today and goals that are unthinkable today may become achievable tomorrow.

Parents have their own, sometimes painful, adjustment to make, perhaps in modifying the long-term aspirations they originally had for their child. At the same time, parents continue to experience great pride when each step forward is made and the child develops a new skill and increasing self-reliance. The ultimate acceptance of each of our children as a unique and integral individual is the basic challenge faced by *all* parents. Keeping an open mind at all times is essential; it is important *not* to lock into any outdated stereotypes, but to keep an open mind to any and all possibilities.

So, what to do? First and foremost (and do not minimize this essential and extremely difficult task), we must *acknowledge our children's right to grow up!* With whatever their limitations ultimately may be, with whatever level of guidance and supervision they may always need, they still will be full-fledged adults, and soon. Understand that they have the same hopes, dreams, goals, and feelings as anybody else. Just the same, they must be recognized and appreciated as *individuals* with the right to experiment and develop their own individual tastes, interests, likes and dislikes, talents, and opinions. They have a right to participate in the decision making and the planning for their future. They should be helped to develop the techniques and opportunities to speak out and advocate for themselves.

They will be social human beings, needing real, meaningful friendships and appropriate leisure activities.

They will work, hopefully in the community.

They will live away from you, again, in their community.

They will be sexual human beings, with the right to have close, intimate relationships, perhaps leading to marriage.

All of these developments require preparation, training, and teaching. All of this training will be taking place while *you* are feeling apprehension, misgivings, and your own special brand of separation anxiety . . . while *their* hormones are going nuts!

Maybe that idea about going to sleep when they are age 13 and waking up when they are 21 wasn't such a bad one!

But, as you did in every other developmental phase as your child was growing up, you will take a deep breath, roll up your sleeves *one more time,* and do whatever is necessary to get the job done. Look, you've bought this book! That's a terrific first step!

In doing that, you have acknowledged that adolescence is a specific stage that must be understood and dealt with. You have realized that no amount of denial and foot dragging and sticking your head in the sand will prevent your child from experiencing the changes (e.g., physical, intellectual, psychological, hormonal, social) that are inevitable.

As always, and most important, you love your child intensely and want your child to have the best possible foundation for what he or she is unequivocally entitled to: a full, rich, productive, happy, and independent life.

Best of luck!

I

HEALTH AND PHYSICAL DEVELOPMENT

1

General Health Issues and Medical Care

Siegfried M. Pueschel
Mária Šustrová

Many volumes have been written on the medical care of people with Down syndrome, and numerous scientific articles have been published on various system involvements including ophthalmologic, otolaryngologic, musculoskeletal, endocrine, and many others (*Caring for Individuals with Down Syndrome,* 1995; Cooley & Graham, 1991; Lott & McCoy, 1992; Pueschel, 1992; Pueschel & Pueschel, 1992; Rogers & Coleman, 1992; Selikowitz, 1990; Storm, 1995; Van Dyke, Mattheis, Eberly, & Williams, 1995). Most publications mention a higher prevalence rate of specific disorders such as hypothyroidism, sleep apnea, and atlantoaxial instability occurring in young people with Down syndrome as compared with a control population. Although it is well known that the frequency of certain medical disorders is increased in people with Down syndrome, the vast majority of adolescents with the disorder usually enjoy good health.

Health supervision and medical issues in people with Down syndrome have been discussed by investigators from various countries (e.g., United States—American Academy of Pediatrics, 1994, and *Caring for Individuals with Down Syndrome,* 1995; Sweden—Pueschel & Annerén, 1995; Denmark—Goldstein, 1988; Australia—Selikowitz, 1992; United Kingdom—Turner, Sloper, Cunningham, & Knussen, 1990). In a British survey of health problems in children with Down syndrome, Turner et al. (1990) observed that vision and hearing impairments as well as respiratory infections were the most common conditions affecting a large percentage of young people with Down syndrome. Goldstein (1988) surveyed the utilization of health services provided to an adolescent population with Down syndrome in Denmark. Compared with a control group, chronic diseases such as cardiac, respiratory, and endocrine conditions were observed more frequently among this group of adolescents. Adolescents with Down syndrome also utilized secondary health services more often than adolescents in the control group. In Australia, Selikowitz (1992) investigated health problems in youngsters with Down syndrome. Again, certain medical conditions including ophthalmologic, otologic, cardiac, respiratory, thyroid, and skeletal disorders were identified to occur more frequently in youngsters with Down syndrome. According to Selikowitz, this factor should be taken into consideration in planning for health supervision in this population.

Although health care checklists for individuals with Down syndrome have been published previously, more recent reports on optimal health maintenance for youngsters with Down syndrome have been prepared in Sweden (Pueschel & Annerén, 1995), in Germany (Storm, 1995), and in the United States (American Academy of Pediatrics, 1994; *Caring for Individuals with Down Syndrome,* 1995).

MEDICAL ISSUES

Physicians caring for adolescents with Down syndrome, as with all individuals, should practice proactive, preventive medicine and promote general health to help avoid illness and potentially incapacitating medical conditions. It is both cost-effective and advantageous for young people with Down syndrome to have regular physical examinations and follow-ups by a physician knowledgeable about Down syndrome. During these checkups, usually scheduled annually or more often if indicated, the physician typically obtains an interim medical history from the individual and his or her parents. For example, if parents report gait abnormalities or that their child is having difficulty walking, this may suggest atlantoaxial instability, hip dislocation, or other musculoskeletal ailments. If a parent has noted that the young person with Down syndrome is always turning the television or radio on full-blast, this may indicate a significant hearing loss. A careful medical history with a complete review of all systems (e.g., visual, auditory, cardiac, respiratory, gastrointestinal, genitourinary, musculoskeletal, neurologic) may uncover specific health concerns leading to appropriate treatment.

Beyond eliciting information on medical issues, other aspects of daily living, such as educational, job-related, behavioral-emotional, nutritional, environmental, and social concerns, need to be explored. Often an adolescent's social and emotional life has a marked effect on his or her physical health. Conversely, an adolescent with specific medical problems may experience significant psychosocial difficulties. The psychosocial history should focus on basic developmental tasks normally mastered during adolescence. Moreover, the physician may want to elicit information on the adolescent's self-image, family relationships, and peer interrelations.

In addition, developmental issues, such as physical growth and sexual maturation, of the growing adolescent with Down syndrome should be explored during visits with the physician. Important information pertaining to health or environmental concerns in the life of the young person with Down syndrome may thus be revealed.

Subsequently, thorough physical and neurologic examinations with accurate anthropometric measurements (i.e., height and weight) should be performed. Although details of such examinations are covered in subsequent chapters in this volume, certain aspects of the physical assessment that are beyond the routine examination are touched upon here. For example, an ophthalmologic examination may reveal keratoconus (i.e., frontal bulging of the cornea), blepharitis (i.e., inflammation of the eyelid margin), or early cataract formation. As another example, enlarged tonsils or adenoids, or both, may be associated with frequent ear infections and fluid accumulation in the middle ear or may cause sleep apnea. If a significant cardiac murmur or a midsystolic click is heard, or both, this may signify mitral valve prolapse and/or mitral or aortic valve involvements. Also, if neurologic abnormalities are uncovered such as brisk deep-tendon reflexes, clonus, and/or a positive Babinski sign, this may suggest atlantoaxial instability or other central nervous system problems. These are but a few examples of specific medical concerns that are experienced at a higher frequency in adolescents with Down syndrome and that demand the physician's attention. If properly focused, the medical examination may not only reveal important areas of dysfunction and disease that should lead to appropriate remediation and treatment but also will initiate a meaningful dialogue and relationship between the health professional and the adolescent and his or her parents.

Once the complete physical and neurologic examinations have been carried out, certain laboratory and X-ray procedures may need to be pursued. Annual thyroid function tests and audiologic assessments should be done. Moreover, X-ray examinations of the cervical spine may be required to rule out atlantoaxial instability.

Depending on the historical information obtained and the results of the physical examination, other investigations may also be necessary. These investigations may reveal or confirm certain clinical conditions that warrant careful monitoring by the physician or medical treatment. If, for example, the medical history reveals that a young person with Down syndrome snores and has episodes when he or she stops breathing during sleep, and the physical examination identifies large tonsils, the physician may request that the adolescent undergo a sleep study to determine whether he or she indeed has sleep apnea as suggested clinically. If an adolescent with Down syndrome has been found to display clinical symptoms of hypothyroidism and specific laboratory investigations should show evidence of thyroid gland dysfunction, then thyroid hormone treatment and close follow-up would be necessary. The subsequent administration of thyroid hormones will enhance the adolescent's central nervous system function, which in turn will improve his or her educational or job performance. Several guidelines for optimal medical care and management for adolescents with Down syndrome have been developed as mentioned above (*Caring for Individuals with Down Syndrome,* 1995; Pueschel & Annerén, 1995).

HEALTH EDUCATION

In General

During the discussion following the physical and neurologic examination, the physician should explore with the adolescent and his or her parents various issues relating to general health education. Health education, of course, does not begin when the individual becomes an adolescent; rather, it is a continuous process from early childhood throughout life and, as such, can significantly contribute to a better quality of life for the individual.

During the health education discussion, the physician should emphasize a healthy lifestyle, including avoidance of tobacco and alcohol; accident prevention; personal safety, including use of seatbelts while in an automobile; self-care, grooming, and dressing; adequate sleep; a well-balanced, low-calorie, but nutritious, diet; regular dental care; adequate physical activity; and a generally favorable living and working environment without undue stress. Other concerns—both medical and nonmedical—pertaining to individual circumstances should also be addressed at this time.

For instance, the adolescent's schooling, career preparation, and involvement in social and leisure-time activities should be explored. Developing a healthy self-esteem and becoming increasingly more independent are important issues to discuss. Hence, the physician should not only deal with medical issues per se but should be concerned with broader aspects of the individual's life, including educational, vocational, behavioral, and recreational. Many of these concerns are discussed in more detail in other chapters in this volume.

In the health education process, it is also vital that adolescents with Down syndrome learn to take responsibility for their own health. For example, they should receive training in choosing food items that are less fattening; in body hygiene; and in preventing infections and accidents. By setting appropriate examples in this regard, parents and other family members can provide excellent role models for the person with Down syndrome.

Seeing his or her mother and father pursuing good health practices and engaging in various preventive measures will encourage the adolescent to pursue a lifestyle of good physical and mental well-being. If children with Down syndrome are raised in a stable home environment and enjoy a happy family life, if gentle discipline is used in a positive way, if guidance toward independence is provided, and if these factors continue throughout adolescence, then serious behavioral and emotional problems may be avoided.

In addition to their experiences in the home environment, adolescents with Down syndrome should also be exposed to health education in school, during recreational activities such as scouting, and other community activities. Youngsters with Down syndrome can also learn from appropriate television programs and specific written materials on health issues.

Sex Education

Social-sexual skill training should also be incorporated into health education. Like other children, adolescents with Down syndrome also need sex education. Sex education is usually carried out in the home or school, or in both settings. Sex education should not only teach facts about male and female anatomy, reproduction, and the act of intercourse but also, perhaps more important, should focus on human relationships, personal feelings, and desires, as well as attitudes and values (Edwards, 1988). The young person with Down syndrome should be taught appropriate social behaviors and how to avoid socially unacceptable behaviors. Such training would include instruction in social interaction, how to initiate contact with others, and how to enjoy togetherness in a rewarding human relationship.

IMMUNIZATION

An important preventive measure that is part of general health care and that should not be neglected relates to immunization. Most often immunization is emphasized during the first 2 years of life with the administration of hepatitis B, diphtheria, tetanus, pertussis, Hemophilus influenza type B, oral poliovirus, measles, mumps, rubella, and varicella zoster virus vaccines. However, it is important to review the immunization schedule from time to time to ensure complete immunization of the adolescent with Down syndrome.

Because not all youngsters are immunized against hepatitis B in the newborn period and early infancy, the American Academy of Pediatrics recommends that unvaccinated children receive, at about 11–12 years of age, three doses of hepatitis B vaccine. (The second dose of hepatitis B vaccine is administered 1 month after the first, and the third dose is given about 5 months later.) Similarly, if varicella zoster virus vaccine has not been given previously and the adolescent has not yet had chickenpox, the varicella zoster virus vaccine should be dispensed. In addition, booster immunizations against diphtheria and tetanus (DT) as well as measles, mumps, and rubella (MMR) are recommended at about 11–12 years of age. If the adolescent did not receive immunizations against tuberculosis and is not tuberculin positive, annual tuberculin tests should be carried out.

Some adolescents with Down syndrome who have cardiac disease, frequent respiratory illnesses, or other chronic medical conditions may benefit from receiving influenza or pneumococcal vaccinations, or both. Influenza vaccines are usually administered in the fall shortly before the flu season. Again, since new vaccines may be developed and future investigations may necessitate revising the recommended immunizations, the adolescent's immunization schedule should be regularly reviewed and altered as appropriate.

DENTAL CARE

Regular dental care and appropriate dental hygiene are equally important in the overall health maintenance scheme. Like other children, adolescents with Down syndrome should be examined by a dentist annually, semiannually, or more often if indicated. Moreover, thorough dental cleaning by a dental hygienist should be performed regularly. Of great significance is proper toothbrushing, flossing, and gum care. The main reason for pursuing appropriate dental care and meticulous dental hygiene is to prevent periodontitis and gingivitis (gum disease), which are reported to occur at a high frequency in adolescents with Down syndrome.

In addition, because of the small oral cavity observed in most young people with Down syndrome, crowding of teeth and malocclusion are common, often requiring orthodontic care. Sometimes palate expansion, application of braces, and extractions are necessary. By incorporating optimal dental services and good dental hygiene as part of general health care, dental decay and gum disease can be prevented to a large extent.

CONCLUSIONS

In summary, adolescents with Down syndrome require optimal medical and dental care, which has been described in detail in guidelines and health care checklists as mentioned above. During regular follow-up examinations, the physician should obtain a medical history with focus on specific health concerns that occur at a higher frequency in young people with Down syndrome. Also, educational, behavioral, environmental, social, and physical examination may uncover specific bodily dysfunctions. In addition, issues of health education and sex education as well as updating immunization should be emphasized.

REFERENCES

American Academy of Pediatrics—Committee on Genetics. (1994). Health supervision for children with Down syndrome. *Pediatrics, 93,* 855–859.

Caring for individuals with Down syndrome and their families. (1995). Report of the Third Ross Roundtable on Critical Issues in Family Medicine. Columbus, OH: Abbott Laboratories, Ross Products Division.

Cooley, W.C., & Graham, J.M. (1991). Down syndrome—An update and review for the primary care physician. *Clinical Pediatrics, 30,* 233–253.

Edwards, J. (1988). Sexuality, marriage, and parenting for persons with Down syndrome. In S.M. Pueschel (Ed.), *The young person with Down syndrome: Transition from adolescence to adulthood* (pp. 173–186). Baltimore: Paul H. Brookes Publishing Co.

Goldstein, H. (1988). Utilization of health services over a one year period by an adolescent population with Down syndrome. *Danish Medical Bulletin, 35,* 585–588.

Lott, I.T., & McCoy, E.E. (1992). *Down syndrome: Advances in medical care.* New York: Wiley-Liss.

Pueschel, S.M. (1992). The child with Down syndrome. In M.D. Levine, W.B. Carey, & A.C. Crocker (Eds.), *Developmental-behavioral pediatrics* (2nd ed., pp. 221–228). Philadelphia: W.B. Saunders.

Pueschel, S.M., & Annerén, G. (1995). Committee Report: Guidelines for optimal medical care of persons with Down syndrome. *Acta Paediatrica Scandinavica, 84,* 823–827.

Pueschel, S.M., & Pueschel, J.K. (Eds.). (1992). *Biomedical concerns in persons with Down syndrome.* Baltimore: Paul H. Brookes Publishing Co.

Rogers, R.T., & Coleman, M. (1992), *Medical care in Down syndrome.* New York: Marcel Dekker.

Selikowitz, M. (1990). *Down syndrome: The facts.* Oxford, England: Oxford University Press.

Selikowitz, M. (1992). Health problems and health checks in school aged children with Down syndrome. *Journal of Paediatrics and Child Health, 28,* 383–386.

Storm, W. (1995). *Das Down-Syndrom: Medizinische Betreuung vom Kindes bis zum Erwachsenenalter [Down syndrome: Medical care from childhood to adulthood].* Stuttgart, Germany: Wissenschaftliche Verlagsgesellschaft GmbH.

Turner, S., Sloper, P., Cunningham, C., & Knussen, C. (1990). Health problems in children with Down's syndrome. *Child Care, Health, & Development, 16,* 83–97.

Van Dyke, D.C., Mattheis, P., Eberly, S., & Williams, J. (1995). *Medical and surgical care for children with Down syndrome: A guide for parents.* Rockville, MD: Woodbine House.

2

Nutritional Concerns

Mária Šustrová
Siegfried M. Pueschel

Do adolescents with Down syndrome have the same nutritional needs as age-equivalent children without this disorder? This question is often asked by parents and professionals caring for young people with Down syndrome. In general, adolescents with Down syndrome, like youngsters without Down syndrome, require a balanced diet consisting of food items from the four basic food groups including 1) meats, fish, and eggs; 2) fruits and vegetables; 3) cereals and bread; and 4) milk and milk products. However, if adolescents primarily eat "fast food" or "junk food," they may not get a balanced diet.

ENERGY REQUIREMENTS

The basic metabolic rate of adolescents with Down syndrome does not differ from that of individuals without Down syndrome if corrected for surface area and lean body mass. However, the total energy allowance of youngsters with the disorder is less than that of adolescents without the disorder (Schapiro & Rapoport, 1989). There are several possible reasons for this reduced caloric requirement. First, specific genes may be located on chromosome 21 that, in a triple dose, may be responsible for the reduced energy expenditure in people with Down syndrome. Second, youngsters with Down syndrome usually have a smaller body mass and a slower rate of growth as compared with age-equivalent children without the disorder (Pipes, 1992). Third, the intracellular energy expenditure is significantly lower in youngsters with Down syndrome ($39.93 \text{ m}^2/\text{hr}^{-1}$) than in individuals without the syndrome ($44 \text{ m}^2/\text{hr}^{-1}$) (Chad, Jobling, & Frail, 1990).

Sharav and Bowman (1992) investigated dietary practices, physical activity, and body-mass index in a selected population of children with Down syndrome and their siblings. The authors reported that the caloric intake as a percentage of recommended allowance for height was somewhat less in youngsters with Down syndrome (88.7%) when compared with their siblings (95%). The authors postulated that, even though adolescents with Down syndrome have been shown to be at risk for obesity, familial and other environmental factors also have an influence on the occurrence of obesity in these youth.

Chad et al. (1990) reported that body height had the strongest correlation with the resting metabolic rate in people with Down syndrome, and body fat the weakest correlation. Therefore, it makes sense to base the calculations of the caloric intake of adolescents with Down syndrome on height rather than weight. Culley, Goyle, Jolly, and Mertz (1965) observed that young boys with Down syndrome who were shorter and heavier than their peers of the same age consumed 16.1 ± 0.8 kcal/cm/day and girls 14.3 ± 1.1 kcal/cm/day. Apparently, this was the same energy expenditure as for age-equivalent controls. These data support recommendations that the total caloric intake of young people with Down syndrome should be less than that of children who do not have Down syndrome (National Research Council, 1989). Although the average caloric intake for individuals with Down syndrome should be reduced, it is paramount that the intake of protein, vitamins, minerals, and other essential nutrients be adequate. The average nutritional intake in the study by Chad et al. (1990) was 1,434 calories and consisted of 16% protein, 42% fat, and 49% carbohydrates. Table 2.1 lists the recommended dietary allowances for healthy adolescents in the United States as provided by the Food and Nutrition Board of the National Academy of Sciences National Research Council (1989).

Much has been written about the biochemical aspects of food components, including protein, fat, carbohydrates, vitamins, and minerals. Although minor abnormalities in protein, fat, and carbohydrate metabolism of individuals with Down syndrome have been reported by some investigators, others have not confirmed these findings (for a detailed discussion of this topic, see Pueschel and Annerén, 1992). By and large, people with Down syndrome do not have significant derangements of protein, fat, and carbohydrate metabolism.

PREVENTION OF OBESITY

In addition to reduced caloric intake, adolescents with Down syndrome should engage in physical activity. This can take the form of family outings, a stroll through the woods with friends or family, routine adaptive physical education activities in school, skiing, swimming, preparation for and participation in Special Olympics events, various forms of workouts, and other recreational activities (see also Chapters 23 and 24). Such activities should help to burn calories, to keep the young person with Down syndrome in shape, and to prevent a sedentary lifestyle.

Table 2.1. Recommended dietary allowances for healthy adolescents: United States

	Age of males (in years)			Age of females (in years)		
	11–14	15–18	19–24	11–14	15–18	19–24
Protein (g)	45	59	58	46	44	46
Vitamin A (μg RE)	1,000	1,000	1,000	800	800	800
Vitamin D (μg)	10	10	10	10	10	10
Vitamin E (mg TE)	10	10	10	8	8	8
Vitamin K (μg)	45	65	70	45	55	60
Vitamin C (mg)	50	60	60	50	60	60
Thiamin (mg)	1.3	1.5	1.5	1.1	1.1	1.1
Riboflavin (mg)	1.5	1.8	1.7	1.3	1.3	1.3
Niacin (mg NE)	17	20	19	15	15	15
Vitamin B_6 (mg)	1.7	2.0	2.0	1.4	1.5	1.6
Folate (μg)	150	200	200	150	180	180
Vitamin B_{12} (mg)	2.0	2.0	2.0	2.0	2.0	2.0
Calcium (mg)	1,200	1,200	1,200	1,200	1,200	1,200
Phosphorus (mg)	1,200	1,200	1,200	1,200	1,200	1,200
Magnesium (mg)	270	400	350	280	300	280
Iron (mg)	12	12	10	15	15	15
Zinc (mg)	15	15	15	12	12	12
Iodine (μg)	150	150	150	150	150	150
Selenium (μg)	40	50	70	45	50	55

Data are adapted from National Research Council (1989).

Because of the propensity of young people with Down syndrome to become overweight during childhood and adolescence, nutritional counseling should be provided to parents from early childhood on. It is important to monitor the longitudinal growth and weight gain of these youngsters to identify those children who may be gaining more than expected. Early recognition of increased weight gain should result in appropriate intervention.

Once a child with Down syndrome is significantly overweight, it is difficult to reduce the excess weight. Severely restricting food intake is rarely successful. A rational behavior modification approach to weight control, together with a low caloric intake and increased exercise, are often more effective (Warren, 1982).

To prevent children with Down syndrome from becoming overweight, their food intake must be controlled not only in the home environment but also in school and when they are with friends or relatives. Moreover, eating high-calorie snacks while watching television, as well as eating meals high in fat and carbohydrates, should be avoided. In addition, offering food items as a reward in the context of behavior modification activities is not conducive to weight control.

There are numerous reasons why people with Down syndrome should avoid increased weight gain. The adverse effects of obesity on an individual's health are well known. They include increased blood pressure, heart disease, a higher frequency of diabetes, and a reduced life expectancy. There are also other non–health-related concerns. If adolescents with Down syndrome are significantly overweight, they may not want to engage in physical education and recreational activities, choosing instead to watch television and be sedentary. Being overweight may thus limit a person's exposure to experiences that enhance general development. In addition, an adolescent's physical appearance may be an important factor in being socially accepted. In summary, weight control is advantageous because young people with Down syndrome who are of average weight will have fewer health problems and be better accepted by society, and their self-image will be significantly enhanced.

Another reason a low-fat diet during adolescence and beyond may be beneficial was pointed out by Pueschel, Craig, and Haddow (1992). These investigators examined lipids and lipoproteins in 23 young people with Down syndrome and reported significantly higher triglyceride levels in youngsters with Down syndrome when compared with controls (brothers and sisters of individuals with Down syndrome). This study revealed an important finding in that high-density lipoprotein, cholesterol, apolipoprotein AI, and the ratio of high-density lipoprotein cholesterol to total cholesterol all were significantly decreased in the study population. Based on these investigations, there is a possibility that people with Down syndrome may be prone to coronary artery disease, although previous studies have not reported such findings (Murdoch, Rodger, & Rao, 1977).

FOOD PURCHASE AND MEALTIME

Young people with Down syndrome need to be taught how to select and purchase food. Trips to the grocery store or supermarket can be valuable educational experiences for adolescents. They can learn how to read labels for specific ingredients and caloric content. They can learn not only how to shop independently but also how to choose nonfat foods wisely. For example, adolescents with Down syndrome can be taught that, although lean meat and fish may be more expensive, nutritionally, they may be a better choice. Pork, hamburgers, hot dogs, and other high-fat–containing meats and meat products should be avoided. Similarly, high-carbohydrate foods such as pasta, snack foods, ice cream, and other high-calorie foods should be consumed in limited amounts only. Youngsters with Down syndrome can also learn that a nonfat salad dressing has significantly fewer calories than regular salad dressings. They should become aware that fresh vegetables and fruits have important vitamins and minerals and are generally low in calories per serving. Also, foods that are high in fiber may be preferred over those low in fiber to avoid or control constipation.

Once adolescents have chosen healthy foods, they also need to learn how to pay for the food items, including giving the right amount of money to the cashier, counting the change, and so on. Similar learning experiences occur when adolescents eat in restaurants. They may be able to study the menu and learn how to choose specific foods low in fat content. Also, socially acceptable mealtime behavior can be practiced here as well as in the home environment.

Beyond concerns about what constitutes a balanced diet and the educational experiences just mentioned, it is also important that adolescents enjoy their meals together with family and friends. Mealtime experiences should be happy ones.

Among the many reports that have been published on nutrition and related topics in regard to people with Down syndrome, four controversial issues that have been brought to the attention of parents and professionals are discussed here, including celiac disease, alleged vitamin deficiencies, megavitamin therapy, and zinc and selenium therapy.

CELIAC DISEASE

Since the first description of celiac disease (an inability to digest a certain protein [gluten] found in flour) in a person with Down syndrome (Bentley, 1975), numerous reports have focused on the association between celiac disease and Down syndrome. Most articles on celiac disease in young people with Down syndrome have been written by European investigators (e.g., Castro et al., 1993; Nowak, Ghishan, & Schulze-Delrieu, 1983; Santer, Sievers, & Oldigs, 1991; Zubillaga, Vitoria, Arrieta, Echaniz, & Garcia-Masdevall, 1993). These reports indicate that the clinical presentation in children with Down syndrome affected by celiac disease may not follow the classic textbook description of the disease. However, many of these children have persistent diarrhea or failure to thrive, or both.

Several studies (Castro et al., 1993; Nowak et al., 1983; Zubillaga et al., 1993) have described increased blood levels of IgA and IgG antigliadin antibodies as well as antiendomysial antibodies in individuals with suspected celiac disease. Although a significant increase of antiendomysial antibodies is said to be more specific than IgA and IgG antigliadin antibodies, the sine qua non for establishing the diagnosis of celiac disease in children with Down syndrome is a jejunal biopsy showing significant villous atrophy of the jejunal mucosa. The previously mentioned etiologic association between Down syndrome and celiac disease may be due to an altered immune system or to the presence of common histocompatibility antigens or to both (Castro et al., 1993).

Although European investigators have reported a higher prevalence of celiac disease in adolescents with Down syndrome when compared with a control population, no large-scale epidemiologic study has been done in the United States to confirm this.

VITAMIN DEFICIENCIES

Some investigators have suggested that children with Down syndrome are vitamin-deficient. For example, low levels of thiamine, ascorbic acid, and niacin have been observed by Matin, Sylvester, Edwards, and Dickerson (1981). Also, malabsorption of various vitamins, in particular vitamin A, has been reported (Sobel, Strazzulla, & Burton, 1958).

Despite these and other reports on vitamin deficiencies in people with Down syndrome, the majority of adolescents who eat a balanced diet with ample fruits and vegetables will usually not be vitamin-deficient (Pipes, 1992). It should be noted that previous studies were often carried out on people in institutions who were receiving suboptimal nutrition. Antiquated laboratory methods were also sometimes used in the earlier investigations, and caution needs to be exercised in interpreting certain studies done decades ago. For example, when Pueschel et al. (1990) investigated vitamin A absorption in 40 young people with Down syndrome, they found the vitamin A absorption curve to parallel that of controls without Down syndrome. Also, Storm (1990) noted normal vitamin A levels in individuals with Down syndrome. In contrast, previous reports had mentioned decreased vitamin A absorption in people with this disorder (e.g., Auld, Pommer, Houck, & Burke, 1959; Sobel et al., 1958). If adolescents with Down syndrome do not receive a balanced diet with the recommended amounts of vitamins, they may be in need of supplemental vitamins.

MEGAVITAMIN THERAPY

Some authors have claimed that large doses of various vitamins would benefit individuals with Down syndrome. In 1981, Harrell, Capp, and Davis reported significant gains in IQ in children with developmental delays, including five children with Down syndrome, after megavitamins had been administered over a 4-month period. Subsequently, several groups of investigators attempted to replicate the Harrell et al. study (Bennett, McClelland, Kriegsman, Andrus, & Sells, 1983; Ellis & Tomporowski, 1983; Smith, Spiker, Peterson, Cicchetti, & Justin, 1983; Weathers, 1983). None of these studies, however, showed a significant increase in cognitive functioning, motor performance, or communicative abilities as a result of the megavitamin treatment. Although evidence is accumulating that megavitamin treatment is ineffective, there are still professionals who continue to offer false hope to parents of children with Down syndrome by promoting megavitamin therapy.

ZINC AND SELENIUM THERAPY

It has been reported that the administration of zinc sulphate and selenium may benefit children with Down syndrome. Napolitano et al. (1990) observed that 15 of 22 children with Down syndrome who had received zinc sulphate reached a higher percentile in their growth rate, whereas the remaining 7 children did not show any change. The authors concluded that zinc sulphate therapy, when provided to children with Down syndrome, will accelerate their longitudinal growth and will improve their immune function. Also, Björksten et al. (1980), who administered zinc supplements to 12 young people with Down syndrome, noted that the children's immune function improved and that their serum zinc concentration normalized. Similarly, Francheschi et al. (1988) gave zinc to 18 people with Down syndrome who subsequently had higher zinc plasma levels than age-matched controls. The authors also observed a dramatic increase in serum thymic factor, a reduction in respiratory illnesses, and fewer skin infections in 13 out of 18 individuals. Further investigations and research efforts are necessary to shed more light on zinc metabolism in people with Down syndrome.

Selenium therapy has been advocated following the finding of selenium deficiency in people with Down syndrome (Antila, Nordberg, Syvaoja, & Westermarck, 1990). Antila and colleagues observed an increase in erythrocyte glutathione peroxidase activity in young people with Down syndrome after selenium administration. The authors concluded that children with Down syndrome would benefit from selenium supplementation. Annerén, Magnusson, and Nordvall (1990) studied the concentration of four IgG subclasses in 29 children with Down syndrome and observed a significant augmentative effect of selenium on the serum concentration of IgG2 and IgG4, but not on IgG1 and IgG3. Annerén and his co-workers suggested that selenium has an immunoregulatory effect that might be important in clinical practice.

CONCLUSIONS

In summary, young people with Down syndrome have similar nutritional needs and require a balanced diet with sufficient vitamins and trace metals as age-equivalent children who do not have this chromosome disorder. However, their resting metabolic rate and their energy allowances are less; therefore, the caloric intake of youth with Down syndrome should be reduced to prevent increased weight gain and obesity. Parents need nutritional counseling from early on, and regular physical activity for young people with Down syndrome should be encouraged.

REFERENCES

Annerén, G., Magnusson, C.G.M., & Nordvall, S.L. (1990). Increase in serum concentrations of IgG2 and IgG4 by selenium supplementation in children with Down's syndrome. *Archives of Diseases in Childhood, 65,* 1353–1355.

Antila, E., Nordberg, L., Syvaoja, E., & Westermarck, T. (1990). Selenium therapy in Down syndrome (DS): A theory and a clinical trial. In I. Emerit (Ed.), *Antioxidants in therapy and preventive medicine* (pp. 183–186). New York: Plenum.

Auld, R.M., Pommer, A., Houck, J.C., & Burke, F.G. (1959). Vitamin A absorption in mongoloid children. *American Journal of Mental Deficiency, 63,* 1010–1015.

Bennett, F.C., McClelland, S., Kriegsman, E.A., Andrus, L.B., & Sells, C.J. (1983). Vitamin and mineral supplements in Down's syndrome. *Pediatrics, 72,* 707–713.

Bentley, D.A. (1975). A case of Down's syndrome complicated by retinoblastoma and coeliac disease. *Pediatrics, 56,* 131–133.

Björksten, B., Back, O., Gustavson, K.H., Hallmans, G., Hagglof, B., & Tarnvik, A. (1980). Zinc and immune function in Down's syndrome. *Acta Paediatrica Scandinavica, 69,* 183–189.

Castro, M., Crino, A., Papadatou, B., Purpura, M., Glannotti, A., Ferretti, F., Colistro, F., Mottola, L., Digilio, M.C., Lucidi, V., & Borrelli, P. (1993). Down's syndrome and celiac disease: The prevalence of high IgA-antigliadin antibodies and HLA-DR and DQ antigens in trisomy 21. *Journal of Pediatric Gastroenterology and Nutrition, 16,* 265–268.

Chad, K., Jobling, A., & Frail, H. (1990). Metabolic rate: A factor in developing obesity in children with Down syndrome? *American Journal on Mental Retardation, 95,* 228–234.

Culley, W.J., Goyle, K., Jolly, D.H., & Mertz, E.T. (1965). Calorie intake of children with Down's syndrome. *Journal of Pediatrics, 66,* 772–775.

Ellis, N.R., & Tomporowski, R.D. (1983). Vitamin/mineral supplements and intelligence of institutionalized mentally retarded adults. *American Journal of Mental Deficiency, 88,* 211–214.

Francheschi, C., Chiricolo, M., Licastro, F., Zannotti, M.M., Mocchegini, E., & Fabris, N. (1988). Oral zinc supplementation in Down's syndrome: Restoration of thymic endocrine activity and some immune defects. *Journal of Mental Deficiency Research, 32,* 169–181.

Harrell, R.J., Capp, R.H., & Davis, D.R. (1981). Can nutritional supplements help mentally retarded children? *Proceedings of the National Academy of Sciences of the United States of America, 78,* 574–578.

Matin, M.A., Sylvester, P.E., Edwards, P., & Dickerson, J.W.T. (1981). Vitamin and zinc status in Down's syndrome. *Journal of Mental Deficiency, 25,* 121–126.

Murdoch, J.C., Rodger, C.J., & Rao, S.S. (1977). Down's syndrome: An atheroma-free model? *British Medical Journal, ii,* 226–228.

Napolitano, G., Palka, G., Grimaldi, S., Giuliani, C., Laglia, G., Calabrese, G., Satta, M.A., Neri, G., & Monaco, F. (1990). Growth delay in Down syndrome and zinc sulphate supplementation. *American Journal of Medical Genetics Supplement, 7,* 63–65.

National Research Council, National Academy of Sciences. (1989). *Recommended dietary allowances* (10th ed.). Washington, DC: National Academy Press.

Nowak, T.V., Ghishan, F.K., & Schulze-Delrieu, K. (1983). Celiac sprue in Down's syndrome: Considerations on a pathogenetic link. *American Journal of Gastroenterology, 78,* 280–283.

Pipes, P.L. (1992). Nutritional aspects. In S.M. Pueschel & J.K. Pueschel (Eds.), *Biomedical concerns in persons with Down syndrome* (pp. 39–46). Baltimore: Paul H. Brookes Publishing Co.

Pueschel, S.M., & Annerén, G. (1992). Metabolic and biochemical concerns. In S.M. Pueschel & J.K. Pueschel (Eds.), *Biomedical concerns in persons with Down syndrome* (pp. 273–287). Baltimore: Paul H. Brookes Publishing Co.

Pueschel, S.M., Craig, W.Y., & Haddow, J.E. (1992). Lipids and lipoproteins in persons with Down syndrome. *Journal of Intellectual Disability Research, 36,* 365–369.

Pueschel, S.M., Hillemeier, C., Caldwell, M., Senft, K., Mers, C., & Pezzullo, J.C. (1990). Vitamin A gastrointestinal absorption in persons with Down's syndrome. *Journal of Mental Deficiency Research, 34,* 269–275.

Santer, R., Sievers, E., & Oldigs, H.D. (1991). Celiac disease in Down's syndrome. *Journal of Pediatric Gastroenterology and Nutrition, 13,* 121–128.

Schapiro, M.B., & Rapoport, S.I. (1989). Basal metabolic rate in healthy Down's syndrome adults. *Journal of Mental Deficiency Research, 33,* 211–219.

Sharav, T., & Bowman, T. (1992). Dietary practices, physical activity, and body-mass index in a selected population of Down syndrome children and their siblings. *Clinical Pediatrics, 37,* 314–344.

Smith, G.F., Spiker, D., Peterson, C., Cicchetti, D., & Justin, P. (1983). Failure of mineral and vitamin supplementation in Down's syndrome. *Lancet, ii,* 41.

Sobel, A.E., Strazzulla, M., & Burton, S. (1958). Vitamin A absorption and other blood composition studies in mongolism. *American Journal of Mental Deficiency, 62,* 642–656.

Storm, W. (1990). Hypercarotenemia in children with Down's syndrome. *Journal of Mental Deficiency Research, 34,* 283–286.

Warren, L. (1982). *Development and implementation of an obesity treatment model for developmentally delayed clients.* Unpublished master's thesis, University of Washington, Seattle.

Weathers, C. (1983). Effect of nutritional supplementation on IQ and certain other variables associated with Down syndrome. *American Journal of Mental Deficiency, 88,* 214–217.

Zubillaga, P., Vitoria, J.C., Arrieta, A., Echaniz, P., & Garcia-Masdevall, M.D. (1993). Down's syndrome and celiac disease. *Journal of Pediatric Gastroenterology and Nutrition, 16,* 168–171.

3

Physical Growth

Christine E. Cronk

Studies of growth and size of people with Down syndrome agree that by adulthood, the height of these individuals is reduced by an average of about 2 standard deviations. That is, the average adult with Down syndrome is shorter than the shortest normal adult (Benda, 1939; Dutton, 1958; Gustavson, 1964; Oster, 1953; Rarick & Seefeldt, 1974; Roche, 1965). Both studies of institutionalized individuals (Benda, 1939; Dutton, 1958; Gustavson, 1964; Roche, 1965) and of children reared at home (Cronk, 1978; Cronk & Pueschel, 1984; Pueschel, 1984) indicate that the largest growth delays occur in the first years of life.

GROWTH BEFORE ADOLESCENCE

At birth, the length and weight of babies with Down syndrome are slightly less than normal. By 3 years of age, the absolute difference in the average size between children without disabilities and toddlers with Down syndrome is about 3.5 cm. The growth rate in children with Down syndrome is less than 75%–90% that of children without disabilities (around the 10th–25th percentile). The average child with Down syndrome grows about 38.2 cm in the first 3 years of life, whereas the average child without disabilities grows 46 cm during this period. Rate of weight gain is 22% less than that expected for children without disabilities until about age 18 months but is normal between ages 18 months and 36 months. Because gains for height continue to be less than normal, many children with Down syndrome become overweight beginning in late toddlerhood.

This chapter was supported by Maternal and Child Study Project 928, National Institute of Child Health and Human Development grant HDO 5341-03, by March of Dimes grant 6-449, and by funds raised by parents of children with Down syndrome.

27

Most studies have suggested that the growth rate during childhood (ages 4–10 years) in those with Down syndrome is closer to that of children without disabilities (Ershow, 1986; Ikeda, Higurashi, Hirayama, & Ishikawa, 1977; Rarick & Seefeldt, 1974; Roche, 1965). However, evaluation of a larger sample (Cronk et al., 1988) suggests that childhood growth rates in youngsters with Down syndrome continue to be slower than average (between the 10th and 25th percentiles compared to normal).

GROWTH DURING ADOLESCENCE (10–18 YEARS OF AGE)
As with childhood values, the average height of adolescents with Down syndrome is reduced by 2–4 standard deviations below the "normal mean" (i.e., teens with Down syndrome are shorter than most teens of the same age without disabilities). Figures 3.1 and 3.2 show scatterplots for height (cm) for boys and girls, respectively, from the Boston Children's Hospital and Rhode Island Hospital samples of home-reared adolescents with Down syndrome (reported in Cronk et al., 1988). These are mixed longitudinal data (i.e., some, but not all, children were measured and are represented multiple times across the age span), and they include children with heart problems. The National Center for Health Statistics (NCHS) has constructed growth charts that are employed by most pediatricians for children and adolescents without disabilities. The 5th and 50th percentiles from the NCHS are plotted on these charts for reference (Hamill, Johnson, Reed, Roche, & Moore, 1979). At age 10 years, most children with Down syndrome are less than the NCHS 5th percentile. By 17 years of age, virtually

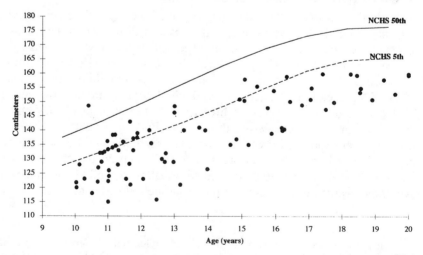

Figure 3.1.   Scatterplot of height (cm) by age (years) for Boston Children's Hospital and Rhode Island Hospital boys with Down syndrome 10–20 years old with the NCHS 5th and 50th percentiles plotted for reference.

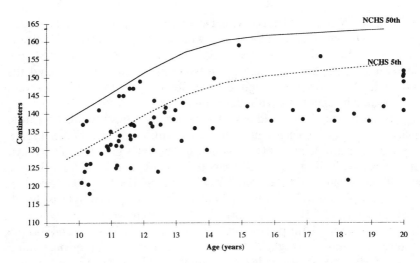

Figure 3.2.   Scatterplot of height (cm) by age (years) for Boston Children's Hospital and Rhode Island Hospital girls with Down syndrome 10–20 years old with NCHS 5th and 50th percentiles plotted for reference.

no boys and only a few girls are taller than the NCHS 5th percentile. Growth rates extrapolated from these data suggest that growth is in the lower percentiles (25th–50th percentiles) for "normal" in each sex throughout the adolescent years.

Roche (1965) found that 90% of an institutionalized group of adolescents with Down syndrome had an adolescent growth spurt (i.e., growth ≥ 4 cm in a single year). These spurts ranged from 5 cm to about 13 cm per year, which is similar to growth spurts in teens without disabilities. Moreover, these growth spurts occurred at about the same age ranges as those of children without disabilities. Cessation in height growth for Roche's sample occurred a little earlier than in teens without disabilities (15.5 years in boys, ranging from 13.9 to 18 years; 14.3 years in girls, ranging from 12.1 to 16 years). Bone maturation at the time of growth cessation was not fully completed. Findings by Rarick and Seefeldt (1974) differed somewhat from those of Roche. Growth in their sample of institutionalized boys with Down syndrome was a little less than in adolescents without disabilities. However, their sample of girls with Down syndrome had normal growth rates. When they subdivided adolescence into two time periods (10–14 years of age and 15–18 years of age), they found the girls had a later pubertal growth spurt than girls without disabilities. There was no parallel finding for boys, however. The maximum size of the growth spurt in adolescents with Down syndrome was about 8 cm for boys (compared with 9 cm for boys without disabilities) and 6.61 cm for girls (compared with 7.8 cm for girls without disabilities). On average, the growth spurt for both boys and girls with Down syndrome was found to occur about a year later than in adolescents without disabilities (Rarick, Wainer, Thissen, & Seefeldt, 1975). Using data on body water determined from deuterium oxide dilution, Culley, Chilko, and Coburn (1974) noted that boys with Down syndrome begin their adolescent growth spurts at a shorter average height than boys without disabilities.

None of the studies addressing height growth has provided a careful analysis of weight changes in adolescents with Down syndrome. Figures 3.3 and 3.4 show scatterplots of weight in boys and girls with Down syndrome, respectively, ages 10–20 years from the Boston Children's Hospital and Rhode Island Hospital samples with the NCHS 5th, 50th, and 95th percentiles plotted for reference. In contrast with height, weight is distributed across the NCHS percentiles. For boys, more values fall below the 5th and above the 95th percentiles than for girls. Figures 3.5 and 3.6 plot weight in relation to height in these same adolescents. The median values from NCHS data are provided for reference. At all heights and in both sexes, weights for virtually all of the children with Down syndrome are greater than the normal median, indicating that many children are overweight. As suggested previously, the onset of being overweight probably occurs in early childhood for many children with Down syndrome. At smaller heights, adolescents with Down syndrome are actually being compared with prepubescent children without disabilities who have not experienced the spurt in lean body mass and fat typical for adolescents. Thus, the degree of excess weight represented by these weights at smaller heights

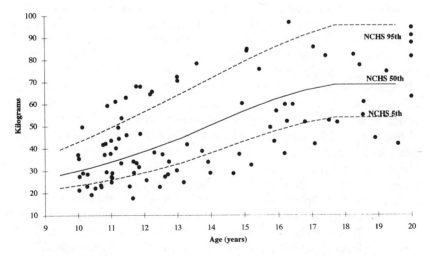

Figure 3.3. Scatterplot of weight (kg) by age (years) for Boston Children's Hospital and Rhode Island Hospital boys with Down syndrome 10–20 years old with NCHS 5th, 50th, and 95th percentiles plotted for reference.

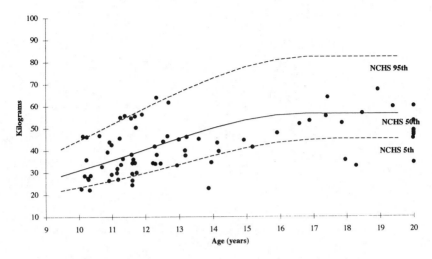

Figure 3.4. Scatterplot of weight (kg) by age (years) for Boston Children's Hospital and Rhode Island Hospital girls with Down syndrome 10–20 years old with NCHS 5th, 50th, and 95th percentiles plotted for reference.

may be exaggerated. However, for heights greater than about 145 cm, body composition for adolescents without disabilities and for adolescents with Down syndrome should be similar. In both boys and girls, values at taller heights (older ages) appear to be farther above the normal median, sug-

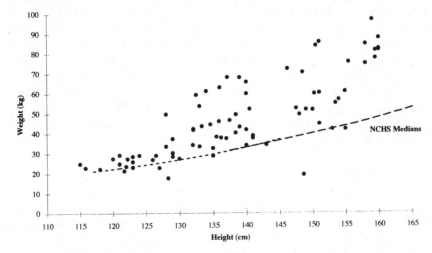

Figure 3.5. Scatterplot of weight (kg) by height (cm) for Boston Children's Hospital and Rhode Island Hospital boys with Down syndrome 10–20 years old with NCHS median plotted for reference. Median values for children without disabilities from 115 cm through 145 cm are based on observed height for weight of prepubescent children. Values for ≥145 cm are extrapolated from median heights and weights of adolescents.

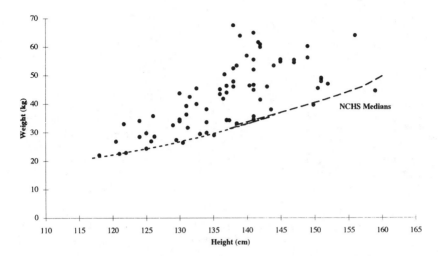

Figure 3.6. Scatterplot of weight (kg) by height (cm) for Boston Children's Hospital and Rhode Island Hospital girls with Down syndrome 10–20 years old with NCHS median plotted for reference. Median values for children without disabilities from 115 cm through 145 cm are based on observed height for weight of prepubescent children. Values for ≥145 cm are extrapolated from median heights and weights of adolescents.

gesting that teens with Down syndrome may be at risk for onset or enhancement of being overweight.

Assessment of height for adolescents with Down syndrome should be done using the growth charts published by Castlemead Publications (12 Little Mundells, Welwyn Garden City, Herts AL7 1EW, ENGLAND). Evaluation of weight status, however, should involve using the Down syndrome growth charts in combination with a measure such as the body mass index (BMI) which is computed by dividing the weight (in kg) by the squared value for height (in cm) and multiplying by 100,000 (Cronk & Roche, 1982). For a child 10–13 years of age, a BMI greater than 200–220 (85th percentile for children without disabilities) suggests that the youngster is overweight. For an adolescent 14 years or older, a BMI greater than about 240 indicates the individual is overweight.

CONCLUSIONS

The average child with Down syndrome arrives at early adolescence already small for his or her age and with a good possibility of being overweight. The adolescent growth spurt occurs a little later for adolescents with Down syndrome. The size of the growth spurt is also less than that seen in teens without disabilities. Because weight gain is about average, the already-present tendency for teens with Down syndrome to be overweight is enhanced as they experience the changes of adolescence. Growth of teens with Down syndrome should be evaluated by using both the special Down syndrome growth charts and reference data for adolescents without disabilities.

REFERENCES

Benda, C.E. (1939). Studies in mongolism: Growth and physical development. *Archives of Neurological Psychiatry, 41,* 83–95.

Cronk, C.E. (1978). Growth of children with Down's syndrome: Birth to age 3 years. *Pediatrics, 61,* 564–568.

Cronk, C.E., Crocker, A.C., Pueschel, S.M., Shea, A.M., Zackai, E., Pickens, G., & Reed, R.B. (1988). Growth charts for children with Down syndrome: 1 month to 18 years of age. *Pediatrics, 81,* 102–110.

Cronk, C.E., & Pueschel, S.M. (1984). Anthropometric studies. In S.M. Pueschel (Ed.), *The young child with Down syndrome* (pp. 105–142). New York: Human Sciences Press.

Cronk, C.E., & Roche, A.F. (1982). Race- and sex-specific reference data for triceps and subscapular skinfolds and weight/stature^2. *American Journal of Clinical Nutrition, 35,* 347–353.

Culley, W., Chilko, J., & Coburn, S. (1974). Body water content of boys with Down's syndrome. *Journal of Mental Deficiency Research, 18,* 25–29.

Dutton, G. (1958). The physical development of mongols. *Archives of Disease in Childhood, 34,* 46–50.

Ershow, A.G. (1986). Growth in black and white children with Down syndrome. *American Journal of Mental Deficiency, 90,* 507–512.

Gustavson, K.-H. (1964). *Down's syndrome: A clinical and cytogenetical investigation.* Uppsala, Sweden: Alonquist & Wiksell.

Hamill, P.V., Johnson, C.L., Reed, R.B., Roche, A.F., & Moore, W.M. (1979). Physical growth: National Center for Health Statistics percentiles. *American Journal of Clinical Nutrition, 32,* 607–629.

Ikeda, Y., Higurashi, M., Hirayama, M., & Ishikawa, N. (1977). A longitudinal study on the growth of stature, lower limb, and upper limb length in Japanese children with Down's syndrome. *Journal of Mental Deficiency Research, 21,* 139–151.

Oster, J. (1953). *Mongolism.* Copenhagen, Denmark: Danish Science Press.

Pueschel, S.M. (1984). The study population. In S.M. Pueschel (Ed.), *The young child with Down syndrome* (pp. 39–58). New York: Human Sciences Press.

Rarick, G.L., & Seefeldt, V. (1974). Observations from longitudinal data on growth in stature and sitting height of children with Down's syndrome. *Journal of Mental Deficiency Research, 18,* 63–78.

Rarick, G.L., Wainer, H., Thissen, D., & Seefeldt, V. (1975). A double logistic comparison of growth patterns of normal children and children with Down's syndrome. *Annals of Human Biology, 2,* 339–346.

Roche, A.F. (1965). The stature of mongols. *Journal of Mental Deficiency Research, 9,* 131–145.

4

Adolescent Development and Sexual Maturation

Siegfried M. Pueschel

The transition from childhood to adulthood—passing through adolescence—
is a challenging time in the lives of young people with Down syndrome.
During this time, significant changes in growth and development occur. For
many youngsters with Down syndrome, these changes can be bewildering.

SEXUAL DEVELOPMENT IN FEMALES

Only limited information is available in the medical literature on the physical and sexual maturation of female adolescents with Down syndrome.
Some of the early literature is based on studies conducted in institutions
for people with mental retardation, and the results of those studies are
frequently not applicable to adolescents with Down syndrome growing up
today. For example, Bleyer (1937) reported that the labia majora are frequently oversized and that the labia minora are enlarged and protruding.
However, such observations were not made by Scola and Pueschel (1992).
Smith, Warren, and Turner (1963) reported delayed development of axillary
hair in females with Down syndrome. Also, Shelley and Butterworth
(1955) noted underdevelopment or absence of axillary apocrine glands as
well as diminished axillary hair.

Tricomi, Valenti, and Hall (1964) studied ovulatory patterns of 13
institutionalized women with trisomy 21 by means of vaginal smears over
two menstrual cycles. The authors concluded that 38.5% of the women in
their study cohort showed a definite pattern of ovulation, 15.4% probably
ovulated, and another 15.4% possibly ovulated. There was no evidence of
ovulation in the remaining 30.7% of females. Scola and Pueschel (1992)
examined menstrual cycles and basal body temperature curves in adolescent girls with Down syndrome. Based on their extensive investigations,

the authors concluded that almost all young women with Down syndrome in their study ovulated. In addition, investigations of pituitary and ovarian hormones revealed that adolescent females with Down syndrome have normal concentrations of follicle-stimulating hormone and of luteinizing hormone, as well as adequate levels of estradiol when compared with a control population. The expected rise in follicle-stimulating and luteinizing hormones in Scola and Pueschel's (1992) study population also occurred during the time period of sexual maturation similar to that observed in adolescents without Down syndrome.

The age of onset of menstruation and characteristics of the menstrual cycle were studied by Bellone, Tanganelli, LaPlaca, and Daneri (1980). These investigators found the average age of onset of the menstrual period to be 13 years, 1 month in females with Down syndrome. They noted that the menstrual cycles occurred every 26–34 days in about two thirds of the study population. More recently, Scola and Pueschel (1992) reported that the average onset of the first menstrual cycle in young females with Down syndrome was 12 years, 6 months, compared with their sisters whose average menarche was at 12 years, 1 month. In this study, of the 38 adolescent females with Down syndrome who had menstruated at least once, 29 were described as having regularly occurring menstrual cycles. The nine females with irregular cycles included three who had their first period in the preceding month, two who had spotted several times without an established pattern, and four who had very irregular patterns but a normal to heavy flow rate. The authors also reported that the average length from the first day of the cycle to the first day of the next cycle varied from 22 days to 33 days. The menstrual flow lasted, on average, 4 days. The amount of flow was described as normal for 22 females, heavy for 5 youngsters, and light for 2. The vast majority of young women with Down syndrome in this study did not require help with menstrual hygiene, and only 6 of the 29 females needed assistance at times with changing pads (Scola & Pueschel, 1992).

The question often arises whether females with Down syndrome are fertile and whether they will be able to bear children. A review of the literature indicates that numerous females with Down syndrome have given birth to children. Bovicelli, Orsini, Rizzo, Montacuti, and Bacchetta (1982) reported 30 pregnancies occurring in 26 women with Down syndrome; about half of their offspring also had Down syndrome. A similar report of 31 pregnancies to mothers with Down syndrome was published by Rani, Jyothi, Reddy, and Reddy (1990) (see also Chapter 5).

SEXUAL DEVELOPMENT IN MALES

Previous studies by Benda (1960), who reported that 50% of males with Down syndrome have undescended testicles, and Oster (1953), who found cryptorchidism (i.e., failure of the testes to descend into the scrotum) in 40% of young males, have not been confirmed by investigations carried out since the mid-1980s. For example, when Pueschel, Orson, Boylan, and Pezzullo (1985) examined adolescent development in males with Down syndrome, they did not find an increase in undescended testicles when compared with a control population. Pueschel et al. (1985) also studied the development of primary and secondary sex characteristics as well as specific pituitary and testicular hormones. The investigators found that the pubic hair development of male individuals, which usually starts at between 11 and 13 years of age, did not differ significantly from that of "normative" data (Alsever & Gotlin, 1978). Moreover, like adolescents without Down syndrome, youngsters with trisomy 21 also showed initial darkening of the villous hair at the base of the penis, then hair growth at the inguinal region, the mons pubis, and adjacent areas of the lower abdominal wall, later extending to the umbilical area, forming the typical male pubic hair pattern.

Pueschel et al. (1985) measured the size of the genitalia of the 45 young males in this study and did not find any statistically significant differences when compared with that of an age-appropriate population without disabilities (Scholfeld, 1943). The authors noted that the testes of the study population were slightly but not significantly larger than those reported in a population without disabilities (Scholfeld, 1943). These observations contradict Benda's (1960) as well as Rundle and Sylvester's (1962) findings of significantly reduced testicular size. Pueschel et al. (1985) also noted that the mean penile length of youngsters with Down syndrome was less, and that the penile circumference was slightly increased; however, these differences were not statistically significant.

Concerning specific pituitary and testicular hormones, Pueschel et al. (1985) observed that follicle-stimulating hormone, luteinizing hormone, and testosterone levels of adolescents with Down syndrome were increasing with advancing age similar to those seen in adolescents without disabilities (Alsever & Gotlin, 1978). When the respective hormone levels were compared with normative data (Alsever & Gotlin, 1978), no significant difference was noted. However, Campbell, Lowther, McKenzie, and Price (1982) and Horan, Beitins, and Bode (1978) found in their respective studies that the serum follicle-stimulating hormone and luteinizing hormone levels were significantly higher in males with Down syndrome when compared with controls. Since most of the subjects in the latter studies (Campbell et al., 1982; Horan et al., 1978) were residents in state institutions and were much older than the individuals in Pueschel et al.'s (1985) cohort, it is possible that testicular failure, including germinal cell hypoplasia and decreased Leydig cell function, may have been responsible for the increased hormone levels in these older individuals.

With regard to fertility in males with Down syndrome, there has been only one report in the literature documenting a young man with Down syndrome fathering a child (Sheridan et al., 1989). Thus, the results of Pueschel et al.'s (1985) investigations of biologic parameters as well as of specific hormones of young maturing males with Down syndrome compare well with normative data from the literature. Although Pueschel and co-workers' studies indicate that adolescents with Down syndrome display normal sequential development of primary and secondary sex characteristics and that their pituitary–gonadal axis appears to be intact, there are still many unanswered questions relating to these adolescents' sexual function, sperm production, and fertility.

REFERENCES

Alsever, R.N., & Gotlin, R.W. (1978). *Handbook of endocrine tests in adults and children*. Chicago: Yearbook Medical Publishers.

Bellone, F., Tanganelli, E., LaPlaca, A., & Daneri, C. (1980). Menarca e fisiopatologia menstrua Down. *Minerva Ginecologica, 32*, 579–588.

Benda, C.E. (1960). *The child with mongolism*. New York: Grune & Stratton.

Bleyer, A. (1937). Theoretical and clinical aspects of mongolism. *Journal of the Missouri Medical Association, 34*, 222–231.

Bovicelli, L., Orsini, L.F., Rizzo, N., Montacuti, V., & Bacchetta, M. (1982). Reproduction in Down syndrome. *Obstetrics and Gynecology, 59*, 13S–17S.

Campbell, W.A., Lowther, J., McKenzie, I., & Price, W.H. (1982). Serum gonadotropin in Down's syndrome. *Journal of Medical Genetics, 19*, 98–99.

Horan, R.F., Beitins, I.Z., & Bode, H.H. (1978). LH-RH testing in men with Down's syndrome. *Acta Endocrinologica, 88*, 594–600.

Oster, J. (1953). *Mongolism*. Copenhagen, Denmark: Danish Science Press.

Pueschel, S.M., Orson, J.M., Boylan, J.M., & Pezzullo, J.C. (1985). Adolescent development in males with Down syndrome. *American Journal of Diseases of Children, 139*, 236–238.

Rani, A.S., Jyothi, A., Reddy, P.P., & Reddy, O.S. (1990). Reproduction in Down's syndrome. *International Journal of Gynecology and Obstetrics, 31*, 81–86.

Rundle, A.T., & Sylvester, P.E. (1962). Endocrinological aspects of mental deficiency: II. Maturational status of adult males. *Journal of Mental Deficiency Research, 6*, 87–95.

Scholfeld, W.A. (1943). Primary and secondary sexual characteristics: Study of their development in males from birth throughout maturity, with biometric study of penis and testis. *American Journal of Diseases of Children, 65*, 535–549.

Scola, P.S., & Pueschel, S.M. (1992). Menstrual cycles and basal body temperature curves in women with Down syndrome. *Obstetrics and Gynecology, 79*, 91–94.

Shelley, W.B., & Butterworth, T. (1955). The absence of the apocrine glands and hair in the axilla in mongolism and idiocy. *Journal of Investigative Dermatology, 25*, 155–160.

Sheridan, R., Ilerena, J., Matkins, S., Debenham, P., Cawood, A., & Bobrow, M. (1989). Fertility in a male with trisomy 21. *Journal of Medical Genetics, 26*, 294–298.

Smith, G.S., Warren, S.A., & Turner, D.R. (1963). Hair characteristics in mongolism (Down's syndrome). *American Journal of Mental Deficiency, 68*, 362–371.

Tricomi, V., Valenti, C., & Hall, J.E. (1964). Ovulatory patterns in Down's syndrome. *American Journal of Obstetrics and Gynecology, 89*, 651–656.

5

Gynecologic Concerns

Janet D. Lawson
Thomas E. Elkins

The gynecologic concerns of adolescents with Down syndrome are essentially the same as those for young women without Down syndrome. Unfortunately, as important as gynecologic evaluation is for these young women, this area of medical care has not been emphasized (Elkins, 1995). Access to gynecologic care for young women with Down syndrome may be problematic for several reasons. Parents or caregivers are often apprehensive about taking a young woman for a gynecologic evaluation (especially for her first pelvic examination). Some physicians are uncomfortable dealing with issues of the reproductive system and sexuality in a patient with Down syndrome and other disabilities, particularly if she has complex medical problems or has limited ability to communicate. Moreover, the young woman herself may be fearful and anxious about being examined. These factors and others that limit access to care must be overcome so that the adolescent can receive timely and appropriate care.

In this ever-changing medical climate, where managed care is becoming a dominant force, providing cost-effective and efficient health care should include a program of preventive care. Gynecologic concerns should be addressed as part of a comprehensive health care program.

APPROACH TO GYNECOLOGIC EVALUATION

A parent discovering the signs that one's little girl is developing breasts or growing pubic and axillary hair may become distressed. Previously, the daughter's health care concerns had involved general care, immunizations, and prophylaxes (for childhood diseases), as well as screening (particularly for conditions seen more often in children with Down syndrome). With these normal signs of puberty may come a realization that this innocent and childlike person is emerging into a young woman who will need to deal with a different set of problems and concerns. How will she manage menstrual hygiene? Will she have problems with cramps, heavy bleeding, or other menstrual difficulties? How will she express her sexuality? Will there be those who take advantage of her giving nature or her desire to please? Can she get pregnant? If she can, will the baby be born without Down syndrome or other disabilities? Suddenly, there are so many questions to answer.

Physicians and other health care providers add other questions to this list. When is a gynecologic evaluation indicated? Who should provide this evaluation? When and how often should a pelvic examination be performed? What about PAP smears?

By 18 years of age, most women in the United States should have received their first pelvic examination. Menstrual irregularities, dysmenorrhea (i.e., menstrual cramps) or pelvic pain, premenstrual syndrome symptoms, vaginal discharge, odor or itching, initiation of sexual activity, possible sexual abuse or assault, and precocious or delayed puberty are conditions that may indicate the need for an earlier evaluation. Any physician, physician assistant, or nurse practitioner who is skilled in caring for patients with developmental disabilities and is comfortable with gynecologic issues can perform the examination. Pelvic examinations should be performed when certain disorders or problems are suspected (discussed later in more detail). PAP smears are indicated when risk factors are present for cervical dysplasia or cancer. These risk factors include

- Early age at onset of sexual activity, multiple sexual partners, nonbarrier contraception, history of sexually transmitted diseases or human immunodeficiency virus (HIV) infection
- History of genital human papilloma virus (HPV) infection
- Smoking
- Failure to obtain regular cytologic screening, lack of access to health care, and inadequate public education
- Immunosuppression
- Lower socioeconomic status (American College of Obstetricians & Gynecologists, 1996)

A practitioner experienced in caring for patients with developmental disabilities should be sought for the first gynecologic evaluation. It is extremely important that this individual be patient, empathetic, and flexible. No set pattern or methodology works for all patients. Prior to the first visit, the nurse can contact a responsible family member or caregiver to request that pertinent information be provided at the time of the visit. This could include a current list of medications, drug allergies, previous illness or surgery, and a menstrual calendar, if available.

The initial interview should be unhurried, with the patient fully clothed. Whenever possible, the patient should be addressed directly because the practitioner is establishing rapport with her. While taking a complete history, special attention should be paid to the menstrual history (i.e., age of first period, frequency, duration and amount of flow), age of thelarche (i.e., breast budding), and pubarche (i.e., development of pubic and axillary hair).

To decrease anxiety, the examination should first be carefully explained, using visual aids (e.g., charts, diagrams, models, instruments) whenever possible. If the patient is very anxious, the examination may be delayed. The patient may visit several times over the course of a few days or even weeks, allowing her to become more familiar and more comfortable with the office and personnel. It is also helpful if the patient can participate in the examination. A mirror may be made available so that the patient can see what is being done.

Positioning the patient for the pelvic examination is one important example where flexibility and creativity are helpful. Most patients can comfortably be examined in a frog-legged position if they cannot tolerate the lithotomy position in stirrups. If the patient has difficulty flexing her knees, two people can assist by holding the legs up straight and exposing the perineum to be viewed.

Visual inspection of the external genitalia should be documented, including the appearance of the hymen. Any evidence of trauma, bruising, tears, or separations should be noted. The shape of the hymen can be described as circumferential smooth rim, posterior rim, or fimbriated rim (Pokorny, 1994). If evaluation of the internal organs is indicated, a rectoabdominal examination is often better tolerated than a bimanual or rectovaginal examination. Pelvic ultrasound is a more expensive, but often a less traumatic and more humane means of assessing the pelvic structures. Many patients tolerate a Huffman or Pedersen speculum. When a speculum examination is not possible and a PAP smear is indicated, this may be accomplished with a saline-moistened Q-Tip, guided to the cervical os with a single digit. The blinded PAP smear is not always optimal, but often provides adequate information.

EVALUATION OF COMMON GYNECOLOGIC CONDITIONS

Vulvovaginitis

Often it is the caregiver who notices a stain in the panties or a foul-smelling odor that indicates a vulvar irritation or a vaginal discharge (Jones, 1989). Occasionally, the patient may scratch her perineal area or complain of itching, burning, or other discomfort. Most often the cause of the vaginal discharge is physiologic (i.e., normal hormone-related secretions) or is related to a monilial (i.e., yeast) infection or poor hygiene. Occasionally, the patient may have placed a foreign body within the vagina. Alternatively, she may be experiencing an allergic reaction to a soap, powder, spray, or lotion she is using. Vaginal discharge can also indicate a more serious problem, including a sexually transmitted disease. Checking the pH and a wet mount (in saline and potassium hydroxide) of the vaginal secretions examined under a microscope can be helpful in diagnosing the problem (see Table 4.1) (Rau, Jones, & Muram, 1994). If there is a history of sexual activity or sexual abuse, testing for chlamydia, gonorrhea, and other bacteria also should be done.

Counseling about appropriate hygiene and sexuality is often an important component of prevention and treatment and may need to be repeated at regular intervals. A diagnosis of a sexually transmitted disease, including bacterial vaginosis, *Trichomonas vaginalis*, gonorrhea, condyloma (i.e., venereal warts), or syphilis warrants consideration of possible sexual abuse.

Menstrual Abnormalities

Several problems or conditions may be associated with the menstrual cycle. These include amenorrhea or oligomenorrhea, menorrhagia or metrorrhagia, premenstrual syndrome symptoms, and dysmenorrhea (i.e., menstrual cramps) and pelvic pain. These are discussed in the following subsections.

Amenorrhea   Primary amenorrhea (i.e., lack of periods) is defined as no spontaneous menses by age 16.5 years or within 2 years of thelarche (i.e., breast budding). Evaluation is also begun if there is no breast development by age 14 years. This is not a common problem among females with Down syndrome.

Secondary amenorrhea, which is more common, is defined as no spontaneous menses for 6 months—in a patient with previous regular menses—or for 1 year, in patients with previous oligomenorrhea (Davajan & Kletzky, 1991). *Oligomenorrhea* is defined as cycle lengths (i.e., interval from the first day of one period to the first day of the next period) of more than 35 days (Mishell, 1987a).

Once a careful history is taken and an appropriate physical examination is performed, pregnancy should be ruled out by obtaining a pregnancy test. Other causes of amenorrhea include thyroid disease (not uncommon in individuals with Down syndrome) (Pueschel, Rynders, Tin-

Table 4.1.   Diagnosing vulvovaginitis

Pathogen	Saline	KOH	pH
Bacterial vaginosis	Clue cells (stippled vaginal epithelial cells)	—	> 4.5
Trichomonas vaginalis	Motile, flagellated tear-shaped organisms	—	> 5
Candida (i.e., yeast)	Fungal hyphae or buds	Fungal hyphae or buds	< 4.5

KOH, potassium hydroxide.

gey, Crocker, & Crutcher, 1987), polycystic ovary syndrome, physiologic ovarian cysts, and prolactinomas (i.e., noncancerous tumor of the pituitary in the brain). Tests to evaluate the patient can include a progesterone challenge (or progesterone withdrawal) test, thyroid-stimulating hormone level (TSH), prolactin level, follicle-stimulating hormone level (FSH), and CT scan of the head to evaluate the size of the sella turcica.

Any underlying medical problem should be treated. If the adolescent with Down syndrome is hypothyroid, thyroid replacement would be indicated. If present, diabetes should be brought under control. Also, seizure medication may have to be titrated to therapeutic levels.

Menorrhagia and Metrorrhagia   Menorrhagia (i.e., prolonged or excessive periods) and metrorrhagia (i.e., frequent and irregular periods) (Mishell, 1987b) are common presenting complaints in females with Down syndrome (Jones & Douglass, 1989). Causes to be included in the differential diagnosis are thyroid disorders, ovarian or adrenal dysfunction, pregnancy-related disorders, certain medications, and uterine problems such as leiomyoma (i.e., fibroids), adenomyosis, endometrial polyps, endometrial hyperplasia, or endometrial cancer (i.e., adenocarcinoma).

If the adolescent with Down syndrome has menorrhagia or metrorrhagia, the following tests should be done: a pregnancy test, complete blood count, thyroid-stimulating hormone level, prolactin level, and coagulation studies to evaluate for bleeding disorders. If she has had a longstanding history of irregular periods, endometrial sampling, which involves obtaining a sample of the lining of the uterus, may be indicated. Thyroid disorders occur more commonly in people with Down syndrome than in the general population. Many tend to be overweight (Odell, 1988), and obesity can be associated with irregular and heavy periods. Again, underlying medical conditions should be treated appropriately. The patient can then be cycled with medroxyprogesterone or an oral contraceptive agent. Occasionally, periods can be decreased or stopped with Depomedroxyprogesterone acetate.

Premenstrual Syndrome and Dysmenorrhea   Premenstrual syndrome includes a spectrum of symptoms, including bloating, headaches, irritability, depression, and so on, that usually occur from mid-cycle to just before each menses and usually last only through the first 1 or 2 days of the menses. A number of situations (e.g., fatigue, depression and other psychiatric problems not related to menses, dysmenorrhea, occasionally endometriosis) can mimic premenstrual syndrome. Therefore, it is important to document the relationship of any symptoms with the menstrual cycle by keeping a careful calendar. Dysmenorrhea (i.e., menstrual cramps) usually occurs with the menses and subsides within 12–72 hours. The patient may be acting out or may seem depressed or withdrawn because of premenstrual syndrome symptoms or because she is experiencing discomfort.

If the patient has difficulty communicating, these two problems can be confused—it is not uncommon to have both dysmenorrhea and premenstrual syndrome symptoms. The patient can become withdrawn, more aggressive, or combative. Sometimes a patient can become self-abusive, verbalize discomfort, or display a rocking behavior (Jones & Douglass, 1989). Seizure activity can occasionally increase prior to menses.

Because premenstrual syndrome seems to be a spectrum of symptoms, treatment is usually based on the specific symptoms identified. A mild diuretic is used for symptoms of bloating and fullness. Diuretics can also be helpful in some patients with increased premenstrual irritability. Analgesics are used for discomfort and headaches. Antidepressants are given for any significant depression. An exercise program, particularly prior to the onset of symptoms, adjustment of the diet, and manipulation of hormones with oral contraceptive agents or progesterone suppositories have all been used in an attempt to control the symptoms.

The administration of nonsteroidal anti-inflammatory drugs (e.g., ibuprofen, naprosyn) is used to control the discomfort of menstrual cramps. It may be helpful to decrease or stop the menses with Depo-medroxyprogesterone. If medical management is not successful, laparoscopy to examine the pelvic structures directly can be done. Endometriosis or pelvic adhesive disease may be discovered in this manner. It should be remembered that just as in the general population, not all pelvic pain is related to the pelvic organs. Evaluation of the urinary and gastrointestinal systems may also be appropriate.

SEXUALITY AND CONTRACEPTION

As indicated previously, it is difficult for many parents to see their daughters becoming sexual beings. Once the menses are established, usually within the first 6–18 months of menarche (the first period), most adolescents with Down syndrome have regular periods. The average age of the first period is usually between 11 and 13 years old for this population, whereas it is typically between 10.2 and 11.2 years in the general population (Elkins, 1995) (see also Chapter 4). Many patients may confine their sexual expression to masturbation. The adolescent may begin exploring her feelings, some of which can be quite confusing for her. This is the time when she will need careful counseling on appropriate behavior (private versus public behavior) and guidance to decrease the risk of sexual abuse (see also Chapter 7). Approximately 20%–40% of individuals with mental retardation requiring intermittent to limited supports are sexually abused in their lifetime. This problem is not limited to patients with Down syndrome; it includes all individuals with developmental disabilities (Elkins, 1995).

Pregnancy can occur in women with Down syndrome, whose off-spring also have an increased risk of having Down syndrome (Elkins, 1995). To prevent unintended pregnancies, these young women should have appropriate counseling and, when indicated, should be provided with appropriate contraceptive methods. An oral contraceptive agent can provide excellent protection for this population, but the individual must be compliant in taking the medication. Oral contraceptive agents give other benefits, including regulation of the menstrual flow, decreased amount of flow and therefore less anemia (i.e., low blood count), decreased ovarian cysts, decreased risk of ovarian and endometrial cancer (when compared to women not using an oral contraceptive agent), lower incidence of breast cysts, and decreased dysmenorrhea. Depo-medroxyprogesterone injections and the levonorgestrel implants offer alternatives to oral contraceptive agents. Both provide excellent contraceptive effectiveness. The implants require a minor surgical procedure for placement and removal, and therefore a general anesthetic may be used. Most patients will tolerate an injection of Depo-medroxyprogesterone once every 3 months. Intrauterine devices are usually not an optimal contraceptive choice for females with Down syndrome. The devices may be associated with heavier vaginal bleeding (adding to any problems associated with menstrual hygiene), increased dysmenorrhea, and increased risk for pelvic infections. It is recommended that the string of the intrauterine device be checked for placement after each period; this would therefore be a poor choice in a patient where communication may not be optimal. Likewise, barrier methods (e.g., condoms with or without spermicide, diaphragm) are rarely appropriate.

There is fear that a young woman with Down syndrome will either enter into a consensual sexual relationship or be sexually abused and thus exposed to an unwanted pregnancy. Because of this concern many of these young women in the past were sterilized by bilateral tubal ligation or hysterectomy (Elkins, 1995). However, oral contraceptive agents, Depo-medroxyprogesterone, and the levonorgestrel implant system are each relatively safe and effective. Given the effectiveness of these options, along with the increased risk of surgical complications for young women with Down syndrome, hysterectomy or bilateral tubal ligation is rarely believed to be appropriate. These options should be considered only after all others have been thoroughly explored.

Of course, although bilateral tubal ligation or hysterectomy would address the concern of unwanted pregnancy or aid menstrual hygiene problems, any concern about sexual abuse or inappropriate sexual behavior would still need to be addressed. Appropriate counseling, particularly involving avoiding high-risk situations, is critical at this stage of development and often needs to be repeated over time (see also Chapter 7).

CONCLUSIONS

Routine gynecologic care is essential to the physical, mental, and emotional health of the adolescent with Down syndrome. Although this premise is well accepted, appropriate gynecologic care has not been emphasized in this population. The concerns and problems noted in this group are often the same as those seen in young women without Down syndrome. A flexible approach to examination is important to the evaluation of the adolescent with Down syndrome.

Counseling is a crucial component of care and is most effective when repeated at regular intervals. Helping to prepare parents and caregivers for this complex stage of life is as important as counseling the adolescent.

REFERENCES

American College of Obstetricians & Gynecologists. (1996). *Guidelines for women's health care.* Washington, DC: Author.

Davajan, V., & Kletzky, O.A. (1991). Secondary amenorrhea without galactorrhea or androgen excess. In D. Mishell, V. Davajan, & R. Lobo (Eds.), *Infertility, contraception and endocrinology* (3rd ed., pp. 372–395). Boston: Blackwell Scientific Publications.

Elkins, T. (1995). Medical issues related to sexuality and reproduction. In D.C. Van Dyke, P. Mattheis, S. Eberly, & J. Williams (Eds.), *Medical and surgical care for children with Down syndrome: A guide for parents* (pp. 253–266). Bethesda, MD: Woodbine House.

Jones, K., & Douglass, J. (1989). Gynecologic problems. In I. Rubin & Croker (Eds.), *Developmental disabilities: Delivery of medical care for children and adults* (pp. 276–281). Boston: Lea & Febiger.

Mishell, D. (1987a). Abnormal uterine bleeding. In W. Droegemueller, A. Herbst, D. Mishell, & M. Stenchever (Eds.), *Comprehensive gynecology* (pp. 965–993). St. Louis: C.V. Mosby.

Mishell, D. (1987b). Reproductive endocrinology. In W. Droegemueller, A. Herbst, D. Mishell, & M. Stenchever (Eds.), *Comprehensive gynecology* (pp. 3–127). St. Louis: C.V. Mosby.

Odell, J. (1988). Medical considerations. In C. Tingey (Ed.), *Down syndrome: A resource handbook* (pp. 33–45). Boston: College-Hill Press.

Pokorny, S. (1994). Genital examination of prepubertal and peripubertal females. In J. Sanfilippo, D. Muram, P. Lee, & J. Dewhurst (Eds.), *Pediatric and adolescent gynecology* (pp. 170–186). Philadelphia: W.B. Saunders.

Pueschel, S.M., Rynders, J.E., Tingey, C., Crocker, A.C., & Crutcher, D.M. (Eds.). (1987). *New perspectives on Down syndrome.* Baltimore: Paul H. Brookes Publishing Co.

Rau, E., Jones, C., & Muram, D. (1994). Vulvovaginitis. In J. Sanfilippo, D. Muram, P. Lee, & J. Dewhurst (Eds.), *Pediatric and adolescent gynecology* (pp. 187–201). Philadelphia; W.B. Saunders.

6

Selected Medical Conditions

Siegfried M. Pueschel
Mária Šustrová

Numerous medical disorders have been described in people with Down syndrome (Pueschel & Pueschel, 1992). It is not possible within the scope of this volume to cover all of these medical conditions or to dwell in depth on the many health-related concerns seen in individuals with this chromosome disorder. Rather, selected medical conditions that are observed at an increased frequency during adolescence are briefly discussed here. Readers are referred to other texts for more detailed descriptions of medical disorders in Down syndrome (e.g., Pueschel & Pueschel, 1992; Pueschel & Rynders, 1982; Storm, 1995).

DERMATOLOGIC DISORDERS
Numerous skin abnormalities have been reported in young people with Down syndrome. The skin in adolescents with Down syndrome is usually described as dry and rough. There is a high prevalence of xerosis (i.e., abnormally dry skin), localized hyperkeratotic lesions, elastosis perforans serpiginosa (i.e., an elastic tissue defect), and alopecia areata (i.e., patchy loss of hair) (Benson & Scherbenske, 1992; Carter & Jegasothy, 1976).

The skin of infants with Down syndrome is usually soft and velvety; but, in later childhood and during the teenage years, more than 70% of people with Down syndrome show mild to moderate generalized xerosis (Burton & Rook, 1986). Management of xerosis usually includes the use of nondrying or oilated soaps and adding oil to the bath water. Also lubrication with creams, moisturizers, and emollients may be used after the bath (Benson & Scherbenske, 1992).

Kersting and Rappaport (1958) studied 232 people with Down syndrome and found that 173 (74.6%) had localized hyperkeratotic skin lesions. The most frequent site of these skin lesions was the dorsum of the upper arms. Such lesions were also found on the anterior thighs, the flexor aspects of the ankles, and the wrists. These lesions were fairly well-defined plaques of thickened, corrugated, lichenified, and slightly reddened skin with a firm gray scale.

Cheilitis, which consists of vertical fissures with mild scaling of lips, also occurs at a higher prevalence in adolescents with Down syndrome when compared with the general population (Butterworth, Leoni, Beerman, Wood, & Strean, 1960). Cheilitis is more often observed in boys than in girls. Regular use of lip moisturizers can often prevent cracking of the lips.

During adolescence, youngsters with Down syndrome often develop skin infections, primarily in the perigenital area as well as at the buttocks and upper thighs. These skin lesions are usually follicular in nature; however, they may develop into abscesses. These infected skin areas are more often observed in adolescents who are significantly overweight. Weight control, frequent bathing, and the application of antibiotic ointment as soon as the follicular eruptions are noted usually control the infection. However, skin infections may recur in spite of appropriate hygienic measures and antibiotic treatment.

Alopecia areata and alopecia totalis (i.e., partial or total absence of scalp hair) are also more often observed in young people with Down syndrome than in youngsters without the disorder. For example, DuVivier and Munro (1974) noted alopecia areata in 6 out of 1,000 adolescents with Down syndrome. Also, Carter and Jegasothy (1976) reported a high prevalence of alopecia areata in a cohort of people with Down syndrome. These authors suggested that immunologic factors may contribute to the increased prevalence of both alopecia areata and vitiligo (i.e., depigmentation of the skin) in youngsters with Down syndrome. Although the etiology of alopecia is unknown, autoimmune and genetic factors are thought to play a role in its pathogenesis.

When only one or a few patches of alopecia areata are present, complete regrowth of hair usually occurs within about a year in 95% of individuals with Down syndrome. However, if alopecia totalis is already present at an early age, complete and permanent recovery occurs in less than 30% of patients (Hurwitz, 1981). Numerous therapeutic modalities have been suggested for the treatment of alopecia areata. Often topical steroids can be of benefit if spontaneous recovery does not occur.

In addition, fungus infections, in particular on the feet, are frequently seen in adolescents with Down syndrome. Other, less-often-observed skin disorders in individuals with Down syndrome are discussed by Benson and Scherbenske (1992).

OPHTHALMOLOGIC CONDITIONS

Structural abnormalities occurring in almost every tissue of the eye have been described in people with Down syndrome by Catalano (1992). A frequently noted eyelid problem is blepharitis (i.e., inflammation of the eyelids) (Shapiro & France, 1985). Gaynon and Schimeck (1977) reported that more than 50% of adolescents with Down syndrome had at least one documented occurrence of blepharitis during a 10-year period. Daily wiping of the eyelid margins with cotton swabs dipped in baby shampoo can reduce the prevalence of blepharitis. Also, the application of a clean, wet washcloth will remove some of the scaling at the eyelid margins. If an acute infection is present and inflammation with purulent (i.e., pus-containing) discharge is observed, then treatment with ophthalmic antibiotic ointment is indicated.

Another ocular concern relates to keratoconus, which involves the anterior bulging of the cornea. The prevalence of keratoconus in individuals with Down syndrome has been estimated at between 5% and 8% (Catalano, 1992). Cullen and Butler (1963) found acute keratoconus to be the second most common cause of blindness in young people with Down syndrome. Therefore, it is important to identify and treat effectively those individuals who have this disorder.

Cataracts are also known to occur more frequently in people with Down syndrome than in the general population. Although the majority of cataracts are identified in adults with Down syndrome, the gradual development of cataracts usually starts during adolescence. Jaeger (1980) reported that "senile" cataracts occur at a younger age in people with Down syndrome, which apparently is a manifestation of the early aging process in this population.

The prevalence of strabismus (i.e., crossed eyes) in people with Down syndrome has been estimated at between 23% and 44% (Cullen & Butler, 1963; Jaeger, 1980; Shapiro & France, 1985). Accommodative esotropia accounts for most of the strabismus observed in adolescents with Down syndrome. However, Jaeger (1980) did not find an association between esotropia (i.e., inward turning of the eyes) and hyperopia (i.e., farsightedness). He noted myopia (i.e., nearsightedness) as frequently as hyperopia in people with esotropia. Whereas strabismus is common in youngsters with Down syndrome, amblyopia (i.e., decreased vision or visual acuity in one eye) has been reported to be less frequent. Pueschel and Giesswein (1993) observed amblyopia in about 12% of adolescents with Down syndrome. Occlusive therapy is usually the treatment of choice for amblyopia.

The most often occurring ocular disorder relates to refractive errors. Myopia has been reported at between 35% and 40%, and hyperopia is noted in 20%–25% of young people with Down syndrome (Jaeger, 1980). In addition, astigmatism of greater than 2.50–3.00 diopters has been observed in about 18%–25% of individuals with Down syndrome (Jaeger, 1980; Shapiro & France, 1985).

Because ophthalmologic conditions in people with Down syndrome are common, it is paramount that children with Down syndrome be examined regularly by an ophthalmologist. For the adolescent with Down syndrome to succeed both educationally and vocationally, it is important that his or her sensory functions, including vision, be optimal.

OTOLARYNGOLOGIC AND AUDIOLOGIC CONCERNS

A number of otolaryngologic and audiologic disorders are commonly observed in people with Down syndrome (Dahle & Baldwin, 1992). Although an increased frequency of middle-ear infections is noted during early childhood, some adolescents with Down syndrome also may have otitis media, or fluid accumulation in the middle ear, and their hearing may be impaired.

Considering the numerous structural and functional concerns related to the ears of children with Down syndrome, it is not surprising that there is a relatively high prevalence of hearing impairment. Whereas prior to 1970 there were only sporadic reports of hearing loss in children with Down syndrome, the advent of acoustic impedance audiometry (i.e., sound reflected by the ear drum), in addition to more refined audiologic assessment, has uncovered a prevalence of hearing impairment in children with Down syndrome of about 60% (Schwartz & Schwartz, 1978). The vast majority of children with hearing deficits have a conductive hearing loss. Impacted cerumen (i.e., wax) in the ear canal, tympanic membrane abnormalities, and middle-ear disease contribute to the high frequency of conductive hearing impairment. Moreover, some youngsters have a sensorineural hearing loss (about 10%–15%), and other adolescents with Down syndrome may have a mixed hearing loss. In adolescents and young adults with Down syndrome, a high-frequency hearing loss has also been described (Buchanan, 1990).

Since anatomic and functional disorders of the ear may result in hearing deficits, which in turn affect language development, it is of utmost importance that hearing assessments in adolescents with Down syndrome be carried out routinely. If otolaryngologic pathology is identified, appropriate treatment should ensue. The goal in treating hearing and otolaryngologic problems in adolescents with Down syndrome is to maximize the youngster's ability to hear and thus to enhance his or her learning potential.

SLEEP APNEA

Sleep apnea occurs when the inspiratory air flow from the upper airway to the lungs is impeded for 10 seconds or more, often resulting in hypoxemia and/or hypercarbia (Howenstine, 1992). Young people with Down syndrome are predisposed to obstructive sleep apnea because of anatomic, functional, and neurologic problems. Usually, the midfacial area in people with Down syndrome is hypoplastic and the hypopharynx is narrow. Also, choanal stenosis, congestion of mucous membranes of nose and throat, and/or increased adenoid tissue may contribute to the narrowing of the airway. Furthermore, if adolescents with Down syndrome are significantly overweight, they will have increased fat tissue in the pharyngeal area, which further compromises the airway. If adolescents sleep in a supine position (i.e., on their back), their tongue may move posteriorly, thus, partially occluding their hypopharynx and potentially resulting in sleep apnea.

Adolescents with sleep apnea may be restless during sleep and snore frequently, being difficult to arouse in the morning, exhibiting daytime somnolence, behavioral changes, and school problems. To identify whether the adolescent has significant sleep apnea, he or she should undergo a sleep study with polysomnography, which involves a multichannel recording of nasal and oral air flow, pulse rate, electrocardiographic pattern, and thoracic and abdominal impedance. If sleep apnea is identified, numerous treatment modalities are available, including weight reduction, avoiding the supine position during sleep, tonsillectomy and adenoidectomy, uvulopalatopharyngoplasty, continuous positive airway pressure, and, as a last resort, tracheostomy.

If adolescents with Down syndrome and sleep apnea are not identified and treated appropriately, poor oxygen supply to the brain and other vital structures may ensue and symptoms as mentioned above may be observed. In addition, some of these individuals may develop pulmonary artery hypertension and heart failure.

CARDIAC CONDITIONS

Congenital heart disease, which is present in about 40%–50% of children with Down syndrome, is usually uncovered in the newborn period. Most of these children undergo surgical repair of the cardiac defect during the first year of life. Therefore, the majority of adolescents with Down syndrome do not have significant cardiac problems. However, some children with complex congenital heart defects will require continuing cardiac care into their adolescent years and beyond (Marino, 1992).

Several reports have been published indicating that young people with Down syndrome often have mitral valve prolapse, and some may have aortic regurgitation and mitral valve insufficiency (Goldhaber, Brown, & St. John Sutton, 1987; Pueschel & Werner, 1994). If the latter two conditions are present, regular follow-up and the use of antibiotic prophylaxis prior to dental and surgical procedures are recommended (Goldhaber et al., 1987).

Fortunately, most individuals with mitral valve prolapse are asymptomatic and do not show any clinical manifestations. However, individuals with mitral valve prolapse who, in addition, have arrhythmias (i.e., variation from normal rhythm of the heartbeat), episodes of fainting, electrocardiographic abnormalities, palpitations, or chest pain should refrain from participating in vigorous sports activities and strenuous exercises.

THYROID DYSFUNCTION

There are numerous reports in the literature of thyroid disorders in people with Down syndrome (Pueschel & Bier, 1992; Šustrová & Štrbak, 1994). The reported prevalence of thyroid disorders has varied from 3% to 50%, depending on the type of study, whether children were examined clinically, whether specific thyroid function studies were performed, and the age group studied. For example, if current methodologies are used to assess thyroid function, or if an older population of people with Down syndrome is tested, a higher prevalence of thyroid disorders will likely be uncovered. Although some youngsters present with hyperthyroidism, hypothyroidism is the most frequently observed thyroid disorder in adolescents with Down syndrome. Pueschel and Pezzullo (1985) examined a large cohort of young people with Down syndrome and found that 10 of the 151 people had both significantly elevated thyroid-stimulating hormone and significantly low thyroxine levels, 21 had only increased thyroid-stimulating hormone levels, 7 had only markedly elevated thyroxine levels, and 3 had only significantly decreased thyroxine levels. Although autoimmune phenomena may play a role in the development of thyroid dysfunction in individuals with Down syndrome, the underlying pathogenic mechanisms are not well understood.

In a subsequent study, Pueschel, Jackson, Giesswein, Dean, and Pezzullo (1991) provided evidence that both thyroxine and triiodothyronine levels gradually decrease during the adolescent years. Thus, thyroid dysfunction may become more apparent during adolescence, and there is a higher risk for individuals with Down syndrome to become hypothyroid during the growing years. Because hypothyroidism affects central nervous system function adversely, it is conceivable that the reported decline of IQ in people with Down syndrome over time may be due in part to undetected inadequate thyroid function.

Because many physical features of Down syndrome are similar to those observed in patients with hypothyroidism, it is difficult at times to recognize hypothyroid adolescents with Down syndrome clinically. Therefore, it is recommended that periodic (annually or more often, if indicated) thyroid function tests be performed. In particular, during adolescence, regular screening for thyroid dysfunction should be carried out because early detection of hypothyroidism and prompt treatment prevents intellectual deterioration and should improve the individual's overall functioning, academic achievement, and vocational skills.

ATLANTOAXIAL INSTABILITY

Another medical condition that occurs more often during adolescence in people with Down syndrome relates to a ligament-skeletal disorder known as *atlantoaxial instability*. Atlantoaxial instability is primarily due to laxity of the ligaments that ordinarily hold the first two neck bones together. During a large-scale study, atlantoaxial instability was identified in nearly 15% of youngsters with Down syndrome (Pueschel & Scola, 1987). These investigators found that 59 of 404 young people with Down syndrome had atlantoaxial instability, 53 (13.1%) had the asymptomatic form, and 6 (1.5%) had symptomatic atlantoaxial instability. Individuals with asymptomatic atlantoaxial instability do not display neuromotor dysfunctions. However, adolescents with asymptomatic atlantoaxial instability should take precautions during physical activities. Special Olympics (1983) recommends that individuals with Down syndrome who have atlantoaxial instability not participate in gymnastics, butterfly stroke in swimming, diving start in swimming, high jump, pentathlon, or soccer. It is also suggested that youngsters with asymptomatic atlantoaxial instability not engage in contact sports, somersaults, flips, trampoline exercises, and other activities that potentially could cause cervical spine injury.

Some orthopedic surgeons recommend operative stabilization of the upper cervical spine in patients with asymptomatic atlantoaxial instability. The authors favor a conservative approach because these individuals do not have any neurologic symptoms, there is no evidence of significant increase of the atlanto-dens interval (i.e., the space between the first two neck bones or between the anterior arch of the atlas and the adjacent odontoid process) over time, and the operation involves major surgery. However, these youngsters should be followed closely and should undergo periodic reexaminations.

In the symptomatic form of atlantoaxial instability, individuals with Down syndrome usually have specific neuropathologic findings, including brisk deep-tendon reflexes, positive Babinski sign, ankle clonus, muscle weakness, abnormal gait, difficulty walking, increased muscle tone, and/ or neck discomfort. Patients with symptomatic atlantoaxial instability require surgical correction, the main goal of which is to reduce the atlantoaxial subluxation as much as possible, to stabilize the upper segment of the cervical spine, and to prevent further spinal cord damage. It is important to emphasize that about 85% of individuals with Down syndrome do not show evidence of atlantoaxial instability and may participate in all physical education programs and sports activities.

Some investigators recommend radiologic reexamination of the cervical spine of adolescents with Down syndrome because there is a higher risk of developing symptomatic atlantoaxial instability during the adolescent years. As mentioned previously, close follow-up of children with asymptomatic atlantoaxial instability is indicated. In particular, a thorough neurologic assessment should be carried out and a repeat radiograph should be obtained, if indicated, during follow-up examinations.

It is important that atlantoaxial instability in young people with Down syndrome be identified early because of its relatively high prevalence, the possibility of its leading to significant neurologic deficits, and its potential for remediation. Because many of these individuals may have difficulty verbalizing specific complaints relating to neck discomfort and/or neuromotor difficulties, regular examinations are paramount to diagnose those youngsters with atlantoaxial instability early. A delay in recognizing this condition may result in irreversible spinal cord damage.

OTHER MEDICAL CONDITIONS

Other medical conditions are observed at an increased frequency in young people with Down syndrome (Pueschel & Pueschel, 1992). Moreover, neurologic, immunologic, hematologic, gastrointestinal, genitourinary, and other disorders may occur from childhood to adulthood (Pueschel & Pueschel, 1992). However, these medical conditions are not discussed here, owing to space limitations. Nonetheless, it should be emphasized that people with Down syndrome need optimal medical and dental care so that they not only can enjoy good health and a high quality of life while on the threshold to adulthood but also can contribute more fully to society.

REFERENCES

Benson, P.M., & Scherbenske, J.M. (1992). Dermatologic findings. In S.M. Pueschel & J.K. Pueschel (Eds.), *Biomedical concerns in persons with Down syndrome* (pp. 209–215). Baltimore: Paul H. Brookes Publishing Co.

Buchanan, L.H. (1990). Early onset of presbycusis in Down syndrome. *Scandinavian Audiology, 19,* 103–110.

Burton, J.L., & Rook, A. (1986). Genetics in dermatology. In A. Rook, F.J.G. Ebling, D.S. Wilkinson, R.H. Champion, & J.L. Burton (Eds.), *Textbook of dermatology* (pp. 115–129). Oxford, England: Blackwell Scientific Publications.

Butterworth, T., Leoni, E.P., Beerman, H., Wood, M.G., & Strean, L.P. (1960). Cheilitis of mongolism. *Journal of Investigative Dermatology, 35,* 347–352.

Carter, D.M., & Jegasothy, B.V. (1976). Alopecia areata and Down syndrome. *Archives of Dermatology, 112,* 1397–1399.

Catalano, R.A. (1992). Ophthalmologic concerns. In S.M. Pueschel & J.K. Pueschel (Eds.), *Biomedical concerns in persons with Down syndrome* (pp. 59–68). Baltimore: Paul H. Brookes Publishing Co.

Cullen, J.F., & Butler, H.G. (1963). Mongolism (Down's syndrome) and keratoconus. *British Journal of Ophthalmology, 47,* 321–330.

Dahle, A.J., & Baldwin, R.L. (1992). Audiologic and otolaryngologic concerns. In S.M. Pueschel & J.K. Pueschel (Eds.), *Biomedical concerns in persons with Down syndrome* (pp. 69–80). Baltimore: Paul H. Brookes Publishing Co.

DuVivier, A., & Munro, D.D. (1974). Alopecia areata, autoimmunity and Down's syndrome. *British Medical Journal, i,* 191–192.

Gaynon, M.W., & Schimeck, R.A. (1977). Down's syndrome: A ten-year group study. *Annals of Ophthalmology, 9,* 1493–1497.

Goldhaber, S.Z., Brown, W.D., & St. John Sutton, M.G. (1987). High frequency of mitral valve prolapse and aortic regurgitation among asymptomatic adults with

Down's syndrome. *Journal of the American Medical Association, 228,* 1793–1795.

Howenstine, M.S. (1992). Pulmonary concerns. In S.M. Pueschel & J.K. Pueschel (Eds.), *Biomedical concerns in persons with Down syndrome* (pp. 105–118). Baltimore: Paul H. Brookes Publishing Co.

Hurwitz, S. (1981). *Clinical pediatric dermatology.* Philadelphia: W.B. Saunders.

Jaeger, E.A. (1980). Ocular findings in Down's syndrome. *Transactions of the American Ophthalmologic Society, 158,* 808–845.

Kersting, D.W., & Rappaport, E.F. (1958). A clinicopathological study of the skin in mongolism. *Archives of Dermatology, 77,* 319–323.

Marino, B. (1992). Cardiac aspects. In S.M. Pueschel & J.K. Pueschel (Eds.), *Biomedical concerns in persons with Down syndrome* (pp. 91–103). Baltimore: Paul H. Brookes Publishing Co.

Pueschel, S.M., & Bier, J.-A. (1992). Endocrinologic aspects. In S.M. Pueschel & J.K. Pueschel (Eds.), *Biomedical concerns in persons with Down syndrome* (pp. 259–272). Baltimore: Paul H. Brookes Publishing Co.

Pueschel, S.M., & Giesswein, S. (1993). Ocular disorders in children with Down syndrome. *Down Syndrome: Research and Practice, 1,* 129–132.

Pueschel, S.M., Jackson, I.M.D., Giesswein, P., Dean, M.K., & Pezzullo, J.C. (1991). Thyroid function in Down syndrome. *Research in Developmental Disabilities, 12,* 287–296.

Pueschel, S.M., & Pezzullo, J.C. (1985). Thyroid dysfunction in Down syndrome. *American Journal of Diseases of Children, 139,* 636–639.

Pueschel, S.M., & Pueschel, J.K. (Eds.). (1992). *Biomedical concerns in persons with Down syndrome.* Baltimore: Paul H. Brookes Publishing Co.

Pueschel, S.M., & Rynders, J. (1982). *Down syndrome: Advances in biomedicine and the behavioral sciences.* Cambridge, MA: Ware Press.

Pueschel, S.M., & Scola, F.H. (1987). Atlantoaxial instability in individuals with Down syndrome: Epidemiologic, radiographic, and clinical studies. *Pediatrics, 80,* 555–560.

Pueschel, S.M., & Werner, J.C. (1994). Mitral valve prolapse in persons with Down syndrome. *Research in Developmental Disabilities, 15,* 91–97.

Schwartz, D.M., & Schwartz, R.H. (1978). Acoustic impedance and otoscopic findings in young children with Down's syndrome. *Archives of Otolaryngology, 104,* 652–656.

Shapiro, M.B., & France, T.D. (1985). The ocular features of Down's syndrome. *American Journal of Ophthalmology, 99,* 659–663.

Šustrová, M., & Štrbak, V. (1994). Thyroid function and plasma immunoglobulins in subjects with Down's syndrome during ontogenesis and zinc therapy. *Journal of Endocrinological Investigation, 17,* 385–390.

Special Olympics. (1983, March 31). *Special Olympics bulletin: Participation by individuals with Down syndrome who suffer from atlantoaxial dislocation.* Washington, DC: Author.

Storm, W. (1995). *Das Down-Syndrom: Medizinische Betreuung vom Kindes bis zum Erwachsenenalter [Down syndrome: Medical care from childhood to adulthood].* Stuttgart, Germany: Wissenschaftliche Verlagsgesellschaft GmbH.

II

BEHAVIORAL, PSYCHOLOGIC, AND PSYCHIATRIC ISSUES

7

Growing into a Social-Sexual Being

Jeanie P. Edwards

Adolescence and young adulthood bring special concerns and challenges for young people with Down syndrome. It is a time of emotional and social change as well as physical development and sexual maturation. This is true for all youngsters, but for young people with Down syndrome, the stage of adolescence may be intensified. Physical changes are often dramatic as these children experience a growth spurt and sexual awakening. Faced with the tasks of becoming a social-sexual person, learning to live independently, and separating from their families, these young people often still need protection and guidance from their family unit. Thus, possible conflicts arise between the desire for freedom and independence and the need for security coupled with the reality of dependence.

A SEXUAL PERSON

The rapid changes that occur during adolescence in physical growth and appearance mean that the youngster with Down syndrome must develop a new self-image and learn to cope with a new physical appearance and new biologic drives. The attention of many parents and professionals has been drawn to the social-sexual development of people with Down syndrome. Chapters 4 and 5 of this volume cited important studies related to sexual development of adolescents with Down syndrome, which confirm that these youngsters' social-sexual needs are more like those of their "normal" peers than they are different (e.g., Elkins, 1995; Pueschel, Orson, Boylan, & Pezzulo, 1985). Social-sexual development, however, is often more problematic for the person with Down syndrome because U.S. society delivers conflicting messages and ambiguous demands about sexuality. This situation is compounded by the fact that social-sexual information is sometimes left to incidental learning. However, the person with Down syndrome does not learn well incidentally; he or she needs concrete learning experiences. State-of-the-art curricular approaches encourage parents and professionals to provide sex education early in their child's life. It is important to inform the young person of body changes he or she can anticipate before these occur.

The sexual development of an adolescent girl with Down syndrome follows the pattern of development typical for all girls. She needs helpful instruction about why females menstruate, as well as proper care of herself during her period. Although she may be smaller in stature, the adolescent girl with Down syndrome will most likely begin to menstruate near the same time as other girls her age (Scola & Pueschel, 1992). Advance preparation should be given to avoid fears. Resources for parents are available to help with specific language, as well as direct instructions, much in the way that parents teach skills like dressing and toileting (Edwards & Elkins, 1990). Most girls with Down syndrome can learn to manage menstruation and should be told that it is a positive part of becoming a woman.

In adolescent boys, wet dreams are a common experience. Boys need to be told that wet dreams are natural and normal but are something private. Likewise, masturbation is a normal response to the physiologic changes of adolescence. Just as it is for their "normal" peers, masturbation by youth with Down syndrome should be a private behavior. Although a youth with Down syndrome may begin to masturbate in public, the adolescent should not be shamed or punished; rather, he should be told that his feelings are normal and natural but that masturbation should occur only in socially acceptable, private places.

SOCIAL-SEXUAL SKILLS TRAINING

Again, provision for socialization and sex education should be ensured. To avoid exploitation, it is critical to teach the concept of privacy to a person with Down syndrome. This concept should be taught early and reinforced at home. Social skills training (e.g., appropriate ways to meet and greet strangers and to show others we care) should also occur at an early age. Appropriate social skills are critical to integration, to peer acceptance, and to taking one's place in the community as an adolescent and young adult. Encouraging assertive behavior, buddy system activities, and avoiding contact with strangers are also important concerns.

Difficulties encountered in instituting social-sexual training programs frequently stem not from problems with course content or teaching methods, but instead from the reluctance of parents, teachers, and the public to admit that people with Down syndrome and other forms of mental retardation are social-sexual beings. It has been well established that people with mental retardation requiring limited or even extensive supports are capable of understanding and being taught social-sexual information (Edwards & Elkins, 1990; Fujira, Wagner, & Pion, 1970; Hingsburger, 1993; Kempton, 1971).

Characterizing young people with Down syndrome as unable to learn about social-sexual competence is inaccurate and accomplishes nothing. It is more accurate to say that their mental retardation merely insulates them from peer experiences and from the core of information that other adolescents without retardation accumulate through incidental learning experiences. In other words, young people with Down syndrome are "like all other people" in regard to the occurrence of sexual development. It is true that stages of social-sexual development may be briefly delayed for them, but, as adolescents, they do exhibit the same needs for belonging and intimacy experienced by "normal" adolescents. They tend to emulate their peers in their clothing styles and speech, and their behavior is molded by internal excitations associated with puberty and by common external environmental interactions. Because of their mental retardation and the restrictions that may be imposed on them, however, they do not always experience the group satisfaction, partying, telephone socialization, community experiences, and all of the other interpersonal exposures needed to augment their knowledge of, and skills in, social-sexual relationships. The consequences of this are inept development and ineffectual and often embarrassing interpersonal experiences.

Irregularities in development may also lead to gaps in maturation that may cause additional anxiety for the adolescent with Down syndrome. These irregularities may emerge on the physical level as interference with growth and development of secondary sex characteristics resulting from a heart condition, early sterilization, or a birth anomaly. On a psychologic level, irregularities may emerge as a lack of well-defined body image, unsatisfactory self-concept, indifference to environment, sensory and environmental deprivation (especially for those who are isolated), the inability to shift thinking, or a lack of strong personal identity.

Thus, part of the adjustment problem for people with Down syndrome may relate to physical or psychologic deficiencies; however, a more important aspect, if for no other reason than that it is avoidable, is that these young people are typically deprived of opportunities to experiment in activities with other adolescents. To reiterate, social-sexual skills training is essential for all young people, but it is especially crucial for young people with Down syndrome. This is because the latter often do not have opportunities to acquire this awareness through typical channels of socialization, and they do not learn well incidentally.

Effective social-sexual behavior involves the intricate application of motor, cognitive, and affective skills that are carefully displayed according to the circumstances, environment, and the person (Eisler, 1976; Herson & Bellack, 1976; Trower, Bryant, & Argyle, 1978). Trower et al. (1978) analyzed these components and noted that effective social behavior consists of the following skills and behaviors:

1. Nonverbal motoric behaviors (e.g., facial expressions, gestures, appearance)
2. Verbal behaviors (e.g., greeting people, making small talk, asking questions appropriately)
3. Affective behaviors (e.g., expressing attitudes and feelings, recognizing internal emotional cues, empathic responding)
4. Social cognitive skills (e.g., interpersonal problem solving, role taking, thinking empathically, discriminating among social cues, understanding social norms, linking together a sequence of thoughts and behaviors)

In his book, *The Cloak of Competence*, Edgerton (1967) discussed the irritation aroused in community members by the social incompetence of those with mental retardation. As a result of Edgerton's leadership, independent living programs are increasingly focusing on social skills competence training. Since 1970, more than 50 significant social skills training research projects have incorporated young people with Down syndrome into their training populations. The results show that although social skills training is an extremely complicated task involving a combination of motoric, cognitive, affective, verbal, and nonverbal skills, it is nonetheless possible to teach these behaviors to people with Down syndrome (Davies & Rogers, 1986). Technologies are available to teach these skills to populations with varying degrees of mental retardation. It is also significant that these research reports indicate that the most successful teaching methods seem to include a combination of active rehearsal, parental feedback, and consistent behavior management (Edwards & Elkins, 1990). This conclusion supports the tremendous need for parent–professional partnerships in teaching appropriate social-sexual skills.

Other researchers have demonstrated success with behavioral rehearsal (role playing), primary reinforcement, instruction, demonstration, positive guided practice, corrective feedback via videotape, social reinforcement, and parental reinforcement. For young people with Down syndrome, the most frequently used and successful of these methods consist of visual modes of instruction, positive practice (active role playing and rehearsal), and contingent reinforcement (Edwards & Elkins, 1990; Senatore, Matson, & Kazdin, 1982).

A state-of-the-art social skills curriculum teaches skills to people with Down syndrome that help lighten the burden of moving in the mainstream of the community. Some characteristics of such a curriculum have proven tremendously helpful in this respect, namely, suitable communications skills, normalized appearance, social coping behaviors (including assertiveness), and comfortable interrelationships based on sensitivity and responsiveness to other people's needs. These four characteristics, or personal attributes, are not all-inclusive, but they are fundamental to social acceptance. Two of them, in particular, merit elaboration here.

Normalized Physical Appearance

A person's degree of visible deformities has great implications for social acceptance. Clothing is an individual's artificial second skin and has a two-sided effect: It is a reflection of the individual's self-image and self-confidence (Frank & Edwards, 1986), and it creates a strong first impression on others. Peer-appropriate clothing, with as normalizing an effect as possible, and appropriate contemporary hairstyling are two major aspects that contribute to the physical attractiveness of people with Down syndrome. Although young people with Down syndrome may appear different in some ways, if they dress like their peers without disabilities, there is a greater chance of their being accepted by them.

Shushan (1974) conducted a study in which he obtained data from respondents' reactions to "before-and-after" photographs of a group of adolescents and young adults with Down syndrome and other forms of mental retardation compared to photographs of eight "normal" people. The subjects with mental retardation selected for this study had been judged to have deficits in physical appearance. After pictures were taken of both groups of test participants, those with Down syndrome and other forms of mental retardation were subjected to intervention procedures that included the following:

- *For females*: Eye shadow, mascara to highlight eyelashes, eyeglass frames, wigs, hairstyling, and sunglasses
- *For males*: Hair styling, eyeglass frames, wigs, and sunglasses
- *For both men and women*: Clothes with necklines complementary to their faces

The participants were given simple verbal training and were instructed in how to hold their heads and how to make their facial expressions around their eyes and mouth appear typical. A finger applied lightly to the side of the individual's mouth guided him or her in following directions. Assistance was given for appropriate mouth movements for smiling.

Shushan's (1974) intervention efforts resulted in significantly fewer deficits in physical appearance, as determined by the respondents' reactions to the "after" photographs of people with Down syndrome. These intervention procedures also favorably influenced social and work relationships for these young people. The point, then, is that prejudice against individuals who do not fit the current mold of physical attractiveness in society greatly interferes with many aspects of satisfactory living and community acceptance.

Social Coping Behavior

The cultivation of social coping skills depends on recurrent, diversified, and satisfying interpersonal experiences. In any social encounter, reciprocal interactions (i.e., mutual influences) occur. These interactions are initiated when people first meet; thus, first impressions are extremely important. The ability to meet and greet people appropriately, to respond warmly to greetings, to appear nicely dressed and well groomed, and to display proper eating habits can be keystones to community acceptance. The young person with Down syndrome best learns these coping behaviors in the real world of community exposure with its attendant interactions with people without disabilities. Risks are involved in this situational programming, of course, but without taking such risks, habilitation is only a pretense. Shushan (1974) clearly showed the need for training in social copy behavior, and Davies and Rogers (1986) demonstrated the success of such training for people with Down syndrome.

Several state-of-the-art social skills programs are available for parents and teachers, which incorporate the teaching of social coping behaviors, communication skills, normalizing of one's appearance, and relationship building. These programs include *Life Horizons* (Stanfield, 1990), *Life Facts* (Cowardin, 1990), *Being Me* (Edwards, 1979), *ACCESS* (Close, 1982), *TIPS* (Alexander, 1983; Kempton, 1974), and *Circles* (Champagne & Walker-Hirsh, 1983). Methods used in these curricula support Davies and Rogers's (1986) findings.

An examination of these curricula reveals that each author shares a commitment to three essential goals—heightened expectations, normalization, and human dignity. Each curriculum supports the notion that it is not only "normal" for a child with Down syndrome to grow up, to leave his or her parents, and to choose a living partner, but also his or her right. For some, this might mean taking a roommate in a group home or sharing an apartment, whereas for others it may mean selecting a marriage partner. Some people may also prefer to live alone. Most important, however, is the *right to choose.*

Both parents and professionals struggle with this issue of choice. The following discussion illuminates many of the difficulties, real and imagined, that they face.

Training Role of Parents and Professionals

Parent participants in the "Living Options Workshop" at the National Down Syndrome Congress in 1995 overwhelmingly supported the notion of independent living as a convention goal; however, follow-up research addressing the attitudes of many of the same families indicated that, when talking specifically about their own child, parents felt the notion was frightening, inappropriate to their child's level of functioning, and ultimately something outside the realm of possibility for their child. Although one can find many parents and professionals committed to teaching "living skills" to people with Down syndrome, most stop at the thought of independence or marriage, especially for their own child.

The possibility exists that this fear or misconception on the part of parents and professionals indeed creates more inappropriate sexual behaviors in young people with Down syndrome. It is normal in U.S. society for young adults to socialize, date, and pair off, thus channeling their social-sexual life into a context that enjoys the blessing of society. However, this is more often not the case for individuals with Down syndrome. Instead, they frequently face the frustration of segregated social environments in which they live in residential programs or group homes, or they remain with their parents beyond the typical age. Without an appropriate sexual outlet, these young people often express their normal needs by touching strangers, standing "too close for comfort," or confusing relationships—perhaps calling a staff member a boyfriend or girlfriend—in effect, presenting themselves as socially and sexually immature. This inappropriate behavior occurs because these people have not had an opportunity for normal expression of real and present needs. Without an early and deep commitment to the principles of normalization (helping the child to obtain a life as close to typical as possible; making available to him or her early and lifelong patterns of everyday life [Bank-Mikkelsen, 1971]), neither parents nor professionals will deal directly with the social-sexual skills training so vitally necessary if the person with Down syndrome is to fully realize his or her humanity

The need to experience such social reactions in a caring relationship knows no boundaries, regardless of the presence of Down syndrome or the degree of mental retardation. For some young people with Down syndrome, life together may someday mean a carefully worked-out marriage supported by family, friends, or advocates. For others, it may be life together in a mixed-group home or supported living apartment where young people are encouraged and allowed to form deep, warm relationships that provide an opportunity for touching, caring, and emotional expression, all of which are basic to each human being. Such facilities are rare in the United States, although they are more prevalent in northern Europe and have been very successful and humanizing. For those with Down syndrome, such efforts toward a normalized and independent lifestyle and the possibility of eventually living with a partner represent a great step forward. Both parents and professionals must work together, and concertedly, however, for this to happen.

A DIFFERENT PERSPECTIVE

Although this chapter has affirmed the right of young people with Down syndrome to grow up, marry, have a sexual relationship, and possibly have children, it is not the sexual side of these issues that is of prime importance. Of far greater significance is the basic need of people with Down syndrome for approval: in short, the need to be liked. The wish to avoid loneliness—to have friends, to do things and go places together—is much more important to most people than sex. To gain friendship, individuals with Down syndrome thus need to make themselves both physically and socially attractive so that they can be accepted by others. A current hair-style, using cosmetics (for females), wearing jewelry, and establishing an identity as a young adult are far more important than sex. Only when it seems that no other vehicle is available for establishing social relationships will sex become overly important to the person with Down syndrome. However, to experience the feeling of "togetherness" is one of the deepest, indeed most "normal," of human needs.

Most of our social-sexual needs can be met outside a physical relationship; yet it, too, is one component of human relationships. Out of sexual togetherness, a warm feeling of solidarity can grow and become the foundation of the finest, most mutually rewarding relationship human beings experience. Some people with Down syndrome quite normally grow and desire this kind of solidarity. Others meet each other and become lifelong friends without any sexual element. But either kind of relationship can bring freedom from loneliness and new meaning to life.

Young people with Down syndrome want what young people without disabilities want:

- *A friend*—someone to talk to, someone with whom they can share "important things"
- *Warmth*—someone to touch, someone who will put their hand on their shoulder in a way that says, "I like you"
- *Approval*—some message from others that tells them, "You're okay"
- *Affection*—love and the feeling that they are loved; not necessarily involving sex
- *Dignity*—communication from others that makes them feel that they have worth
- *Social outlets*—to avoid loneliness
- *Sexual satisfaction*—the purely biologic need for sexual contact and stimulation

This last need is small in comparison to the other needs listed here, but is genuine nonetheless. There is a wide range of intellectual function in people with Down syndrome, and numerous non–sex-related variables need to be taken into account when approaching issues of sexuality, marriage, and parenting. Nevertheless, it is essential that the issue of sexual fulfillment be addressed.

CONCLUSIONS

This chapter has contended that a discussion of sexuality and relationships is incomplete if separated from a consideration of social skills training and competence building. Therefore, social skills developed through a community-based, "real-life," situation-programming training program reinforced by parents and caregivers are fundamental to the fulfillment of the sexual needs of the person with Down syndrome. In spite of the recognized importance of the ability of people with Down syndrome to learn to function with others, only recently have concerted efforts been directed toward relationship and sexuality training within the social skills context. Skills in identity formation, self-acceptance, awareness of others, problem solving, decision making, communication, and assertiveness form the backbone of such training. Learning social amenities such as how to meet and greet people, how to show others we care, proper eating, and conversational cues and tips are suitable skills for initial community contacts. These capacities have been researched and have proven to be dependent on opportunities for recurrent, diversified, and satisfying interactions with other people. Young adults with Down syndrome are frequently shut off from such interactions, however.

Although "the enlightened" may deny that first impressions actually do impress, the fact remains that physical appearance is a crucial component of interpersonal contact for people with Down syndrome. Young people with Down syndrome who do not fit into the prevailing criteria for physical attractiveness because of facial or body expression and form, gait, or speech become the victims of their labels (e.g., retarded, childlike) and therefore are assigned lowered expectations. Intervention procedures to normalize their appearance help to break down some of the barriers to their social integration.

Sexual activity and marriage are probably the most controversial and feared aspects of social skills training. Likewise, to deny these rights and behaviors cancels out the humanness of sex. Sex, sexuality, and sexual activities are important facets of social skills training. To bypass the teaching of appropriate social-sexual facts is to deny people with Down syndrome a large measure of their personal rights. The expression of sexual needs and the self-control important in sexual expression can be taught and are critical to the development of the self-concept and self-esteem in people with Down syndrome (Frank & Edwards, 1986).

Young people with Down syndrome need social-sexual skills training even more than "normal" people do, both because the former are often shut off from typical learning opportunities in society and because they do not learn well incidentally. The scope of this training must include social amenities, decision making, interpersonal satisfaction, relationships, marriage, antifertility methods, parenthood, and the meaning of sexual relations. Numerous state-of-the-art curricular materials are available that utilize proven methods of training for people with Down syndrome. But successful training seems to depend on parents and professionals forming a partnership, affording normalizing experiences with heightened expectations, and sustaining a commitment to ensuring the right to human dignity and decision making.

REFERENCES

Alexander, D. (1983). *TIPS: Teaching interpersonal skills to the mentally handicapped* [Audiovisual material and training manual]. Santa Monica, CA: James Stanfield Film Associates.

Bank-Mikkelsen, N.E. (1971, September 21). *Meeting particular problems of normalization.* Paper presented at the National Convention of the International Council for Exceptional Children, Boston.

Champagne, M., & Walker-Hirsh, L. (1983). *Circles* [Audiovisual material and training manual]. Santa Monica, CA: James Stanfield Film Associates.

Close, D. (1982). Access. *Oregon Department of Education's Interact, 8.*

Cowardin, S. (1990). *Life facts.* Santa Monica, CA: James Stanfield Film Associates.

Davies, R., & Rogers, E.S. (1986). Social skills training with persons who are mentally retarded. *Mental Retardation, 23*(4), 186–193.

Edgerton, R.B. (1967). *The cloak of competence: Stigma in the lives of the mentally retarded.* Berkeley: University of California Press.

Edwards, J.P. (1979). *Being me: Social/sexual skills training guide.* Austin, TX: PRO-ED.

Edwards, J.P. (1983). *My friend David: A sourcebook about Down syndrome.* Portland, OR: Ednick Communications.

Edwards, J.P., & Elkins, T.E. (1990). *Just between us: Social sexual guide for parents* (2nd ed.). Austin, TX: PRO-ED.

Eisler, R.M. (1976). The behavioral assessment of social skills. In M. Herson & A.S. Bellack (Eds.), *Behavioral assessment: A practical handbook* (pp. 369–396). New York: Pergamon Press.

Elkins, T. (1995). Medical issues related to sexuality and reproduction. In D.C. Van Dyke, P. Mattheis, S. Eberly, & J. Williams (Eds.), *Medical and surgical care for children with Down syndrome: A guide for parents* (pp. 185–191). Rockville, MD: Woodbine House.

Frank, R.A., & Edwards, J.P. (1986). *Building self-esteem in those with retardation.* Portland, OR: Ednick Communications.

Fujira, B., Wagner, N.N., & Pion, R.J. (1970). Sexuality, contraception, and the mentally retarded. *Social Medicine, 47*, 193–197.

Herson, K., & Bellack, A.S. (1976). Social skills training for chronic psychiatric patients: Rationale, research findings, and future directions. *Comprehensive Psychiatry, 17*, 559–580.

Hingsburger, D. (1993). *I openers: Questions parents ask about sexuality and disability.* Vancouver, British Columbia, Canada: Family Support Press.

Katz, E. (Ed.). (1972). *Mental health services for the mentally retarded.* Springfield, IL: Charles C Thomas.

Kempton, W. (1971). *Guidelines for planning a training course on the subject of human sexuality for the retarded.* Philadelphia: Planned Parenthood Association of Southern Pennsylvania.

Kempton, W. (1974). *TIPS* [Audiovisual material and training manual]. Santa Monica, CA: James Stanfield Film Associates.

Perske, R. (1973). About sexual development. *Mental Retardation, 11*(1), 6–8.

Pueschel, S.M., Orson, J.M., Boylan, J.M., & Pezzulo, J.C. (1985). Adolescent development in males with Down syndrome. *American Journal of Diseases of Children, 139*, 236–238.

Scola, P.S., & Pueschel, S.M. (1992). Menstrual cycles and basal body temperature curves in women with Down syndrome. *Obstetrics and Gynecology, 79*, 91–94.

Senatore, V., Matson, J.L., & Kazdin, A.E. (1982). A comparison of behavioral methods to train social skills to mentally retarded adults. *Behavior Therapy, 13*, 313–324.

Shushan, R.D. (1974). *Assessment and reduction of deficits in the physical appearances of mentally retarded people.* (Doctoral dissertation, University of California at Los Angeles, 1974). *Dissertation Abstracts International, 35*, 5974A.

Stanfield, J. (1990). *Life horizons.* Santa Monica, CA: James Stanfield Film Associates.

Trower, P., Bryant, B., & Argyle, M. (1978). *Social skills and mental health.* Pittsburgh, PA: University of Pittsburgh Press.

8

Promoting Adolescent Self-Competence

Laurie E. Powers
Darryn M. Sikora

Adolescence is typically a period of expanding personal awareness, autonomy, independence, and social relationships. For adolescents with disabilities such as Down syndrome, adjustment during this period can be more difficult. However, having a disability is only one aspect of adolescents' life experience, which combines myriad typical child-related and contextual factors to predict adjustment (Sinnema, 1991). Factors related to a child's disability, such as level of functional challenge (Breslau, 1985) and personal perceptions of disability (Drotar & Bush, 1985), appear to be important predictors of adjustment. Generic factors such as attributional style and temperament have an impact on adjustment for all children, including those with disabilities (Schoenherr, Brown, Baldwin, & Kaslow, 1992). Contextual factors such as poverty, family discord, and social isolation also interact with disability to substantially increase risk for impaired adjustment (Cadman, Boyle, Szatmari, & Offord, 1987).

Although the majority of the literature on disability and psychosocial adjustment is focused on adolescence, little validated information is available on the adjustment of youth with Down syndrome. Therefore, conclusions must be generalized from information available on the adjustment of children with disabilities in general and, more specifically, of those with cognitive and health challenges. The validity of generalizing findings across disabilities is strengthened by information suggesting that there is

This chapter was supported in part by grant H086U20006 from the U.S. Department of Education. The opinions expressed herein are exclusively those of the authors, and no official endorsement should be inferred.

much similarity in the impact of adjustment factors across different disabling conditions (Stein & Jessop, 1989). Thus, it is reasonable to expect that most findings and strategies related to youth with disabilities can be applied to youth with Down syndrome.

Historically, the disability literature has emphasized maladjustments associated with disability. Since the mid-1980s, however, a growing body of literature suggests that the development of self-competence among children with ongoing health conditions and physical disabilities is very similar to that of children who do not experience disability (e.g., Perrin, Ramsey, & Sandler, 1987). *Self-competence* is conceptualized as the interrelationship of self-perception of personal worth and efficacy. High levels of self-competence are demonstrated by children who exhibit self-esteem, self-determination, and effective coping strategies (Powers, Singer, & Sowers, 1996). In the case of youth with cognitive challenges, disability and self-competence have traditionally been regarded as oxymorons. Little attention has been focused on acknowledging either that adolescents with developmental disabilities are *foremost* typically developing human beings or that adolescents with developmental disabilities can and do demonstrate self-competence. As a result, youth with developmental disabilities have had few opportunities to engage in behaviors that promote self-competence—that is, setting personal goals, making choices, solving problems, or developing advocacy skills (Abery, 1994).

The developmental disabilities field is beginning to direct increasing attention to adjustment and resilience among youth with disabilities. This shift reflects, in part, a similar evolution in understanding and attitudes in regard to other populations at risk (Werner & Smith, 1992), as well as increasing achievement and advocacy among people with disabilities (Shapiro, 1993). It is becoming clear that all youth, regardless of level of challenge, are capable of expressing self-competence in a multitude of ways (Wehmeyer, 1996). This chapter outlines the central factors underlying adolescent self-competence and discusses strategies for promoting the self-competence of teenagers with cognitive and health challenges such as Down syndrome.

ESSENTIAL FACTORS UNDERLYING SELF-COMPETENCE

Research indicates that children typically perceive their competence in two primary domains: task related and social (Harter, 1981). This dichotomy becomes even stronger as adolescence approaches and as youth become focused on peer-group relations and performance of autonomous activity (Schinke & Gilchrist, 1984). Perceptions of efficacy and of worthiness appear to be the primary factors contributing to child self-competence (Powers, Singer, & Sowers, 1996). Perceptions of efficacy tend to be behaviorally based, whereas perceptions of worthiness are more affectively derived. Self-efficacy generally refers to beliefs about one's capabilities to attain desired outcomes or to manage undesirable circumstances (Bandura, 1986). Worthiness refers to self-evaluations of personal regard and value as a human being (Rosenberg, 1965). Perceptions of efficacy cannot be isolated from perceptions of worthiness; efficacy promotes self-worth, and self-worth facilitates striving toward efficacy (Branden, 1969).

Conditions that promote self-perceptions of worthiness include positive family climate, gender, birth order, and being valued by others (Bednar, Wells, & Peterson, 1989; Harter, 1990; Mruk, 1995). Conditions that promote perceptions of efficacy include mastery experiences, successful management of challenges, vicarious learning, social influence, and positive physiologic feedback (Bandura, 1986; Harter, 1985). As a product of both efficacy and worthiness, self-competence is manifested in *self-esteem, self-determination,* and *successful coping.*

Self-Esteem

Self-esteem is a multidimensional construct with many different definitions. Mruk (1995) defined self-esteem based on perceptions of worthiness and competence: "the lived status of one's individual competence and personal worthiness at dealing with the challenges of life over time" (p. 21). High self-esteem appears to be associated with self-confidence, effective coping, and psychosocial well-being (Bednar et al., 1989; Harter, 1993; Wells & Marwell, 1976). In contrast, low self-esteem is associated with depression, substance abuse, and delinquency (Harter, 1993; Jung, 1994; Kaplan, Martin, & Johnson, 1986). The evidence is mixed regarding the impact of disability on self-esteem. For example, Zeltzer, Kellerman, Ellenberg, Dash, and Rigler (1980) found that adolescents with disabilities did not exhibit different levels of self-esteem from those of their typical peers. However, adolescents' perceptions of the impact of disability on their lives were inversely related to their self-esteem. Magill and Hurlbut (1986) found that disability was significantly associated with impaired self-esteem among adolescents. Detailed analysis revealed that the finding was due to low levels of self-esteem shown by the young women in the study and, when the effect of gender was removed, disability was not a significant predictor of low self-esteem. Other studies have associated disability with lowered self-esteem, particularly for children with cognitive, emotional, or learning challenges (Heyman, 1990; Prout, Marcal, & Marcal, 1992). Factors cited previously, such as predictability of disability, demographics, family stress, functional impact, atypical physical appearance, and social isolation, appear to put children with disabilities at increased risk for low self-esteem.

Self-Determination

Self-determination is an emerging construct within the disability literature. Wehmeyer (1992) defined self-determination as "acting as the primary causal agent in one's life and making choices and decisions regarding one's quality of life, free from external influence or interference" (p. 305). Powers, Sowers, et al. (1996) describe self-determination as

> personal attitudes and abilities that facilitate an individual's identification and pursuit of goals . . . reflected in personal attitudes of empowerment, active participation in decision making, and self-directed action to achieve personally valued goals. (p. 292)

To express self-determination is most basically to decide and act on one's own behalf.

Evidence suggests that people with high levels of self-determination behave more autonomously, are more effective social problem-solvers, are more assertive, and exhibit higher levels of self-efficacy and self-esteem than do individuals with low levels of self-determination (Wehmeyer, Kelchner, & Richards, 1995). Likewise, adolescents who learn skills essential to the development of self-determination, such as decision making, problem solving, and interpersonal negotiation, exhibit significantly higher levels of empowerment, psychosocial adjustment, and goal setting than do their peers who do not learn self-determination skills (Powers, Turner, et al., 1995).

Successful Coping

Coping generally refers to the individual's responses to stressful situations (Compas, 1987; Lazarus & Folkman, 1984). Coping can encompass many different types of responses, such as direct efforts to manage the stressor, managing feelings stimulated by the stressor, or thinking differently to reduce the threat of the stressor. As such, coping responses are generally classified as problem focused, emotion focused, or perception focused. Coping is a highly complex, situationally specific process: The same coping response (i.e., avoidance) may reduce perceived stress in one situation but worsen it in another situation. Generally, problem-focused responses are most useful in situations in which the threat can be managed, whereas emotion-focused or perception-focused responses are most useful in stressful situations that cannot be controlled (Folkman & Lazarus, 1980). Generally, coping responses that emphasize situational, depersonalized, and temporary interpretations of stressful events promote resilience (Seligman, 1990). Coping becomes increasingly differentiated as children develop. Youth who possess the broadest repertoires of different coping strategies generally are most prepared to effectively respond to stress (Compas, 1987).

Family Factors

In General   Family climate and parenting practices are major factors underlying the development of child self-competence. Scant information is available regarding the family factors and parenting practices that help to promote self-competence among youth who experience disability. One of the most informative studies of the impact of family climate and parenting practices on the adaptation of children with cognitive disabilities to the school and community was conducted by Mink, Nihira, and Meyers (1983). From their analysis, two family types emerged as providing the conditions that help children with moderate cognitive challenges develop high self-esteem, community independence skills, and positive psychosocial adjustment. Both of these family types were characterized by family climates that were *high in cohesion* and relatively *low in conflict*. Both had households that provided a variety of *active stimulation* for the children and used parenting practices that were characterized by high levels of *involvement* and *pride in the children*.

Dyson, Edgar, and Crnic (1989) also found that children with disabilities and their siblings from families marked by high cohesion, low conflict, and relatively high expressiveness were most likely to have positive self-concepts and fewer behavior problems than children from less cohesive and more conflicted families. Parent stress also was found to be a contributor to children's adaptation. Children with disabilities and their siblings from families in which parents experienced stress associated with parenting a child with a disability were more likely to have negative self-concepts. The more intensively parents reported that they experienced stress associated with parenting a child with disability, the more the siblings and child with a disability were likely to have negative self-concepts.

Little research has been conducted relating to the impact of divorce and single parenthood on children with disabilities. Considerable evidence from the general literature on families suggests that children in single-parent families are at risk of doing less well in school and of having more emotional and behavioral problems than children in two-parent families (Hernandez, 1995). A major cause of these problems is economic distress. In 1992, approximately 45% of families with children headed by single mothers were living below the poverty line, compared with 8.4% of families with two parents (McLanahan & Sandefur, 1994). Because economic disadvantage is a predictor of poorer outcomes for children with disabilities (Mink et al., 1983), it is likely that single parenthood is correlated with poorer outcomes. However, this does not mean that children invariably do worse in single-parent homes. In the Mink et al. (1983) study, one of the family types that was most supportive for children was composed predominantly of single mothers. Extrapolating from related studies, we would expect that single parents who have sufficient economic resources and who are not under severe stress are more likely to do well with their children, particularly if they are able to establish positive parenting practices.

Parenting Practices Zetlin, Turner, and Winick (1987) studied parenting practices in families with adolescents who experienced cognitive challenges. They described the families that they studied as either *supportive, dependency-producing*, or *conflict-ridden*. Supportive families had a warm relationship with their teenager. This relationship was generally manifested by a high degree of interest in the teenager and interactions with a positive, affective tone. The parents in these families were a stable source of support to the young people. In addition, they encouraged them to develop independence and to acquire skills that would promote self-care and community living. Dependency-producing families also had warm relationships with their teenagers, but instead of encouraging development of skills and judgment, their styles of providing support and regulating conduct did not allow for independence. Conflict-ridden relationships, as the name implies, were marked by emotional coldness or anger and by arguments and fights. These parents exercised control over their adolescents that continued into adulthood, but with decreased support.

Grolnick and Ryan (1989) interviewed 96 couples from two-parent families of high school–age students in order to analyze their parenting practices. They found that children from homes that were highly structured and in which parents used controlling and punitive disciplinary practices had more problems in school and were less confident of their own capabilities. Parents whose teenagers at school were the most well adjusted were those who valued their child's autonomy and who used reasoning and empathic limit setting rather than controlling or punitive discipline. These parents involved their children in problem solving, gave them choices, and provided them with consistent structure through their statement of clear rules and expectations for behavior.

Ferguson and Asch (1989) investigated parenting practices by reviewing published accounts by adults with disabilities who wrote about their families of origin. Their analysis yielded four patterns of parent response: 1) parents who were overprotective, 2) parents who ignored or denied their child's disability, 3) parents who tried to fix the disability or minimize its impact, and 4) parents who tried to minimize the disability while ensuring that the child had a full life. Ferguson and Asch found that adults with disabilities who recalled their early relationships with their parents in the most positive light described them as providing accommodations to help them maximize their abilities while helping them to have as full a life as possible in ways that emphasized their multidimensionality. Adults who had to struggle to become more independent and autonomous were likely to have been reared by parents who were excessively focused on their disabilities and who had low expectations for them. Adult distress was also associated with childhood experiences in which parents denied the impact of disability and did not attempt to explain it or to provide adaptive equipment or other accommodations. A final set of adult accounts described parents who tended to push the children too much to try to overcome their disabilities. These parents intensively focused on reducing disability while deemphasizing the other characteristics and strengths of their children.

In another study, Powers, Singer, and Todis (1996) conducted a qualitative study of the retrospective accounts of childhood among successful adults with physical and multiple disabilities. Many of their findings parallel those of Ferguson and Asch (1989), emphasizing the importance of parents focusing on children's strengths while also acknowledging disability-related challenges and providing appropriate accommodation. The adults interviewed by Powers and colleagues also reported that they benefited from their parents' modeling of assertiveness and advocacy and from parental facilitation of their participation in typical peer relationships, recreational activities, and inclusive education.

In summary, parenting practices that promote self-competence in adolescents include: 1) positive, supportive interaction; 2) providing opportunities to practice and develop autonomy; 3) focusing on the individual's strengths; 4) providing accommodation to reduce the restrictiveness of disability; 5) using reasoning and limit setting; and 6) encouraging involvement in typical teenage activities.

STRATEGIES FOR PROMOTING SELF-COMPETENCE

Enhanced focus on competence and resilience among children with disabilities has fueled prevention and promotion efforts. Initiatives in inclusive education, coping skills training, medical self-management, self-determination and leadership development, family support, mentoring, and peer support provide a few examples of emerging approaches aimed at assisting children and families to identify and maximize their personal strengths and adaptive skills. Evidence suggests that such approaches enhance children's psychosocial adjustment and disability management and minimize the adverse impacts of disability (Pantell, Lewis, & Sharp, 1989; Powers, Sowers, & Stevens, 1995; Singer & Powers, 1993; Sinnema, 1991; Ward & Kohler, 1996). Additional prevention and promotion interventions to enhance social problem solving, self-esteem, and stress management have been largely validated with children who do not experience identified disabilities and hold promise for bolstering the self-competence of children with disability (e.g., Dubrow, Schmidt, McBride, Edwards, & Merk, 1993; Henderson, Kelbey, & Engebretson, 1992; Pope, McHale, & Craighead, 1988). Many of these approaches influence self-competence by bolstering four factors: 1) opportunities to attempt new behaviors; 2) information; 3) coping, social, and task-related skills; and 4) access to support.

Opportunities to Attempt New Behaviors

Access to opportunities is a primary factor in bolstering self-competence. Adolescents must have opportunities to make decisions, to communicate ideas, to attempt new activities, to assume responsibilities, to negotiate privileges, and to gain experience managing obstacles to success. Opportunities most facilitate self-competence when they maximize youths' self-attribution of success (Bandura, 1986). It is insufficient to provide enjoyable activities for youth or to ensure their success by performing tasks for them. Opportunities must be provided for youth to exercise their own capabilities and to achieve outcomes they value. Ideally, such opportunities should both encourage self-help and highlight accomplishments (Arborelius & Bremberg, 1991; Hughes, Korinek, & Gorman, 1991).

For children with Down syndrome, opportunities may also include increased responsibility for monitoring the status of their health challenges. Perrin and Shapiro (1985) found that children with chronic health conditions who assumed more responsibility for their health care were better at independent decision making than children who were overly reliant on others for their health management. Youth who experience cognitive disabilities may also benefit from having more opportunities for repeated practice and refinement of skills than adolescents who do not have cognitive challenges (Abery, 1994).

Information

Promoting the future planning and development of youth requires that they have access to information that they can use for self-exploration and informed decision making (Christopher, Kurtz, & Howing, 1989; Powers, Sowers, et al., 1996). Helping youth to explore their future dreams through mapping strategies (Bolles, 1995; see also Chapter 18); encouraging them to clarify their interests through activities such as job shadowing; and assisting them to sort out information about housing options, benefits, sexuality and relationships, crime, and alcohol and other drug use and abuse are all examples of useful methods to aid youth. Much of the information currently available on these topics is not provided in formats that are "friendly" to youth with cognitive challenges. Additional attention should be focused on developing informational materials that are accessible to all youth. Until this happens, youth with cognitive challenges will require support to locate and digest information relevant to their knowledge development and decision making.

Evidence also suggests that the social self-competence of adolescents with Down syndrome may be enhanced when they have accurate information about their disability. Sanger, Perrin, and Sandler (1993) found that children with seizure disorders who had accurate information about their disability were better able to interact with others related to health management than children who were less well informed. Similarly, adolescents with Down syndrome who are able to intelligently discuss their physical and medical differences may be more likely to feel positive about those differences. In addition, all adolescents, including those with Down syndrome, benefit from information regarding hygiene, contemporary dress and hairstyles, and other aspects of appearance that help them make friends and feel good about themselves (Edwards, 1990).

Coping, Social, and Task-Related Skills

Many skills are important for the expression of self-competence. There are specific skills we can impart to youth, including academic knowledge and independence strategies. Other skills are generic in that they provide students with lifelong strategies to achieve success. Generic skills include goal setting, problem solving, assertiveness, coping with challenges, self-regulation, management of helping partnerships, and medical self-care (Olson & Cooley, 1996; Powers, Sowers, et al., 1996; Ward & Kohler, 1996; Wehmeyer, 1992). Skill development typically requires integrated instruction and practice. The authors' experience suggests that youth self-competence is bolstered through the acquisition and application of specific achievement, partnership, and coping skills (Powers, Sowers, et al., 1996). Each of these skills can be broken down into discrete generic steps that youth can apply to achieve current and future goals.

Hopes and dreams fuel the vitality and motivation of most youth. Articulating one's future dreams is a skill that requires creativity, knowledge of life options, and strategies for organizing and integrating the many facets of future life. Some youth, particularly those with fewer life experiences or those who have been economically deprived, have difficulty articulating their dreams. It is essential that these youth be provided opportunities to learn about different life options and to risk developing dreams for a more hopeful future.

Goal Setting   One of the most important skills for expressing self-competence is goal setting (Brotherson, Backus, Summers, & Turnbull, 1986; Gardner, 1986; Mitchell, 1988). Youth typically choose goals that they value; at the same time, they are empowered by goal achievement. Individuals tend to infer high self-efficacy from success achieved through effort on tasks that are perceived to be difficult. In contrast, they infer low self-efficacy if they have to work hard to master easy tasks (de Vries, Dijkstra, & Kuhlman, 1988). Thus, youth should be encouraged to select moderately challenging goals that have a reasonable probability of success.

Adolescents with cognitive challenges will likely require additional assistance in identifying and working toward goals.

Problem Solving Another essential skill for developing self-competence is problem solving. Evidence indicates that individuals with cognitive disabilities can effectively apply problem-solving strategies if they are provided with systematic, in situ training (Hughes & Rusch, 1989). Problem solving is initially difficult for many adolescents. Many youth have a history of limited access to life experiences and information about activity requirements and options for solving problems. Problem-solving skills can be bolstered by assisting youth to learn straightforward steps for identifying parts of activities, those parts that are difficult for them, and strategies for performing the hard parts. Youth who have difficulty with such abstract analysis can be given opportunities to learn the requirements of activities by trying the activities or watching others perform them. They can then identify strategies for accomplishing activities by learning to tell others what they want and then enlisting their aid in pinpointing ways to overcome challenges. Once youth experience problem-solving success, they are likely to demonstrate increased enthusiasm for working toward additional goals as well as to become more resilient when faced with challenges (Seligman, 1990).

Assertiveness Assertiveness refers to the ability to express needs directly and to act with self-confidence (Des Jardins, 1986). Subskills such as establishing positive body language, communicating clearly, and managing others' resistance are important components of assertiveness (Jakubowski & Lange, 1978). Assertiveness training has been used widely with people without disabilities and has also been shown to be effective for individuals with disabilities (Granat, 1978; Heimberg, Montgomery, Madsen, & Heimberg, 1977).

Self-Advocacy Self-advocacy is another important skill for young adults with disabilities (Jones & Ulicny, 1986; McGill, 1978; Turnbull & Turnbull, 1985; Varela, 1986). Participation in advocacy activities appears to be associated with both social and political change (Balcazar, Seekins, Fawcett, & Hopkins, 1990) and enhanced self-esteem for those involved (Halpern, Close, & Nelson, 1986). Advocacy preparation must include instruction in personal rights and responsibilities, information about legislative initiatives, and effective methods for self-advocacy.

Negotiation Negotiation skill is essential for adolescents who are striving for increasing independence and autonomy. Skillful win–win negotiation is a complex and demanding process (Fisher & Ury, 1981). Yet even a skill as sophisticated as negotiation can be learned at a rudimentary level as a series of steps as follows: 1) listen to what they want, 2) decide what you can live with, and 3) compromise. The authors' experience indicates that many youth with cognitive challenges can learn to apply basic negotiation skills if they are provided systematic coaching and support (Powers, Sowers, et al., 1996).

Positive Self-Talk   A growing body of literature indicates that positive self-talk is effective in assisting people to shape their own behavior (Dush, Hirt, & Schroeder, 1989). Self-talk that emphasizes situational, depersonalized, and temporary interpretations of negative events is associated with heightened perseverance in dealing with failure and frustration (Seligman, 1990). Youth should be encouraged to use positive self-talk to reframe their failure as a temporary event. They should also be encouraged to depersonalize their failures by attributing the problem to a flawed game plan rather than to personal failings.

Self-Monitoring   By self-monitoring their accomplishments, people have opportunities to observe their competence; as a result, they begin to view themselves as more competent (Dowrick, 1983). In turn, they begin to demonstrate higher levels of skill (Gonzales & Dowrick, 1983). Youth, like the rest of us, seldom attend to their accomplishments or positive experiences. It is critical that youth be provided strategies for regularly identifying their accomplishments and rewarding their efforts in ways they select. Typically, professionals assist youth to take note of their accomplishments by delivering reinforcement that is professionally referenced (i.e., "I think you did a great job"). Although this form of reinforcement is useful, it is preferable to provide reinforcement that promotes youth self-attribution of competence (i.e., "I hope you feel great about the job you did"). Although the difference between these statements is subtle, the latter statement is more likely to catalyze youth self-reflection and self-attribution of success.

Frustration Management   Frustration is a typical response to situations in which goals are not achieved quickly or effectively. Learning to productively manage frustration is important if youth are to avoid demoralization and maintain their momentum for goal attainment. Youth skilled in the use of problem-focused and emotion-focused coping strategies are optimally prepared to respond to obstacles (Compas, 1987). Problem-focused techniques such as problem solving are appropriate coping strategies for situations in which an obstacle can be overcome, whereas emotion-focused strategies are helpful in instances in which an outcome cannot be controlled (Folkman & Lazarus, 1980). Frustration management can be learned on a variety of levels, using discrete steps (e.g., "stop, think, do something different"). It is important for youth to learn to recognize and manage their frustration, as well as to identify and resist being demoralized by other people's discouragement.

Medical Self-Care   A final skill that can be crucial for teenagers with ongoing health problems is medical self-care. Traditionally, medical self-management has not been emphasized for youth with cognitive challenges.

Yet medical self-care can often be presented as a series of simple routines that most youth can master (Olson & Cooley, 1996). Meeting alone with a teenager during part of the medical visit, demonstrating interest in the teenager's general life in addition to his or her disability, and soliciting the teenager's reactions and ideas regarding self-care strategies are all important methods for promoting medical self-management (see also Chapter 1).

Access to Support

A final major requisite for promoting self-competence is support provided by others. Support can be provided as encouragement, challenge, praise, and partnership. Assisting youth to acknowledge and self-reinforce effort and success, challenging them to take risks, validating their experiences, providing honest feedback, and being available to provide needed assistance are all important support strategies. Perhaps the most important support strategy adults need to use with teenagers is that of listening. Listening and acknowledging what is heard are particularly important with teenagers who experience significant disabilities. A parent of a teenager with communication challenges expressed concern to us that her son's disruptive behavior was usually interpreted as occurring independently of the context in which he became disruptive. She stated that she hoped professionals would notice that his disruptive behavior was sometimes an expression of dissatisfaction or distress with the situation he was facing and that they would thus focus on improving the situation as well as imposing consequences for his behavior.

Promoting child self-competence is not a primary focus of preservice and in-service training for educators or physicians (Field & Hoffman, 1996; Olson & Cooley, 1996). Most educators are required to function within educational structures that emphasize uniformity and compliance ahead of individualized programming, self-direction, and partnership. Many medical professionals are also inadequately informed regarding methods to work with teenagers to maximize their understanding of health issues and their medical self-care. If professionals are to effectively facilitate the self-competence of youth, they must have access to information about adolescent development, communication and support strategies, and methods to promote informed decision making and skill development among youth with challenges.

Many parents are unsure about how to support their children's self-competence. Parents may benefit from acknowledgment of the ways they already support their children, communication of respect for family norms regarding child independence, information about resources and strategies for promoting self-competence, and assistance in managing family stressors that impede parental capacities to support child self-competence (Singer & Irvin, 1989; Summers, Behr, & Turnbull, 1989; Turnbull & Turnbull, 1996).

Friendship It is clear that social support from peers is important for children's mental health (Spivack & Shure, 1982; Trower, Bryant, & Argyle, 1978), self-esteem (Berndt & Hawkins, 1987), and resilience (Garmezy & Rutter, 1983). Children who experience social isolation from their peers tend to be more anxious than children with strong peer networks (Belle, 1989). Furthermore, between 7th and 10th grades, the intimacy and companionship provided by same-sex friends typically surpasses the depth of companionship that adolescents have with their parents (Buhrmester & Furman, 1987). For many adolescents, friendships with peers provide an outlet for sharing hopes and dreams, expressing feelings and ideas, and participating in new activities and experiences. The development of relationships between youth of diverse capabilities generally promotes the well-being of all participants (Bricker, 1978; Gaylord-Ross, Haring, Breen, & Pitts-Conway, 1984).

Establishing friendships can be difficult for many youth with disabilities. Many youth benefit from coaching in specific strategies for establishing friendships, including talking to other youth at school and on the telephone, joining clubs and teams, inviting youth to their homes and to activities in the community, and asking friends to introduce them to other teenagers they know. Vernberg, Beery, Ewell, and Abwender (1993) found that parents of young adolescents without disabilities used four clusters of strategies to encourage their children's friendships: They interacted with parents who also had adolescent children, they created opportunities for their children to spend time with friends, they talked with their children about friendship, and they encouraged their children to participate in activities with peers.

Mentoring Mentoring is a popular approach for promoting youths' living skills, positive attitudes toward disability, knowledge, self-confidence, and motivation (Fredricks, 1988; Jones & Ulicny, 1986; Rhodes, 1994). Powers, Sowers, and Stevens (1995) found that when adolescents with disabilities interacted with adult role models who experience disabilities, their disability-related knowledge and self-confidence as well as their parents' perceptions of the knowledge and capabilities of their children was enhanced. Interaction with successful adult role models with disabilities was also identified as a significant factor contributing to children's self-competence in a qualitative study of the childhood experiences of successful adults with disabilities (Powers, Singer, & Todis, 1996).

Peer Support Peer support between people with disabilities is a powerful way to enhance personal skills, self-acceptance, and leadership (Jones & Ulicny, 1986; Williams & Shoultz, 1984). Through interaction with their peers with disabilities, youth have opportunities to learn and practice self-determination and leadership skills, to share strategies for managing disability-related barriers, and to receive support for self-acceptance. As youth with disabilities are increasingly involved in inclusive settings, it will be important to ensure that they have options for interacting with youth who experience similar disability-related challenges.

CONCLUSIONS

This chapter has provided a brief overview of the foundations of self-competence among adolescents as well as of diverse strategies that may be used to improve the self-competence of children with disabilities. Perhaps the most important conclusion to be drawn from this discussion is that the essence of developing self-competence during adolescence does not have to be substantially affected by disability. Factors that promote self-competence for most adolescents also enhance self-competence for adolescents with challenges, including those with Down syndrome. The extent to which youth who experience disabilities develop self-competence is a function of their exposure both to typical sources for promoting self-competence as well as to opportunities, information, skills, and support that accommodate their unique strengths and needs. If provided these experiences and accommodations, most youth with disabilities will successfully navigate their way toward self-competent adult lives.

REFERENCES

Abery, B.H. (1994). A conceptual framework for enhancing self-determination. In M.F. Hayden & B.H. Abery (Eds.), *Challenges for a service system in transition: Ensuring quality community experiences for persons with developmental disabilities* (pp. 345–380). Baltimore: Paul H. Brookes Publishing Co.

Arborelius, E., & Bremberg, S. (1991). How do teenagers respond to a consistently student-centered program of health education at school? *International Journal of Adolescent Medicine and Health, 5*(2), 95–112.

Balcazar, F.E., Seekins, T., Fawcett, S.B., & Hopkins, B.L. (1990). Empowering people with physical disabilities through advocacy skills training. *American Journal of Community Psychology, 18*(2), 281–296.

Bandura, A. (1986). *Social foundation of thought and action: A social cognitive theory.* Englewood Cliffs, NJ: Prentice Hall.

Bednar, R.L., Wells, M.G., & Peterson, S.R. (1989). *Self-esteem: Paradoxes and innovations in clinical theory and practice.* Washington, DC: American Psychological Association.

Belle, D. (Ed.). (1989). *Children's social networks and social supports.* New York: John Wiley & Sons.

Berndt, T.J., & Hawkins, J.A. (1987). *The contribution of supportive friendships to adjustment after the transition to junior high school.* Unpublished manuscript, Purdue University, Lafayette, IN.

Bolles, R.N. (1995). *The 1995 what color is your parachute? A practical manual for job-hunters and career-changers.* Berkeley, CA: Ten Speed Press.

Branden, N. (1969). *The psychology of self-esteem.* New York: Bantam.

Breslau, N. (1985). Psychiatric disorder in children with physical disabilities. *Journal of the American Academy of Child Psychiatry, 24,* 87–94.

Bricker, D.D. (1978). A rationale for the integration of handicapped preschool children. In M.J. Guralnick (Ed.), *Early intervention and the integrating of handi-*

capped and nonhandicapped children (pp. 3–26). Baltimore: University Park Press.

Brotherson, M.J., Backus, L.H., Summers, J.A., & Turnbull, A.P. (1986). Transition to adulthood. In J.A. Summers (Ed.), *The right to grow up: An introduction to adults with developmental disabilities* (pp. 17–44). Baltimore: Paul H. Brookes Publishing Co.

Buhrmester, D., & Furman, W. (1987). The development of companionship and intimacy. *Child Development, 58,* 1101–1113.

Cadman, D., Boyle, M., Szatmari, P., & Offord, D.R. (1987). Chronic illness, disability, and mental and social well-being: Findings of the Ontario Child Health Study. *Pediatrics, 79,* 805–813.

Christopher, G.M., Kurtz, P.D., & Howing, P.T. (1989). Status of mental health services for youth in school and community. *Children and Youth Services Review, 11,* 159–174.

Compas, B.E. (1987). Coping with stress during childhood and adolescence. *Psychological Bulletin, 101*(3), 393–403.

Des Jardins, C. (1986). Assertiveness is/is not. In F. Weiner (Ed.), *No apologies: A guide to living with a disability, written by the real authorities—people with disabilities, their families and friends* (pp. 122–123). New York: St. Martin's Press.

de Vries, H., Dijkstra, M., & Kuhlman, P. (1988). Self-efficacy: The third factor besides attitude and subjective norm as a predictor of behavioral intentions. *Health Education Research, 3*(3), 273–282.

Dowrick, P.W. (1983). Self modeling. In P.W. Dowrick & S.J. Biggs (Eds.), *Using video: Psychological and social applications* (pp. 105–124). London: John Wiley & Sons.

Drotar, D., & Bush, M. (1985). Mental health issues and services. In N. Hobbs & J.M. Perrin (Eds.), *Issues in the care of children with chronic illness* (pp. 827–863). San Francisco: Jossey-Bass.

Dubrow, E.F., Schmidt, D., McBride, J., Edwards, S., & Merk, F.L. (1993). Teaching children to cope with stressful experiences: Initial implementation and evaluation of a primary prevention program. *Journal of Clinical Child Psychology, 22,* 428–440.

Dush, D.M., Hirt, M.L., & Schroeder, H.E. (1989). Self-statement modification in the treatment of child behavior disorders: A meta-analysis. *Psychological Bulletin, 106*(1), 97–106.

Dyson, L., Edgar, E., & Crnic, K. (1989). Psychological predictors of adjustment by siblings of developmentally disabled children. *American Journal on Mental Retardation, 94*(3), 292–302.

Edwards, J.P. (1990). Adolescence and adulthood. In S. Pueschel, *A parent's guide to Down syndrome: Toward a brighter future* (pp. 259–267). Baltimore: Paul H. Brookes Publishing Co.

Ferguson, P.M., & Asch, A. (1989). Lessons from life: Personal and parental perspectives on school, childhood, and disability. In D. Biklen, D. Ferguson, & A. Ford (Eds.), *Schooling and disability* (pp. 108–140). Chicago: University of Chicago Press.

Field, S., & Hoffman, A. (1996). Increasing the ability of educators to support youth self-determination. In L.E. Powers, G.H.S. Singer, & J.A. Sowers (Eds.), *On the road to autonomy: Promoting self-competence in children and youth with disabilities* (pp. 171–187). Baltimore: Paul H. Brookes Publishing Co.

Fisher, R., & Ury, W. (1981). *Getting to yes: Negotiation agreement without giving in.* New York: Penguin Books.

Folkman, S., & Lazarus, R.S. (1980). An analysis of coping in a middle-aged community sample. *Journal of Health and Social Behavior, 21,* 219–239.

Fredericks, H.D.B. (1988). Tim becomes an Eagle Scout. *National Information Center for Children and Youth with Handicaps: Transition Summary, 5,* 8–9.

Gardner, N.E.S. (1986). Sexuality. In J.A. Summers (Ed.), *The right to grow up: An introduction to adults with developmental disabilities* (pp. 45–66). Baltimore: Paul H. Brookes Publishing Co.

Garmezy, N., & Rutter, M. (Eds.). (1983). *Stress, coping, and development in children.* New York: McGraw-Hill.

Gaylord-Ross, R.J., Haring, T.G., Breen, C., & Pitts-Conway, V. (1984). The training and generalization of social interaction skills with autistic youth. *Journal of Applied Behavior Analysis, 17*(2), 229–247.

Gonzales, F.P., & Dowrick, P.W. (1983, October). *Effects of video self-modeling in "feedforward" training hand/eye coordination.* Unpublished manuscript, University of Alaska, Anchorage.

Granat, J.P. (1978). Assertiveness training and the mentally retarded. *Rehabilitation Counseling Bulletin, 22,* 100–107.

Grolnick, W.S., & Ryan, R.M. (1989). Parent styles associated with children's self-regulation and competence in school. *Journal of Educational Psychology, 81*(2), 143–154.

Halpern, A.S., Close, D.W., & Nelson, D.J. (1986). *On my own: The impact of semi-independent living programs for adults with mental retardation.* Baltimore: Paul H. Brookes Publishing Co.

Harter, S. (1981). A model of mastery motivation in children: Individual differences and developmental change. In S. Collins (Ed.), *Minnesota symposium on child psychology* (Vol. 4, pp. 215–255). Hillsdale, NJ: Lawrence Erlbaum Associates.

Harter, S. (1985). Competence as a dimension of self-evaluation: Toward a comprehensive model of self-worth. In R. Leahy (Ed.), *The development of the self* (pp. 55–118). New York: Academic Press.

Harter, S. (1990). Causes, correlates, and the functional role of global self-worth: A life-span perspective. In R.J. Sternberg & J. Kolligian, Jr. (Eds.), *Competence considered* (pp. 67–97). New Haven, CT: Yale University Press.

Harter, S. (1993). Causes and consequences of low self-esteem in children and adolescents. In R. Baumeister (Ed.), *Self-esteem: The puzzle of low self-regard* (pp. 87–111). New York: Plenum.

Heimberg, R.C., Montgomery, D., Madsen, C.H., & Heimberg, J.S. (1977). Assertion training: A review of the literature. *Behavior Therapy, 8,* 953–971.

Henderson, P.A., Kelbey, T.J., & Engebretson, K.M. (1992). Effects of a stress-control program on children's locus of control, self-concept, and coping behavior. *School Counselor, 40,* 125–130.

Hernandez, D.J. (1995). *America's children: Resources from family, government, and the economy.* New York: Russell Sage Foundation.

Heyman, W.B. (1990). The self-perception of a learning disability and its relationship to academic self-concept and self-esteem. *Journal of Learning Disabilities, 23*(8), 472–475.

Hughes, C., & Rusch, F.R. (1989). Teaching supported employees with severe mental retardation to solve problems. *Journal of Applied Behavior Analysis, 22*(4), 365–372.

Hughes, C.A., Korinek, L., & Gorman, J. (1991). Self-management for students with mental retardation in public school settings: A research review. *Education and Training in Mental Retardation, 26,* 271–291.

Jakubowski, P., & Lange, A.J. (1978). *The assertive option: Your rights and responsibilities.* Champaign, IL: Research Press.

Jones, M.L., & Ulicny, G.R. (1986). The independent living perspective: Applications to services for adults with developmental disabilities. In J.A. Summers (Ed.), *The right to grow up: An introduction to adults with developmental disabilities* (pp. 227–241). Baltimore: Paul H. Brookes Publishing Co.

Jung, J. (1994). *Under the influence: Alcohol and human behavior.* Pacific Grove, CA: Brooks/Cole.

Kaplan, H., Martin, S., & Johnson, R. (1986). Self-rejection and the explanation of deviance: Specification of the structure among latent constructs. *American Journal of Sociology, 92,* 384–441.

Lazarus, R.S., & Folkman, S. (1984). *Stress, appraisal, and coping.* New York: Springer-Verlag.

Magill, J., & Hurlbut, N. (1986). The self-esteem of adolescents with cerebral palsy. *American Journal of Occupational Therapy, 40*(6), 402–407.

McGill, J. (1978). *We are people first: A book on self-advocacy.* Lincoln: Nebraska Advocacy Services.

McLanahan, S., & Sandefur, G. (1994). *Growing up with a single parent: What hurts, what helps.* Cambridge, MA: Harvard University Press.

Mink, I.R., Nihira, K., & Meyers, C.E. (1983). Taxonomy of family life styles: I. Homes with TMR children. *American Journal of Mental Deficiency, 87,* 484–497.

Mitchell, B. (1988). Who chooses? *National Information Center for Children and Youth with Handicaps: Transition Summary, 5.*

Mruk, C. (1995). *Self-esteem: Research, theory, and practice.* New York: Springer Publishing Co.

Olson, A.L., & Cooley, W.C. (1996). The role of medical professionals in supporting children's self-competence. In L.E. Powers, G.H.S. Singer, & J.A. Sowers (Eds.), *On the road to autonomy: Promoting self-competence in children and youth with disabilities* (pp. 257–272). Baltimore: Paul H. Brookes Publishing Co.

Pantell, R.H., Lewis, C., & Sharp, L. (1989). Improving outcomes in asthmatic patients: Results of a randomized trial. *American Journal of Diseases of Children, 143*(4), 433.

Perrin, E., & Shapiro, E. (1985). Health locus of control beliefs of healthy children, children with chronic physical illness and their mothers. *Journal of Pediatrics, 107*(4), 627–633.

Perrin, E.C., Ramsey, B.K., & Sandler, H.M. (1987). Children and adolescents with a chronic illness. *Child: Care, Health and Development, 13,* 13–32.

Pope, A.W., McHale, S.M., & Craighead, W.E. (1988). *Self-esteem enhancement with children and adolescents.* Elmsford, NY: Pergamon Press.

Powers, L.E., Singer, G.H.S., & Sowers, J.A. (1996). Self-competence and disability. In L.E. Powers, G.H.S. Singer, & J.A. Sowers (Eds.), *On the road to autonomy: Promoting self-competence for children and youth with disabilities* (pp. 3–24). Baltimore: Paul H. Brookes Publishing Co.

Powers, L.E., Singer, G.H.S., & Todis, B. (1996). Reflections on competence: Perspectives of successful adults. In L.E. Powers, G.H.S. Singer, & J.A. Sowers (Eds.), *On the road to autonomy: Promoting self-competence in children and youth with disabilities* (pp. 69–92). Baltimore: Paul H. Brookes Publishing Co.

Powers, L.E., Sowers, J., & Stevens, T. (1995). An exploratory, randomized study of the impact of mentoring on the self-efficacy and community-based knowledge of adolescents with severe physical challenges. *Journal of Rehabilitation, 61*(1), 33–41.

Powers, L.E., Sowers, J.A., Turner, A., Nesbitt, M., Knowles, E., & Ellison, R. (1996). Take charge: A model for promoting self-determination among adolescents with challenges. In L.E. Powers, G.H.S. Singer, & J.A. Sowers (Eds.), *On the road to autonomy: Promoting self-competence for children and youth with disabilities* (pp. 291–322). Baltimore: Paul H. Brookes Publishing Co.

Powers, L.E., Turner, A., Wilson, R., Matuszewski, J., Ellison, R., & Rein, C. (1995). *A controlled field-test of the efficacy of a multi-component model for promoting adolescent self-determination.* Lebanon, NH: Hood Center for Family Support, Dartmouth Medical School.

Prout, H.T., Marcal, S.D., & Marcal, D.C. (1992). A meta-analysis of self-reported personality characteristics of children and adolescents with learning disabilities. *Journal of Psychoeducational Assessment, 10,* 59–64.

Rhodes, J.E. (1994, Spring). Older and wiser: Mentoring relationships in childhood and adolescence. *Journal of Primary Prevention, 14*(3), 187–196.

Rosenberg, M. (1965). *Society and the adolescent self-image.* Princeton, NJ: Princeton University Press.

Sanger, M., Perrin, E., & Sandler, H. (1993). Development in children's causal theories of their seizure disorder. *Developmental and Behavioral Pediatrics, 14*(2), 88–93.

Schinke, S.P., & Gilchrist, L.D. (1984). *Life skills counseling with adolescents.* Austin, TX: PRO-ED.

Schoenherr, S.J., Brown, R.T., Baldwin, K., & Kaslow, N.J. (1992). Attributional styles and psychopathology in pediatric chronic-illness groups. *Journal of Clinical Child Psychology, 21,* 380–387.

Seligman, M.E.P. (1990). *Learned optimism.* New York: Pocket Books.

Shapiro, J.P. (1993). *No pity: People with disabilities forging a new civil rights movement.* New York: Times Books.

Singer, G.H.S., & Irvin, L.K. (Eds.). (1989). *Support for caregiving families: Enabling positive adaptation to disability.* Baltimore: Paul H. Brookes Publishing Co.

Singer, G.H.S., & Powers, L.E. (Eds.). (1993). *Families, disability, and empowerment: Active coping skills and strategies for family intervention.* Baltimore: Paul H. Brookes Publishing Co.

Sinnema, G. (1991). Resilience among children with special health-care needs and among their families. *Pediatric Annals, 20*(9), 483–486.

Spivack, G., & Shure, M. (1982). The cognition of social adjustment: Interpersonal cognitive problem-solving thinking. In B. Lahey & A. Kazdin (Eds.), *Advances in clinical child psychology* (Vol. 5, pp. 323–372). New York: Plenum.

Stein, R.E.K., & Jessop, D.J. (1989). What diagnosis does not tell: The case for a noncategorical approach to chronic illness in childhood. *Social Science and Medicine, 29,* 769–778.

Summers, J.A., Behr, S.K., & Turnbull, A.P. (1989). Positive adaptation and coping strengths of families who have children with disabilities. In G.H.S. Singer & L.K. Irvin (Eds.), *Support for caregiving families: Enabling positive adaptation to disability* (pp. 27–40). Baltimore: Paul H. Brookes Publishing Co.

Trower, P., Bryant, B., & Argyle, M. (1978). *Social skills and mental health.* London: Methuen.

Turnbull, A.P., & Turnbull, H.R. (1985). Developing independence. *Journal of Adolescent Health Care, 6*(2), 108–119.

Turnbull, A.P., & Turnbull, H.R., III. (1996). Self-determination within a culturally responsive family systems perspective: Balancing the family mobile. In L.E. Powers, G.H.S. Singer, & J.A. Sowers (Eds.), *On the road to autonomy: Promoting self-competence in children and youth with disabilities* (pp. 195–220). Baltimore: Paul H. Brookes Publishing Co.

Varela, R.A. (1986). Risks, rules, and resources: Self-advocacy and the parameters of decision making. In J.A. Summers (Ed.), *The right to grow up: An introduction to adults with developmental disabilities* (pp. 245–254). Baltimore: Paul H. Brookes Publishing Co.

Vernberg, E.M., Beery, S.H., Ewell, K.K., & Abwender, D.A. (1993). Parents' use of friendship facilitation strategies and the formation of friendships in early adolescence: A prospective study. *Journal of Family Psychology, 7*(3), 356–369.

Ward, M.J. (1988). The many facets of self-determination. *National Information Center for Children and Youth with Handicaps: Transition Summary, 5,* 2–3.

Ward, M.J., & Kohler, P.D. (1996). Teaching self-determination: Content and process. In L.E. Powers, G.H.S. Singer, & J.A. Sowers (Eds.), *On the road to autonomy: Promoting self-competence in children and youth with disabilities* (pp. 275–290). Baltimore: Paul H. Brookes Publishing Co.

Wehmeyer, M.L. (1992). Self-determination and the education of students with mental retardation. *Education and Training in Mental Retardation, 27,* 302–314.

Wehmeyer, M.L. (1996). Self-determination for youth with severe cognitive disabilities: From theory to practice. In L.E. Powers, G.H.S. Singer, & J.A. Sowers (Eds.), *On the road to autonomy: Promoting self-competence in children and youth with disabilities* (pp. 115–133). Baltimore: Paul H. Brookes Publishing Co.

Wehmeyer, M.L., Kelchner, K., & Richards, S. (1995). Individual and environmental factors related to the self-determination of adults with mental retardation. *Journal of Vocational Rehabilitation, 5,* 291–305.

Wells, E.L., & Marwell, G. (1976). *Self-esteem: Its conceptualization and measurement.* Beverly Hills, CA: Sage Publications.

Werner, E.E., & Smith, R.S. (1992). *Overcoming the odds: High risk children from birth to adulthood.* Ithaca, NY: Cornell University Press.

Williams, P., & Shoultz, B. (1984). *We can speak for ourselves: Self-advocacy for mentally handicapped people.* Cambridge, MA: Brookline Books.

Zeltzer, L., Kellerman, J., Ellenberg, L., Dash, J., & Rigler, D. (1980). Psychological effects of illness in adolescence: II. Impact of illness in adolescents—Crucial issues and coping styles. *Journal of Pediatrics, 97,* 132–138.

Zetlin, A.G., Turner, J.L., & Winick, L. (1987). Socialization effects on the community adaptation of adults who have mild mental retardation. In S. Landesman, P.M. Vietze, & M.J. Begab (Eds.), *Living environments and mental retardation: NICHD Mental Retardation Research Centers series* (pp. 293–313). Washington, DC: American Association on Mental Retardation.

9

Cognitive Functioning

Issues in Theory and Practice

Robert M. Hodapp

When evaluating studies of cognitive functioning in adolescents with Down syndrome, the glass can be considered either half-full or half-empty. On the positive side, cognitive functioning—like many aspects of behavior—has been the subject of psychologic studies for more than 50 years (Gibson, 1978). Since the mid-1970s, studies have proliferated on cognitive strengths and weaknesses, symbolic play, effects of different environments and experiences, and the connections between cognition and language (see Cicchetti & Beeghly, 1990, for a review). Such studies of cognitive functioning are much more common in relation to Down syndrome than with respect to any other genetic disorder of mental retardation (Hodapp & Dykens, 1994).

Yet, at the same time, we know surprisingly little about cognitive development in *adolescents* with Down syndrome because most studies concentrate on individuals who are either much younger or much older. During infancy and early childhood, children with Down syndrome have been found to continue developing cognitively, but at slower rates as they get older (see Hodapp & Zigler, 1990, for a review). During adulthood, researchers have attempted to understand IQ changes as adults with Down syndrome age. The issue here has revolved around whether IQ declines in people with Down syndrome occur during the mid-adult years and, if so, whether such declines are a by-product of the aging process, Alzheimer's disease, or some combination of these factors (Devenny, Wisniewski, & Silverman, 1993).

As a result of this emphasis on younger and older individuals, cognitive functioning in adolescence has received much less attention. The few studies available for review provide some basic data, but even these must be considered within a broader context. This context, in turn, provides several important lessons for parents and professionals concerned with adolescents with Down syndrome.

THEORETICAL ISSUES

At least three major issues relate to cognitive functioning during adolescence in individuals with Down syndrome. The first issue concerns the *critical age* for development. Simply stated, there may be a set age span during which development can—and cannot—occur. To cite the strongest example, data from certain groups with disabilities indicate that a critical or sensitive period may exist for the acquisition of grammar. In one study, a severely abused and neglected girl named Genie was first exposed to language only at 13 years of age, after she was discovered (and removed from her abusive parents) (Curtiss, 1977). Genie's subsequent language development was remarkable. She quickly learned large numbers of new words and rapidly developed abilities to use language easily and effectively. But even after intensive intervention, Genie was never able to master grammatical features such as past, present, and future verb forms. In another set of studies, adults who are deaf were found to differ in their ultimate grammatical abilities based on when they had first been introduced to American Sign Language (ASL) (Newport, 1990). Those adults first introduced to sign language in their early childhood years were the most grammatically proficient as adults; those introduced in middle childhood and adolescence (usually after oral training had failed) were less advanced; and those first introduced only as adults were least proficient of all. This gradually decreasing ability to "pick up" grammar does not mean that no child can progress after the early childhood years, but that grammatical development becomes increasingly difficult after that time.

In addition, these studies pinpoint areas that do *not* show critical or sensitive periods. For example, Genie improved markedly in her vocabulary, ability to use language, and general cognitive skills. Similarly, adults who are deaf subsequently learned a variety of cognitive and noncognitive skills, regardless of when they were first introduced to sign language (Newport, 1990). Researchers now feel that children with any disability can continue to develop in most areas.

Continued development also generally occurs in adolescents with Down syndrome. In a 1995 study, Shepperdson examined large numbers of British children with Down syndrome, including one group who had been born from 1964 to 1966 and another born from 1973 to 1975. Although some differences emerged between the two groups, the basic finding was identical: People with Down syndrome continue developing into the adolescent and early adult years. Although development may slow from adolescence (when children were 15–17 years old) until early adulthood (ages 24–26 years), these individuals nevertheless continued developing. Furthermore, development occurred across a variety of areas, including general social competence, overall expressive and receptive language, and some measures of vocabulary (see also Carr, 1988, 1994).

A second issue concerns *strengths and weaknesses,* or what have been called profiles of development. Many years ago, researchers assumed that all children showed development that was generally flat or even from one domain to another. A child at a particular level of language was assumed to be at a similar level in all areas of cognitive development. More recently, however, this view has been questioned, on the basis that many children show pronounced strengths and weaknesses in their intellectual abilities. Children with certain genetic retardation disorders can also show areas of pronounced strengths and weaknesses. For example, children with the rarely occurring Williams syndrome show particularly high levels of language, even though their overall IQs are relatively low (Bellugi, Wang, & Jernigan, 1994). This pattern of "language in the relative absence of thought" is strikingly different from behavioral strengths and weaknesses shown by children with most other disorders.

Down syndrome generally falls in the middle in this regard. Individuals with this disorder show some relative strengths and weaknesses, but rarely as often or as prominently as children with Williams syndrome. For example, language typically has been considered an area of specific weakness in individuals with Down syndrome. Children with this disorder show grammatical abilities that may be lower than their abilities in other aspects of both cognition or language (e.g., Fowler, 1990) (see also Chapter 11). In addition, these children may more often demonstrate related speech and articulation difficulties (Miller, Leddy, Miolo, & Sedey, 1995; Pueschel, 1990).

In other areas of intelligence, no particular strengths or weaknesses are observed. Consider these children's performance on the Kaufman Assessment Battery for Children (K–ABC; Kaufman & Kaufman, 1983). This intelligence test taps three distinct abilities. The first area, Sequential Processing, examines the individual's ability to understand and reproduce information presented in serial or temporal order. The child must repeat a sequence of digits or reproduce a series of hand movements provided by the experimenter. The second area, Simultaneous Processing, tests one's ability to "see the whole," or Gestalt. The child is asked to identify a picture in which certain lines are missing, or to put together a jigsaw puzzle triangle when given the requisite pieces. The third area, Achievement, taps the child's skills in reading, mathematics, and cultural knowledge.

After administering the K–ABC to children with Down syndrome, Pueschel, Gallagher, Zartler, and Pezzullo (1987) found few areas of strength or weakness. The only possible strength and weakness found may involve some tendency to perform better on tasks of visual versus auditory processing, which may help explain some of these children's problems in (orally) comprehending and producing language. Similarly, Hodapp et al. (1992) compared children with Down syndrome to those with fragile X syndrome (the second most common genetic cause of mental retardation). Children with fragile X syndrome demonstrated a clear pattern. For these children, sequential, or bit-by-bit, processing was a clear weakness compared with simultaneous processing or achievement. In children with Down syndrome, again no clear pattern of strength or weakness emerged. On at least some measures, then, children with Down syndrome demonstrate flat or even profiles of development, whereas on others (e.g., grammar, language, possibly visual versus auditory processing), specific strengths or weaknesses characterize many individuals with this disorder.

A third major issue concerns *connections to other skills*. Here again, more recent thinking contradicts earlier ideas. In past years, much emphasis was devoted to the idea of "prerequisite skills," those skills without which the child could not possibly perform other, more complex tasks. It now seems likely that prerequisite skills have been overemphasized. Although prerequisites may exist for certain high-level tasks, children may be able to perform other high-level skills even in the absence of skills previously considered necessary.

The best example involves reading. Given the difficulties children with Down syndrome have in grammar, articulation, and language in general, one might think it unlikely that these children could be taught to read. In the 1990s, however, Buckley and others have intensively intervened to teach reading to children with Down syndrome. Buckley's results, though preliminary, are impressive. According to Buckley, Bird, and Byrne (1996), approximately 50% of children with Down syndrome can achieve some useful degree of literacy. Although some children have been taught to read words at very young ages, even training begun during adolescence may prove beneficial (Buckley, 1995).

Notable, too, is the way in which reading may relate to other skills. Reading may aid children in speaking and understanding language and, possibly, in overcoming articulation difficulties. In addition, given the possible superiority of visual over auditory processing for these children (Pueschel et al., 1987), reading may provide an entryway into oral language (Buckley, 1995). The earlier view, then, that certain levels of receptive and expressive language must be present as prerequisites to later reading abilities, may well be reversed. Reading, previously assumed to be the more complex skill, may instead help children to develop in other areas of language.

LESSONS FOR PARENTS AND PROFESSIONALS

Critical ages, strengths and weaknesses, and connections to other skills provide clear lessons for intervention. Three important messages can be gleaned from these research findings.

Lesson 1: *In most areas, development can continue beyond childhood.*
With the possible exception of grammatical abilities, the large majority of cognitive abilities can continue to develop during and up to the young adult years in people with Down syndrome. As Carr (1994), Shepperdson (1995), and others have noted, cognitive development can continue, although sometimes at slightly slower rates than in the early and middle childhood years. In the same way, development can continue for nearly every academic and adaptive task.

Note, however, the word *can*. In people with Down syndrome, environmental supports are critical. In Shepperdson's (1995) study, the single most important factor determining whether the child, adolescent, or adult advanced cognitively related to the environment. When adolescents and young adults with Down syndrome went on frequent family outings, belonged to clubs, and participated in other age-appropriate activities, they often flourished. In the few people who declined in functioning from the adolescent to the young adult years, no training or very poor training or work programs had been provided. Activities and stimulation are pivotal for the development of adolescents and young adults with Down syndrome.

Lesson 2: *Academic and adaptive skills are separable from purely cognitive abilities.*
When considering conditions of mental retardation, we are accustomed to thinking in terms of cognitive abilities and disabilities. Psychometric tests, IQ scores, mild-moderate-severe-profound mental retardation—these terms are all commonly referred to when discussing children with disabilities.

Although important, cognitive abilities do not tell the complete story of functioning. Especially when considering which behaviors can be performed by a particular adolescent or young adult with Down syndrome, the child's IQ or general level of cognitive abilities only partially predicts functioning on real-world tasks. Buckley's (1995) work is instructive in this regard. If indeed one does not require a certain level of oral language to accomplish primary reading skills, then no necessary connection exists between these two abilities. So too may this connection—or disconnection—occur in other areas. At the least, the example of reading is instructive: It is always better to attempt to teach or train an important skill, as opposed to simply assuming that the skill or behavior is beyond the capabilities of the adolescent with Down syndrome.

Lesson 3: *Cognitive abilities play a limited role in everyday functioning during adolescence and early adulthood.*

Understanding that adolescents continue to develop and that purely cognitive skills do not necessarily relate to academic skills leads to a final lesson concerning the importance of cognitive skills. Although important, cognitive skills comprise only one limited part of an individual's functioning. Indeed, when examining overall functioning during the adult years, one finds only a weak relationship between a person's IQ levels and his or her overall functioning.

Consider independent living and working, probably the two main barometers of everyday functioning during adulthood. Although adults with IQs below 50 may only rarely live independently, many people with IQs from approximately 50 to 70—the IQ levels of most people with Down syndrome—are able to live either independently or semi-independently (Ross, Begab, Dondis, Giampiccolo, & Meyers, 1985). Instead of IQ per se, independent living seems more a function of the type and quality of adaptive training the individual has received, as well as of various personal characteristics.

In the same way, people with disabilities generally succeed in the workplace because of noncognitive—as opposed to cognitive—reasons. When a person is depressed, argumentative, or unable to remain focused on a task, for example, job performance suffers. In one study from Sweden, a subset of people whose IQs were from 55 to 69 had never even been designated as "mentally retarded," because they were able to hold a job and to live a normal life (Granat & Granat, 1978). In work as well as in independent living, then, cognitive abilities play only a small, circumscribed role. Aspects of the person's behavior (e.g., fewer maladaptive behaviors) and environment (e.g., supportive environment) seem much more important.

CONCLUSIONS

In considering cognitive functioning in adolescents with Down syndrome, then, one must take into account both the facts and their implications. Cognitive development does appear to continue throughout the adolescent and early adult years, particularly when individuals enjoy active, stimulating lives. Cognitive skills alone do not directly relate to academic or other adaptive behaviors. In fact, even a complex skill such as reading may not rely on presumably prerequisite skills in oral language. Finally, intellectual abilities play only a limited role in how the adolescent performs in everyday life. In conclusion, one should value—but not overvalue—cognitive abilities in a comprehensive behavioral view of the adolescent and young adult with Down syndrome.

REFERENCES

Bellugi, U., Wang, P., & Jernigan, T. (1994). Williams syndrome: An unusual neuro-psychological profile. In S.H. Broman & J. Grafman (Eds.), *Atypical cognitive development in developmental disorders* (pp. 23–56). Hillsdale, NJ: Lawrence Erlbaum Associates.

Buckley, S. (1995). Teaching children with Down syndrome to read and write. In L. Nadel & D. Rosenthal (Eds.), *Down syndrome: Living and learning in the community* (pp. 158–169). New York: Wiley-Liss.

Buckley, S., Bird, G., & Byrne, A. (1996). The practical and theoretical significance of teaching literacy skills to children with Down's syndrome. In J.A. Rondal, J. Perera, L. Nadel, & A. Comblain (Eds.), *Down's syndrome: Psychological, psychobiological, and socioeducational perspectives* (pp. 119–128). London: Colin Whurr.

Carr, J. (1988). Six weeks to 21 years old: A longitudinal study of children with Down's syndrome and their families. *Journal of Child and Adolescent Psychiatry, 29,* 407–431.

Carr, J. (1994). Annotation: Long-term outcome for people with Down's syndrome. *Journal of Child Psychology and Psychiatry, 35,* 425–439.

Cicchetti, D., & Beeghly, M. (Eds.). (1990). *Children with Down syndrome: A developmental perspective.* New York: Cambridge University Press.

Curtiss, S. (1977). *Genie: A psycholinguistic study of a modern-day "wild child."* New York: Academic Press.

Devenny, D.A., Wisniewski, K.E., & Silverman, W.P. (1993). Dementia of the Alzheimer type among high-functioning adults with Down's syndrome: Individual profiles of development. In B. Corain, K. Iqbal, M. Nicolini, B. Winblad, H. Wisniewski, & P. Zatta (Eds.), *Alzheimer's disease: Advances in clinical and basic research* (pp. 47–53). New York: John Wiley & Sons.

Fowler, A. (1990). Language abilities in children with Down syndrome: Evidence for a specific syntactic delay. In D. Cicchetti & M. Beeghly (Eds.), *Children with Down syndrome: A developmental perspective* (pp. 302–328). New York: Cambridge University Press.

Gibson, D. (1978). *Down's syndrome: The psychology of mongolism.* Cambridge, England: Cambridge University Press.

Granat, K., & Granat, S. (1978). Adjustment of intellectually below-average men not identified as mentally retarded. *Scandinavian Journal of Psychology, 19,* 41–51.

Hodapp, R.M., & Dykens, E.M. (1994). Mental retardation's two cultures of behavioral research. *American Journal on Mental Retardation, 98,* 675–687.

Hodapp, R.M., Leckman, J.F., Dykens, E.M., Sparrow, S.S., Zelinsky, D.G., & Ort, S. (1992). K–ABC profiles in children with fragile X syndrome, Down syndrome, and nonspecific mental retardation. *American Journal on Mental Retardation, 97,* 39–46.

Hodapp, R.M., & Zigler, E. (1990). Applying the developmental perspective to children with Down syndrome. In D. Cicchetti & M. Beeghly (Eds.), *Children with Down syndrome: A developmental perspective* (pp. 1–28). New York: Cambridge University Press.

Kaufman, A.S., & Kaufman, N.L. (1983). *Kaufman Assessment Battery for Children (K–ABC).* Circle Pines, MN: American Guidance Service.

Miller, J., Leddy, M., Miolo, G., & Sedey, A. (1995). The development of early language skills in children with Down syndrome. In L. Nadel & D. Rosenthal

(Eds.), *Down syndrome: Living and learning in the community* (pp. 115–120). New York: Wiley-Liss.

Newport, E. (1990). Maturational constraints on language learning. *Cognitive Science, 14*, 11–28.

Pueschel, S.M. (1990). Clinical aspects of Down syndrome from infancy to adulthood. *American Journal of Medical Genetics, (Suppl. 7)*, 52–56.

Pueschel, S.M., Gallagher, P.L., Zartler, A.S., & Pezzullo, J. (1987). Cognitive and learning processes in children with Down syndrome. *Research in Developmental Disabilities, 8*, 21–37.

Ross, R., Begab, M., Dondis, E., Giampiccolo, J., & Meyers, C. (1985). *Lives of the mentally retarded: A forty-year follow-up study.* Stanford, CA: Stanford University Press.

Shepperdson, B. (1995). Two longitudinal studies of the abilities of people with Down's syndrome. *Journal of Intellectual Disability Research, 39*, 419–431.

10

Language Development

Robin S. Chapman

The development of communicative skill in adolescents and young adults with Down syndrome is many-faceted, is lifelong, and shows a typical progression within most of the domains of communicative skill acquisition. In 1982, Rosenberg's review of comparisons of language development with typically developing children matched for chronological age suggested a *developmental lag* hypothesis—that comprehension and production developed more slowly than age, but at similar rates, in children with Down syndrome. Rosenberg's review also recognized that mental age tended to predict performance on linguistic tasks better than chronological age. Language-learning strategies were thought to be similar among children of similar language levels. At that time, however, Rosenberg concluded that the great variability in skill levels exhibited by youngsters with Down syndrome suggested that the diagnosis of the disorder was not associated with any particular pattern of linguistic performance except poorer articulation.

This chapter examines more recent evidence that alters those conclusions. The author concludes that a large proportion of children with Down syndrome show evidence of specific language impairment compared with mental-age expectations, and that the syndrome is associated with a characteristic pattern in which some areas of language development and cognition are stronger than others. This pattern reveals diverging skills in comprehension and production of language, with significantly better skill in comprehension, as well as diverging skills in vocabulary and sentence structure (syntax), with special strength in vocabulary comprehension.

This chapter and the author's research reported here were supported by National Institutes of Health grant R01-HD23353. The author thanks study participants and their parents for their assistance.

These differences increase as chronological age increases. Chronological age, intelligibility, and hearing status are identified in this chapter as predictors of skill in comprehension and production domains, in addition to mental age. The author furthermore describes ways in which some language-learning strategies differ from those of peers matched for expressive language skill, particularly in the incidental learning of verbs. Reviews of work on which these reformulated conclusions are based can be found in Chapman (1995); Fowler (1990); Hartley (1986); Miller (1988); and Pruess, Vadasy, and Fewell (1987).

Of special interest for understanding language development in adolescents with Down syndrome are proposals by Fowler (1990) that language development plateaus at adolescence, either because there is a *critical period* for language development that has been passed, or because subsequent acquisition of complex sentences is too challenging—the hypothesis that language is limited to *simple syntax*. The work reviewed here suggests, in contrast, that language and speech acquisition continue throughout adolescence and young adulthood and that individuals with Down syndrome produce complex sentences consistent with their overall level of language production (Chapman, in press). This discussion's account of language development in adolescents with Down syndrome is organized into two sections: comprehension (listening) and production (speaking).

LANGUAGE COMPREHENSION

The language comprehension skills of adolescents with Down syndrome are typically better than their language production skills (Chapman, Ross, & Seung, 1993). There is a split, however, between vocabulary and syntax: Adolescents perform better on tests of word comprehension than on tests of syntax comprehension (Chapman, Schwartz, & Kay-Raining Bird, 1991; Rosin, Swift, Bless, & Vetter, 1988; Sommers & Porter, 1994).

Vocabulary Comprehension

Quick, incidental learning to understand a novel word's referent in the context of a hiding game (and to remember where the novel object was hidden) is as effective for adolescents with Down syndrome as for mental age–matched controls (Chapman, Kay-Raining Bird, & Schwartz, 1990). When multiple novel nouns and verbs are encountered in acted-out stories, however, children and adolescents with Down syndrome understand fewer words than controls; by the same token, like the controls, they are less likely to remember the meanings of novel verbs than of novel nouns (Chapman, Kay-Raining Bird, Sindberg, & Seung, 1994).

Vocabulary comprehension, as measured by performance on standardized tests, is typically an area of strength for adolescents with Down syndrome (Chapman, Schwartz, & Kay-Raining Bird, 1991), often exceeding mental age. The greater life experience of these adolescents may account for these results.

Syntax Comprehension

Among individuals with Down syndrome, understanding of sentence structure (including relations between words, word order as a cue to meaning, and grammatical words and inflections) is equivalent to mental-age performance on nonverbal tests (Chapman, Schwartz, & Kay-Raining Bird, 1991) or is less good (Rosin et al., 1988), depending on the tests for mental age. Poorer comprehension of difficult items is associated with shorter auditory memory spans and limitations in language production (Marcell, Croen, & Sewell, 1990).

Reading

Some individuals with Down syndrome develop reading skills when given the opportunity to do so (Buckley, 1993)—estimates range from 33% to 86% of adolescents reared at home. Half the parents of adolescents in Pueschel and Hopmann's (1993) study reported that their children could read sentences, enjoyed books, and could sound out some words. In typically developing children, awareness of speech sounds and their links to letter patterns predicts rate of development; a similar relationship is found in adolescents and young adults with Down syndrome, although sight vocabularies may exceed the levels predicted by sound awareness (Doherty, Fowler, & Boynton, 1993). Learning to read is associated with a significant advantage in language and memory skills (Laws, Buckley, Bird, MacDonald, & Broadley, 1995). (Information for parents on teaching reading to children with Down syndrome can be found in Buckley [1993] and Oelwein [1995].)

LANGUAGE PRODUCTION

When the speaking skills of adolescents with Down syndrome are analyzed and compared to their comprehension skills or their nonverbal problem-solving or spatial skills, there is evidence for specific impairment in language production.

Speech Development

Intelligibility is a particular problem for many individuals with Down syndrome. The development of the ability to produce speech sounds is delayed; indeed, intervention programs for young children often include a period of time when signing is used to achieve effective communication. School-age children with Down syndrome continue to show many more speech errors and inconsistencies than either other children with mental retardation or children of similar mental age (Dodd, 1976).

In adolescents with Down syndrome, intelligibility can be significantly poorer than for children with other disorders associated with mental retardation who are matched for mental age (Rosin et al., 1988). In the Rosin et al. (1988) study, the two groups differed in the percentage of consonants correctly articulated on tests (75% versus 94%). Intelligibility ratings, percentage of intelligible words in speech, and percentage of correct consonants were all significantly related to each other and to the shorter mean length of utterance.

In a survey of parents of adolescents with Down syndrome (Kumin, 1994), 54% reported that their son or daughter had frequent difficulty with intelligibility, and an additional 43% reported difficulty sometimes. Difficulties in chewing (16%), swallowing (18%), and tongue thrusting (25%) were also reported. Pueschel and Hopmann (1993), in a somewhat differently worded survey of parents of adolescents ages 11–16 years old and 17–21 years old, found that 91% of both cohorts' parents reported their children were effective in getting others to understand them; and that 88%–91%, respectively, of parents of the two age cohorts stated that their children were understood by strangers. Problems in speech modulation (too loud: 70%, 39%, respectively; too soft: 49%, 42%; too rapid: 59%, 46%) and fluency (stuttering: 56%, 23%) were also frequent among those who reported. Articulation problems were the most frequent (91% and 71%, respectively).

The speech errors that persist in adolescents and young adults with Down syndrome can include deleting final consonants in words, reducing clusters of consonants in a word to fewer ones, substituting speech sounds made by stopping the air flow for other sounds, and substituting consonant sounds made toward the front of the mouth for those made farther back (Hughes & Ratner, 1989; Van Borsel, 1988). At the same time, intelligibility shows improvement with chronological age in a study of children ages 5 years–20 years (Chapman, Schwartz, & Kay-Raining Bird, 1989). In that cross-sectional study, 30% of the variability in intelligibility was accounted for by chronological age and concurrent performance on a hearing screening.

These findings point to the continued need for adolescents to work on speech skills for communicative effectiveness with speech therapists, including strategies to improve intelligibility, fluency, and speech sound articulation, as well as methods for dealing with the other person's comprehension problems and requests for clarification. Swift and Rosin (1990) have outlined such strategies. The foregoing findings furthermore underscore the continuing need to consider the role of temporary or permanent hearing loss in speech problems. Continued monitoring of hearing ability and treatment of otitis media are important in adolescence as is hearing aid management for those with permanent hearing loss. Crutcher (1993) offers a parent's perspective on how professionals might better meet family and client needs by coordinating efforts and individualizing goals.

Both professionals and parents have asked whether a surgical procedure of tongue reduction, undertaken to alter appearance, might improve articulation and intelligibility. Available evidence suggests not; assessments of speech intelligibility before and after partial glossectomy for cosmetic appearances show no significant change (Margar-Bacal, Witzel, & Munro, 1987).

Although the vast majority of adolescents with Down syndrome are able to express themselves verbally, there were some individuals in the foregoing surveys who had such significant difficulties that augmentative and alternative support for communication would have to be considered. If comprehension skills are relatively good, augmentative systems can support effective communication (Beukelman & Mirenda, 1992). These include both low-tech communication boards with pictures (and words) for particular settings, events, and topics and high-tech computerized systems that provide spoken and written output. If comprehension skills are compromised by hearing impairment, then alternative sources of language input such as signing systems (e.g., total communication, American Sign Language) offer ways to acquire language comprehension and production. The system selected depends on family and school preference and signing skills, as well as the system's future effectiveness for communication. Work on literacy skills—reading and writing—offers another alternative method for supporting language learning and effective use.

Vocabulary Development

The expressive vocabulary development of adolescents with Down syndrome appears more limited than their comprehension of vocabulary but is perhaps less limited than their ability in terms of expressive sentence structure. The number of different words produced in narration is significantly less than that of children matched for mental age (Chapman, Kay-Raining Bird, & Schwartz, 1991), although this difference disappears when referents are provided, as in the task of picture description (Chapman & Swanson, 1996). Among older children and young adults with Down syndrome who are describing pictures, the use of nouns decreases and the use of verbs increases with mental age (Mein, 1961). Ability to describe the function of a concrete noun also increases with mental age (Cornwell, 1974).

As stated previously, the incidental learning to say simple novel words encountered once or a few times in a hiding game is as advanced as that for children matched for mental age (Chapman et al., 1990), although neither group learns enough to produce the words when they stand for novel actions rather than novel objects (Chapman et al., 1994).

Syntax Development

The ability to form grammatical sentences in one's native language is known as *syntax production*. It is in the area of syntax production that adolescents with Down syndrome show their greatest difficulties in language learning. Compared to mental age–matched controls, average length of sentences in narrative tasks is significantly shorter among youngsters with Down syndrome (Chapman et al., 1989; Rosin et al., 1988). In addition, when an individual's skill in expressive syntax is compared with mental-age measures based on spatial tasks or to syntax comprehension, there is significant delay in syntax production (Chapman et al., 1993). Thus, there is evidence of *specific language impairment* in the learning of productive syntax for both younger children and adolescents with Down syndrome.

In a study of the language of Dutch children with Down syndrome ages 8–19 years, with mental ages greater than 3½ years, Bol and Kuiken (1990) found patterns of sentence construction and grammatical morphemes (word inflections) to be more delayed than those of typically developing children ages 1–4 years. The patterns, however, were not atypical of the normal developmental sequence. For example, there was less-frequent use not only of subject-predicate sentences but also of pronouns and of the verb with the subject noun.

Limits to Learning?
Fowler (1990), in her review of her own and others' work, proposed that the picture of language "delayed without deviance" (p. 302) should be modified in recognition of an apparent limit or ceiling to syntax acquisition. She based this proposal on observations of plateauing in average utterance length that was unrelated to mental age. Such limits might arise, she proposed, either as a result of 1) a *critical period* tied to chronological aging or 2) a restriction on the complexity of what can be learned to that of *simple syntax*.

According to the *critical period* hypothesis, maturational events might place a limit on the time during which language could be easily learned. The end of this period could be variously placed as either the onset of adolescence (Lenneberg, 1967) or at about 7 years of chronological age, when there is an apparent shift in ability to learn the motor patterns of a second language.

This author and colleagues' cross-sectional work (Chapman, Schwartz, & Kay-Raining Bird, 1992) has refuted these hypotheses. We found significant increases in the average sentence lengths produced in storytelling by older adolescents (16–20 years of age), compared to those of younger adolescents and children (5–16 years of age). Moreover, these narratives contained instances of complex sentences at rates similar to those of a group of younger preschool controls of similar language level. Some individuals in the group did not show gains (again reflecting the variability in individuals with Down syndrome), but the older group, on average, showed higher syntax production skills. Thus, these data suggest that learning to produce sentences *can* continue in adolescence and young adulthood, as well as that learning does not stop with simple sentence structure, despite the relative difficulty of this learning.

Similar cross-sectional findings have been reported in parents' evaluations of their adolescents' expressive language abilities (Pueschel & Hopmann, 1993): Ninety-seven percent of parents responding reported that their 11- to 16-year-old sons or daughters use sentences and talk about past events and initiate and participate in conversations; 86%–88% of parents of 17- to 21-year-olds responded similarly.

This author and colleagues' work (Chapman et al., 1992) has also suggested a reason for the apparent plateauing that Fowler (1990) found: Other language samples taken by Chapman et al. were based on conversation, rather than narration, and these also indicated such a plateauing in younger adolescents. A language sample more likely to elicit complex sentences, such as telling a story, is needed to provide a sensitive index of more advanced language learning.

Additional Deficits in Grammatical Words?

Children with specific language impairment (but not cognitive delay) have even more difficulty learning the grammatical words and inflections of English than would be expected on the basis of their delay in average sentence length. This author also found this to be true of adolescents with Down syndrome (Chapman, in press). Grammatical words (e.g., prepositions such as *in*, *on*; articles such as *a*, *the*; and conjunctions such as *because*) were omitted more frequently by those with Down syndrome than by preschoolers using similar sentence lengths. Omissions of grammatical inflections (e.g., a noun plural, or *-ing*) also occurred more frequently, but with greater variability.

Intervention for Syntax Production

The implication of these findings for intervention is that adolescents with Down syndrome are still learning important syntactic aspects of language production, and that language therapy is likely to be helpful during this period. The findings suggest that an approach based on targeting the typical developmental sequence in syntax is appropriate, with the expectation that learning of grammatical morphemes will be more delayed. Programs that support the production of more complex sentences in play-based, script-based, familiar story, and theme-based contexts that make meaning clear and event relations predictable are likely to be effective for individuals who are moving beyond the stage of simple syntax (see, e.g., the intervention programs in Kaiser & Gray, 1993). In addition, language intervention goals should take into account the person's communicative needs in everyday life, including social activities, school, work, family, recreation, and activities of daily living.

Pragmatic Development

Knowledge of how to use language in context is called *pragmatics* and includes the development of diverse and socially appropriate communicative goals, as well as the use of varied language structure according to the speaking context. This dual view of pragmatics would lead one to expect adolescents with Down syndrome to reveal their social skill development in the variety of communicative goals pursued and to encounter limits in their language use that are related to limits in expressive syntax rather than to social awareness. The results of studies are consistent with that expectation.

Social sensitivity of young adults with Down syndrome is reflected in their appropriate nonverbal communication with acquaintances and strangers (Leudar, Fraser, & Jeeves, 1981). Adolescents with Down syndrome speak even more often than language-matched (Harris, 1983) or mental age–matched controls (Chapman et al., 1989) in telling a story, possibly in compensation for the limited length of sentences. Conversations of men with Down syndrome and their caregivers often show extended talk on the same topic (Bennett, 1976). Young adolescents, however, show difficulty in making conversational repairs (Bray & Woolnough, 1988).

When asked to describe one among several objects to another person, the success of youngsters with Down syndrome is as great as that of mental age–matched controls in conveying relevant information (Jordan & Murdoch, 1987). At the same time, the limits of expressive language may be revealed. For example, when asked to describe a young woman reading her newspaper (after looking at other pictures of the same woman as well as other people carrying out similar and different actions), the individual with Down syndrome might say "Girl read paper," whereas the child in the control group might say, "It's the mother again, walking with the paper and she's reading." Both versions encode the three elements relevant to picking out the picture. The longer one includes sentence structure that marks each of the elements as new information in context.

SUPPORT FOR LANGUAGE LEARNING

Communication skills are important at any age; in adolescence and beyond, they serve to establish friendships, create community relationships, solve problems, navigate the work world, and negotiate the everyday tasks of living and opportunities for recreation. Adolescents with Down syndrome will encounter expectations for appropriate communication in the worlds of work and recreation. At the same time, they bring their own needs to be understood and to express their own thoughts, experiences, and emotions. Language skills are crucial to the quality of everyday life, and the new worlds encountered in adolescence require new language learning. Continued support for language learning in these new contexts is critical.

In working on pragmatic skills with adolescents with Down syndrome, clinicians can teach strategies for greeting and leave taking, initiating and continuing conversations, telling and listening to stories, making friends, resolving conflict, making requests persuasively, making reference successfully, monitoring one's own and the other's understanding, and requesting and providing clarification. Language skills can also be practiced in the context of communicative events that are important in the person's life at home, in school, in recreation, in the workplace, and in the community. Individualization of work to meet the adolescent's and family's communicative goals is important.

A variety of creative and expressive uses of spoken and written language important to the adolescent can be explored: learning to report events of the day, tell jokes, give instructions, follow a recipe, dictate and write letters or journal entries, relate news reports, prepare class assignments, write lists of things to do, and so on. Techniques for the development of discourse skills come not only from speech-language research but also from social skills research; literacy work including whole-language approaches; and other activities such as working on student newspapers, writing and binding stories and poems, developing and acting out skits, and participating in plays. Always, the focus is on functional—and enjoyable—communication skills, tempered by awareness both of the developmental complexity of the language required and of the ways that simpler language can be made to do more advanced communicative work. Pragmatic approaches for teaching linguistic skills are found in Paul (1992), and recommendations for teaching reading and writing skills are found in Buckley (1993) and Oelwein (1995).

CONCLUSIONS

This review of the speech and language skills of adolescents with Down syndrome has presented evidence for a characteristic pattern of diverging language strengths and deficits that becomes more pronounced with chronological and cognitive growth. In these individuals, comprehension skills are more advanced than production skills, and vocabulary skills are more advanced than skills in grammatical word use and sentence structure. Pragmatic skills that can be accomplished with limited language use are more advanced than those that depend on the mastery of complex structure.

Intelligibility is a continuing problem for adolescents with Down syndrome. None of the evidence presented here can be considered to support claims by previous researchers that language learning stops with simple sentences or with the onset of adolescence. Rather, evidence indicates that language learning continues through adolescence, extending into young adulthood; that it can often include literacy skills; and that it is an important focus for intervention work in adolescence.

REFERENCES

Bennett, T.L. (1976). Code-switching in Down's syndrome. In *Proceedings of the Second Annual Meeting of the Berkeley Linguistic Society*. Berkeley, CA: Berkeley Linguistic Society.

Beukelman, D.R., & Mirenda, P. (1992). *Augmentative and alternative communication: Management of severe communication disorders in children and adults*. Baltimore: Paul H. Brookes Publishing Co.

Bol, G., & Kuiken, F. (1990). Grammatical analysis of developmental language disorders: A study of the morphosyntax of children with specific language disorders, with hearing impairment, and with Down's syndrome. *Clinical Linguistics and Phonetics*, *4*, 77–86.

Bray, M., & Woolnough, L. (1988). The language skills of children with Down's syndrome aged 12 to 16 years. *Child Language Teaching and Therapy*, *4*, 311–324.

Buckley, S. (1993). Developing the speech and language skills of teenagers with Down's syndrome. *Down's Syndrome: Research and Practice*, *1*, 63–71.

Chapman, R.S. (1995). Language development in children and adolescents with Down syndrome. In P. Fletcher & B. MacWhinney (Eds.), *Handbook of child language* (pp. 641–663). Oxford, England: Blackwell Scientific Publications.

Chapman, R.S. (in press). Cognitive development in children with Down syndrome. In J.F. Miller, L.A. Leavitt, & M. Leddy (Eds.), *Communication development in children with Down syndrome*. Baltimore: Paul H. Brookes Publishing Co.

Chapman, R.S., Kay-Raining Bird, E., & Schwartz, S.E. (1990). Fast mapping of novel words in event contexts by children with Down syndrome. *Journal of Speech and Hearing Disorders*, *55*, 761–770.

Chapman, R.S., Kay-Raining Bird, E., & Schwartz, S.E. (1991, November). *Fast mapping in stories: Deficits in Down syndrome*. Paper presented at the American Speech-Language-Hearing Association meeting, Atlanta.

Chapman, R.S., Kay-Raining Bird, E., Sindberg, H., & Seung, H.-K. (1994, June). *Fast mapping of novel nouns and action verbs in story contexts by children and adolescents with Down syndrome*. Poster presented at the Symposium on Research in Child Language Disorders, Madison, WI.

Chapman, R.S., Ross, D.R., & Seung, H.-K. (1993, July). *Longitudinal change in language production of children and adolescents with Down syndrome*. Paper presented at the Sixth International Congress of the Study of Child Language, Trieste, Italy.

Chapman, R.S., Schwartz, S.E., & Kay-Raining Bird, E. (1989, November). *Are children with Down syndrome language delayed?* Paper presented at American Speech-Language-Hearing Association meeting, St. Louis.

Chapman, R.S., Schwartz, S.E., & Kay-Raining Bird, E. (1991). Language skills of children and adolescents with Down syndrome: I. Comprehension. *Journal of Speech and Hearing Research*, *34*, 1106–1120.

Chapman, R.S., Schwartz, S.E., & Kay-Raining Bird, E. (1992, August). *Language production of children and adolescents with Down syndrome.* Paper presented at the 9th World Congress of the International Association for the Scientific Study of Mental Deficiency, Gold Coast, Australia.

Chapman, R.S., & Swanson, B.M. (1996). *Lexical and syntactic differences in Cookie Theft picture descriptions by children with Down syndrome.* Manuscript in preparation.

Cornwell, A.C. (1974). Development of language, abstraction, and numerical concept formation in Down's syndrome children. *American Journal of Mental Deficiency, 79,* 179–190.

Crutcher, D.M. (1993). Parent perspectives: Best practice and recommendations for research. In A.P. Kaiser & D.B. Gray (Eds.), *Communication and language intervention series: Vol. 2. Enhancing children's communication: Research foundations for intervention* (pp. 365–373). Baltimore: Paul H. Brookes Publishing Co.

Dodd, B.J. (1976). A comparison of the phonological systems of mental age matched normal, severely subnormal, and Down's syndrome children. *British Journal of Communication Disorders, 11,* 35–43.

Doherty, B., Fowler, A., & Boynton, L. (1993, March). *Phonological prerequisites to reading in young adults with Down syndrome.* Poster presented at Biennial Meeting of the Society for Research in Child Development, New Orleans.

Fowler, A. (1990). Language abilities in children with Down syndrome: Evidence for a specific syntactic delay. In D. Cicchetti & M. Beeghly (Eds.), *Children with Down syndrome: A developmental perspective* (pp. 302–328). Cambridge, England: Cambridge University Press.

Harris, J. (1983). What does mean length of utterance mean? Evidence from a comparative study of normal and Down's syndrome children. *British Journal of Disorders of Communication, 18,* 153–169.

Hartley, X.Y. (1986). A summary of recent research into the development of children with Down's syndrome. *Journal of Mental Deficiency Research, 26,* 263–269.

Hughes, M., & Ratner, N. (1989, November). *Phonological processes in the speech of Down syndrome adults.* Paper presented at the American Speech-Language-Hearing Association meeting, St. Louis.

Jordan, F.M., & Murdoch, B.E. (1987). Referential communication skills of children with Down syndrome. *Australian Journal of Human Communication Disorders, 15,* 47–59.

Kaiser, A.P., & Gray, D.B. (Eds.). (1993). *Communication and language intervention series: Vol. 2. Enhancing children's communication: Research foundations for intervention.* Baltimore: Paul H. Brookes Publishing Co.

Kumin, L. (1994). Intelligibility of speech in children with Down syndrome in natural settings: Parents' perspectives. *Perceptual and Motor Skills, 78,* 307–313.

Laws, G., Buckley, S., Bird, G., MacDonald, J., & Broadley, I. (1995). The influence of reading instruction on language and memory development in children with Down's syndrome. *Down's Syndrome: Research and Practice, 3,* 59–64.

Lenneberg, E. (1967). *Biological foundations of language.* New York: John Wiley & Sons.

Leudar, I., Frazer, W.I., & Jeeves, M.A. (1981). Social familiarity and communication in Down syndrome. *Journal of Mental Deficiency Research, 25,* 133–142.

Marcell, M., Croen, P.S., & Sewell, D.H. (1990, March). *Language comprehension in Down syndrome and other trainable mentally handicapped individuals.* Paper presented at the Conference on Human Development, Richmond, VA.

Margar-Bacal, F., Witzel, M.A., & Munro, I.R. (1987). Speech intelligibility after partial glossectomy in children with Down's syndrome. *Plastic and Reconstructive Surgery, 79,* 44–49.

Mein, R. (1961). A study of the oral vocabularies of SSN patients: II. Grammatical analysis of speech samples. *Journal of Mental Deficiency Research, 5,* 52.

Miller, J.F. (1988). The developmental asynchrony of language development in children with Down syndrome. In L. Nadel (Ed.), *The psychobiology of Down syndrome* (pp. 167–198). Cambridge, MA: MIT Press.

Oelwein, P. (1995). *Teaching reading to children with Down syndrome.* Rockville, MD: Woodbine House.

Paul, R. (1992). *Pragmatic activities for language intervention.* Tucson, AZ: Communication Skill Builders.

Pruess, J.B., Vadasy, P.F, & Fewell, R.R. (1987). Language development in children with Down syndrome: An overview of recent research. *Education and Training of the Mentally Retarded, 22,* 44–55.

Pueschel, S., & Hopmann, M. (1993). Speech and language abilities of children with Down syndrome. In A.P. Kaiser & D.B. Gray (Eds.), *Communication and language intervention series: Vol. 2. Enhancing children's communication: Research foundations for intervention* (pp. 335–362). Baltimore: Paul H. Brookes Publishing Co.

Rosenberg, S. (1982). The language of the mentally retarded: Development, processes, and intervention. In S. Rosenberg (Ed.), *Handbook of applied psycholinguistics* (pp. 329–392). Hillsdale, NJ: Lawrence Erlbaum Associates.

Rosin, M.M., Swift, E., Bless, D., & Vetter, D.K. (1988). Communication profiles of adolescents with Down syndrome. *Journal of Childhood Communication Disorders, 12,* 49–64.

Sommers, R.K., & Porter, B. (1994). Word skills and measures of syntax and morphemes in children with Down syndrome. *Hearsay, 8,* 20–27.

Swift, E., & Rosin, P. (1990). A remediation sequence to improve speech intelligibility for students with Down syndrome. *Language, Speech, and Hearing Services in Schools, 21,* 140–146.

Van Borsel, J. (1988). An analysis of the speech of five Down's syndrome adolescents. *Journal of Communication Disorders, 21,* 409–421.

11

Behavior Concerns

Monica Cuskelly
Patricia Gunn

Many parents approach their children's adolescence with trepidation, for it is a time that is often characterized by increased difficulties in the parent–child relationship, a change that is generally seen as partly attributable to hormone levels. Although adolescents with Down syndrome may function at a much lower cognitive level than their peers, the timing of their physical maturation, secondary sex characteristics, and changes in hormone levels is similar to that of typical teenagers, and they can be subject to the same feelings and mood swings as their age peers. Many adolescents with Down syndrome choose the same role models (e.g., television stars, popular musicians) as typical teenagers, and they, too, may receive messages about social behaviors that conflict with parental convictions.

Consequently, for parents of adolescents with Down syndrome, concerns related to sexual behavior and exploitation can be accentuated at this time. For instance, a young person may be too friendly with others, a behavior that can be misinterpreted as either an invitation or a threat. One mother described her daughter as follows: "She is so naïve and trusting. She could easily be taken advantage of." Of concern with a son is that a too friendly touch by a young man can lead to fear and complaints by a female stranger. These behaviors can be addressed in sex education or human relationship programs at school, a sheltered workshop, or a medical clinic, but learning appropriate social behavior is developed over time on a foundation built at home. Similarly, girls need to be prepared for menstruation well before adolescence if they are to learn generally acceptable behavior and manage menstruation without distress or anxiety. Mothers are often responsible for this preparation, although educational programs can also contribute (see, e.g., Fegan, Rauch, & McCarthy, 1993). Again, however, acceptable behaviors are developed over time.

Adolescent behaviors do not emerge spontaneously, and many social behaviors have been molded by a decade or more of experience and practice. Experience helps to determine the form and limits of behavior (is it successful?), whereas practice converts behaviors (some desirable, some not) into skills or entrenched habits. The genesis of behavior may lie in temperament characteristics during infancy and early childhood, but the ultimate form develops over time.

TEMPERAMENT

Temperament represents a basic aspect of individual reactivity to the physical and social environment and is regarded as both a component of and a precursor to personality. It describes the style of behavior (e.g., immediate and intense), rather than the content or context of the behavior (e.g., working or playing). Various attributes of temperament such as a predominantly negative mood, withdrawal, poor adaptability to new situations, unpredictable behavior, and intense response to stimulation have been used to describe children with a difficult temperament (Thomas, Chess, & Birch, 1963). It is believed that the relationship will be stormy if caregivers are unable to provide an environment that complements or takes account of these attributes. In contrast are the so-called easy children who show positive mood and low intensity of response and who are predictable, approachable, and adaptable.

The characteristics of easy temperament have special relevance for people with Down syndrome because they seem to relate to the stereotype of a placid, amiable personality that has been promulgated for the syndrome. Yet, despite the perpetuation of this picture of passive amiability, writers from Langdon Down (1887) onward have included obstinacy or stubbornness as a personal characteristic. Gibson (1978) tried to reconcile the contradiction by suggesting a change to the more negative characteristics at adolescence, but the authors' own study of temperament (Cuskelly & Gunn, 1991; Gunn & Cuskelly, 1991) does not support this proposal. If anything, compared with younger children, we found that adolescent participants seemed to show fewer signs of difficult temperament not only to mothers but also to teachers. The authors' studies furthermore support the amiable, placid stereotype in that the study group of adolescents with Down syndrome was more positive in mood than the standardization sample. However, this finding was tempered by an additional finding of lower persistence and higher distractibility among the study group. Although these qualities contraindicate stubbornness, they do have negative connotations for behavioral management, because the mothers had an overall impression that children with low persistence were more difficult than others. We also found that no one pattern of temperament attributes could be used to describe all the children, and most parents will agree that children with Down syndrome have their own unique personalities.

BEHAVIOR PROBLEMS

Temperament is not the sole determinant of behavior. We may expect a child with difficult temperament characteristics to develop negative behaviors, but even a child with an easy temperament can develop oppositional behaviors or conduct disorders in certain environments. For instance, the child who is pampered from an early age can learn to exploit parents with tantrums and aggressive behavior.

Also, young people with Down syndrome have no special protection from the vicissitudes of life and may experience illness, death of a loved one, and so forth, which may act to predispose them to adjustment problems. Individuals with disability may undergo additional experiences that are uncommon in the typically developing population. Among these are the experience of seeing siblings move out of the home and start work—opportunities that may not be afforded the adolescent with Down syndrome. Chicione, McGuire, Hebein, and Gilly (1994) have reported withdrawal, depression, weight management problems, and even despair in young people with Down syndrome on making the transition from school to adult life. These young adults were acutely conscious of the greater opportunities afforded their siblings. At the same time, in contrast to the voluntary moves of siblings, young people with Down syndrome may be moved out of the family home into another living arrangement not of their choosing, as a result of their parents' death, or because the parents can no longer cope or believe it will be best for their child.

It is difficult to compare the rates of behavior disorder reported in various studies of Down syndrome because of the different classifications used. On occasion, behaviors that would appear to be *behavioral problems* in that they do not suggest misperceptions of reality such as hallucinations, delusions, and so on, are referred to as *psychiatric or mental problems*. It would seem useful to differentiate psychiatric diagnoses from behavioral problems, but the American Psychiatric Association (1994) incorporates the severe forms of behavioral disorder under psychiatric labels. (Learning problems and mental retardation are also included as psychiatric disorders.) Buckley and Sacks (1987) have carefully considered this issue. Their survey of adolescents divided difficult behaviors into two types, "basically ordinary" behaviors (annoying, provocative, or attention seeking) and behaviors "more likely to be associated with serious long term difficulties" (p. 90). As Myers (1992) has pointed out, it is important to be specific in diagnosing the problem because some behaviors respond to medication, some are ameliorated by behavioral management, and others require a combination of medical and behavioral or psychotherapeutic treatment.

The overall health of the person with Down syndrome should also be considered in any explanation of behavior. Prasher and Krishnan (1993) have emphasized the need to consider the role of sensory deficits and thyroid functioning. Communication skills should also be evaluated. Many adolescents with Down syndrome have limited speech and language skills, which makes diagnosis of certain psychiatric disorders difficult (Reid, 1982).

Adolescents with Down syndrome who have impaired speech and language skills face many trying situations. What may be regarded as problem behavior may stem from frustration, either because their communication was not understood or because they could not understand a spoken request or command. Indeed, this may be the root of many reports of stubbornness. Hearing difficulties and problems with verbal processing make it imperative that a person with Down syndrome not be overloaded with verbal information; the possibility of sensory deficit should always be considered in cases of poor compliance with requests or with what may seem bizarre behavior.

Several writers have also focused on the possibility that people with severe learning difficulties and few or no verbal competencies will engage in bizarre or challenging behaviors as a form of communication. Approaches that seek to reduce challenging behaviors by teaching communication skills have been documented by Butterfield, Arthur, and Sigafoos (1995). A typical example is the study by Sigafoos and Meilke (1996) in which attention-motivated aggression and self-injury were replaced by the learned gesture of tapping the teacher on the shoulder.

The majority of adolescents with Down syndrome do not exhibit a high level of difficult behaviors, although Myers (1992) concluded that they may be at a higher risk for such behaviors than the general population. Even so, no areas of problem behavior appear to be specific to Down syndrome. In the United Kingdom, Gath and Gumley have examined behavioral difficulties in children with Down syndrome over a number of years. The most common diagnostic category reported in their 1986a study was conduct disorder (11%). Some children in the study were early adolescents, but most were preteens. In the United States, Myers (1992) reported a similar percentage (12%) of outpatients younger than 20 years displaying conduct or oppositional disorders or aggression.

Gath and Gumley (1986b) found an interesting discrepancy between the proportion of children with Down syndrome believed by their parents to have significant behavior problems (15%) and the proportion classified as displaying behavior disorders on measures of the Rutter scale (41%).

Gath and Gumley interpreted this as an indication of parental resignation that a low level of adaptive behaviors was part of the disability.

Gender presents a contradictory picture. Gath and Gumley (1986a) reported that boys were more likely to be classified as having a psychiatric disorder, but in a later study (1987) those authors failed to find differences between the sexes in this regard. In contrast, Cuskelly and Dadds (1992) found that more female than male children were reported by fathers to display conduct disorders. Gath and McCarthy (1996) have suggested that these differences partially reflect historical changes in families with a child with Down syndrome, as well as changes in family structure and patterns of female delinquency in the general community.

Gath and Gumley (1986a) examined the impact of age on the level of problem behavior and found a decrease (on the Rutter scale) in problem behaviors over time. Using a different scale, the Revised Behavior Problem Checklist (Quay & Peterson, 1983), Cuskelly and Gunn (1991) did not find a decrease in problem behavior; however, the adolescents in the study showed a similar number of problems as younger participants. Teachers and parents, however, tended to report different types of behavior problems; compared to parents, teachers reported more problems of a socialized aggression nature (rejecting authority) and of attention problems related to immaturity.

Other studies have not used clinical assessment instruments, but mothers have been interviewed regarding annoying or difficult behaviors and the manageability of adolescents. Buckley and Sacks (1987) reported a decrease with age in the number of difficult behaviors (before and after 14 years of age), and Carr (1988, 1992) found an improvement in behavior among the children in her longitudinal study from ages 11 to 21 years, with a relative lack of management problems at this later age. She reported, however, that sexual safety had become an issue of concern for parents of females who were 21 years of age.

Shepperdson (1984, 1988) reported that 40% of her teenage sample showed some negative behaviors, but that violent and aggressive behavior was uncommon. This is similar to the findings of Buckley and Sacks (1987), who stated that parents reported few problems in managing the behavior of their teenagers with Down syndrome, with no sex differences. Children with ill health were somewhat more likely to be reported as difficult than were healthier children, and there was a significant negative relationship between communication skills and problem behavior. The less-able children were more difficult, with the exception of some who were very passive.

Buckley and Sacks (1987) concluded that although difficult behavior was not a serious problem, swearing, temper tantrums, and annoying behaviors were common. About half the teenagers were affected by phobias, and about half had fantasy friends. Buckley and Sacks's distinction between *annoying* and *difficult* behaviors is interesting because it not only explains why few children were judged to be difficult in comparison with other studies such as those by Gath and Gumley (1986a) and Myers (1992) but also appears to be related to Gath and Gumley's earlier-mentioned report (1986b) of a discrepancy between parental perceptions of difficulty and difficulty as judged by a psychiatric measure. It also seems that some annoying behaviors are immature for chronological age but not for developmental (cognitive) level.

FAMILY DYNAMICS

Marital stress has been associated with an increase in behavior problems in children with intellectual disabilities (Floyd & Zmich, 1991), and Cuskelly and Dadds (1992) found that marital satisfaction was an important predictor of mothers' (but not fathers') reports of problem behavior in children with Down syndrome. Gath and Gumley (1986b) also found that behavior problems in children with Down syndrome were more common in families in which there was marital discord or where parents were having problems with their own mental health. Disagreement over child-rearing practices can be an important aspect of parental disagreements. Block, Block, and Morrison (1981) found that disagreement over child rearing was moderately predictive of both increased behavior problems in boys and, later, marriage breakdown.

Parents' expectations are vitally important in regard to the adolescent's adjustment. In a book by Roger Moody and his adult brother Peter, who has Down syndrome, Roger suggested that adolescent behavior that seems eccentric to parents may be regarded by adolescents as a means of self-expression (Moody & Moody, 1986). If the adolescent has Down syndrome, it can be especially difficult for parents to accept the new behaviors with equanimity: "Having got your child to move in a certain fashion, talk in a certain way acceptable for a child, you become afraid to let him or her develop other modes of interaction" (Moody & Moody, 1986, p. 72). It is also difficult for parents when they find that, with increased physical strength, the adolescent has become more assertive than they expected (Buckley & Sacks, 1987).

If parental expectations are too low, parents will find it hard to accept that many social behaviors and interests of their son or daughter are in synchrony with those of age peers, and that physical changes may bring feelings and emotions similar to those of other teenagers. However, if parental expectations are too high, they may not recognize that although many of their son's or daughter's social behaviors and interests are in synchrony with those of peers, deficits in cognition and communication can impede judgment and reasoning.

The way in which the adolescent was raised during childhood influences his or her behavior in subsequent years. In the worst-case scenario, the adolescent may not have been required to fit in with family schedules, and family routines have been altered instead. This has a negative effect on the adolescent's attainment of personal competence and independence. After considering the way in which his brother had been raised, Roger Moody concluded,

> The family or group can allow a personal space ... meaning, literally, "What you do there is up to you" and can then stick to that concession, emphasizing that the rules of living elsewhere are not fixed but have to be decided mutually, as people go along.... No group should have any of its formative stages monopolized by the requirements of a single member. It is this kind of tyranny which results in the really "handicapped family." (Moody & Moody, 1986, p. 82)

In a study of "normal" families, Lamborn, Mounts, Steinberg, and Dornbusch (1991) found correlations between adolescent adjustment and parenting style. Parental acceptance and involvement contributed to the psychologic well-being of adolescents. Adolescents in indulgent families were self-confident and had a positive self-concept but a higher level of problem behavior than adolescents in families that were more strict and provided more supervision. This parallels the findings of Shepperdson (1984), who found that firm discipline was associated with fewer behavior problems in adolescents with Down syndrome.

Although both Carr (1988, 1992) and Shepperdson (1988) have considered some aspects of parental discipline in regard to adolescents, and Gunn and Berry (1985) have examined the relationship between child temperament and maternal discipline for younger children, no studies have examined systematically the relationship between parental discipline and long-term outcome in children with Down syndrome. Carr (1992) reported only one significant correlation between discipline methods and outcome. Families who used little physical punishment when their child with Down syndrome was 4 years of age had fewer problems at age 21 years. However, the author pointed out that this finding must be treated with caution, as a number of comparisons were made. This increases the likelihood that a relationship will achieve a significant correlation by chance. Carr (1988) discussed management strategies with mothers and found that about half (55%) used techniques such as persuasion, explanation, and reasoning. Only six mothers reported using threats or punishment, whereas some would use firm tones or would insist on the behavior and some used physical prompting. A similar picture emerged from Gunn and Berry's (1985) study with younger children.

STRATEGIES FOR BEHAVIOR MANAGEMENT

Many successful interventions have been developed to provide parents with strategies for managing everyday and extreme behavior problems in children with disabilities (e.g., Kennedy, 1994; Steege, Wacker, Berg, Cigrand, & Cooper, 1989). Numerous books and other publications have also been directed to parents, explaining theories and techniques of behavior management and change (see, e.g., Carr & Collins, 1992), in addition to educational programs for parents of children with disabilities. Many families have found these materials to be extremely important in assisting them to teach their child appropriate behavior.

A lengthy learning period is required for the acquisition of many skills. Especially during childhood, constant attention to a series of skills or rules seems necessary for the management of some behaviors, particularly those Goodman (1992) termed *social-conventional*. Roger Moody described the long period needed for Peter to learn the "what nots" of behavior and their mother's constant, daily application to every detail of the action she required until Peter could comb his hair or fasten his belt (Moody & Moody, 1986). But Roger then went on to perceptively observe that

> whether this was Peter's main mode of learning, rather than following other people's examples, or "modelling," I'm not sure. Someone may copy another person's actions, down to the merest tic. But how do we know whether that person was conditioned into doing this, or scrupulously followed the other's behavior—for reasons of loyalty, love, or simply fascination and play? (p. 32)

Perhaps we need to ask more. What is the value of the skill in the child's mind? Is it associated with fun or relaxation? Does it have social or functional benefits?

In cases of unacceptable behavior, many parents use management strategies such as those outlined by Carr and Collins (1992), Kennedy (1994), or Steege et al. (1989). These strategies are developed after determining the conditions that evoke the problem behavior and that encourage its continuance. It is important to understand the child's motivation for engaging in the problem behavior. Common reasons are to gain attention or to escape a task or situation. Once the motivation is understood, there is a better chance of formulating successful management strategies. One important issue concerns the nature of reinforcement.

Parents and teachers of children with disabilities have been bombarded with information on positive reinforcement. Little information has been given, however, regarding the circumstances under which positive reinforcement is best avoided or strategies for withdrawing these external supports as they become unnecessary.

Nonproductive persistence or perseveration may be associated with inappropriate reinforcement, and children may conclude that pleasing adults is more important than initiating or continuing task activity (Brockman, Morgan, & Harmon, 1988). An overused and indiscriminate "good boy" or "good girl" may result in a child seeking social praise rather than success in an activity (Gunn, 1982). With such a background, perhaps it is not surprising that children with Down syndrome learn to use their social skills to divert attention away from a task they find difficult (Pitcairn & Wishart, 1994).

The effect of extrinsic rewards also needs to be carefully examined. A number of studies have demonstrated that the inappropriate use of extrinsic rewards can lead to a reduction in intrinsic motivation, not just for the behavior that was rewarded (Miller & Hom, 1990), but for other behaviors as well. In part, reinforcement is useful because it provides feedback on one's behavior. Rewards for difficult tasks lead to increased effort, because the rewards tell children that they are competent (Miller & Hom, 1990), but providing a reward for completion of tasks that are well within a child's capabilities can be interpreted by that child as evidence of low ability (Barker & Graham, 1987; Weiner, 1990). This is not to argue that external rewards should be avoided—they should be used precisely in those circumstances where the child (or adolescent) does not have the intrinsic motivation to perform. If, however, they are used in circumstances where the child is prepared to engage in the behavior for the fun or the challenge, the initial motivation may well be undermined. This may well be an important issue with respect to children with intellectual disabilities. Rewards have been found to be worthwhile reinforcers if they are contingent on effort rather than results (Brophy, 1987; Harter, 1981). Again, however, one's reinforcement of effort must be truthful and contingent on real effort; a phoney "good try" is just as meaningless and damaging as a phoney "good boy."

It is common for caregivers, teachers, therapists, and others to set the stage for desired behaviors and to manage behaviors in the young child, but by the time children are adolescents, they are expected to independently manage their own behavior. This is true for adolescents whether they have Down syndrome or not, but the literature on strategies for behavioral management has tended to ignore the self-regulation aspect of behavior.

SELF-REGULATION

The ability to manage one's own behavior is an important issue for adolescents with Down syndrome, given today's espoused goals of independence. Self-regulation is a complex skill with behavioral, cognitive, and motivational components (Kendall, 1990). It consists of many elements that allow individuals to take control of their own behavior. These skills are important for effective learning and enhance the ability to continue to learn throughout life.

Kopp (1982) has cataloged the way in which young children without developmental delays progress in their ability to monitor and modify their own behavior. Compliance and the delay of self-gratification have been found to develop during the early years of life, and Zelazo and Reznick (1991) have emphasized the distinction between knowing rules and being able to apply them. They concluded that rule-governed behavior increased at about 3 years of age. Since most teenagers with Down syndrome could be expected to have achieved this developmental age in other areas of functioning, one may assume that they, too, have developed the ability to apply rules about compliance and delay of self-gratification to their own behavior. Zelazo and Reznick (1991), however, proposed that the ability to systematically use rules depends on aspects of cognitive functioning such as the control of attention, the ability to inhibit competing responses, and proficiency in self-correction. In other words, children must focus on the task requirements, must not be distracted by aspects that are irrelevant to the action required, must monitor the success or failure of their own behavior, and, if necessary, must try an alternative approach. This suggests that impulsive and distractible behavior or difficulty in sustaining motivation will preclude progress in the development of self-controlling behaviors and may need to be addressed before the development of rule-governed behavior can be expected.

Another viewpoint with implications for Down syndrome emphasizes language proficiency as the basis for self-regulation. Whitman (1990) advocated training to establish an ability both to use words for self-control of action, and conversely, to describe the actions in words. However, Pressley (1990) argued that this central role for language is unduly emphasized in Whitman's analysis and suggested alternative strategies using imagery-based approaches.

Adults with intellectual disability have been taught to self-manage their behavior with respect to vocational tasks (e.g., Agran, Fodor-Davis, Moore, & Deer, 1989; Hildebrand, Martin, Furer, & Hazen, 1990). The studies just cited, however, generally teach skills related to monitoring and rewarding one's own performance in meeting goals established by someone else. There have been some attempts to teach self-regulation (using self-instructional techniques) pertaining to academic skills (see Agran & Martella, 1991) and the results are encouraging; however, none of the studies has adequately assessed maintenance over time or generalization to different settings or tasks.

Allowing individuals to exercise choice or control (Kinzie, 1990) is one way to provide a context in which self-regulation can develop. Of course, giving responsibility without support may be insufficient to produce the desired behavior. For example, Goodman (1981) suggested that young children with intellectual disabilities may find it difficult to direct their own behavior in a purposeful way and they may approach problems in a disorganized manner.

In addition to the explicit teaching of self-regulatory mechanisms and behavior, the processes used in the classroom (and in the home) should support the development of self-regulation. It is possible that current instructional practices in both integrated and segregated settings directly impede self-regulation. Too much adult direction may hinder the development of self-regulatory behaviors, and there may be a greater need to encourage responsibility by providing more opportunities for turn taking and making choices.

It has been proposed that mastery motivation is one attribute that impels human beings toward competency (White, 1959). The urge toward competency may be a necessary precursor to development of effective self-regulatory behavior. Central to a mastery goal is the belief that effort is related to outcome; that is, the conviction that the more one tries, the greater one's success (Ames, 1992). This belief acts to maintain behaviors that are directed at achievement over time (Weiner, 1986), even in the face of failure. Orientation toward mastery is associated with a positive attitude toward learning (Ames & Archer, 1988). Although the children who have participated in these research studies are typically developing without cognitive delays, there seems to be no reason why the general thrust of the findings should not apply to adolescents with Down syndrome.

Factors that are believed to enhance mastery motivation are challenge, interest, student choice of the goal (Lepper & Hodell, 1989; Malone & Lepper, 1987), and task structures that focus more on self-improvement and less on competition with others (Marshall & Weistan, 1984). It has been suggested that, for young children, comparison with others is compatible with mastery learning (Butler, 1989), but that prolonged experience in the achievement-oriented environment of school leads older children to evaluate their own performance in terms of an innate capability that cannot be changed rather than in terms of effort (Stipek & MacIver, 1989). This has special implications for students in inclusive settings. Students who believe they are not capable in specific learning activities choose less-challenging tasks and use self-regulatory behaviors less frequently (Dweck, 1986; Pintrich & de Groot, 1990).

Factors that are likely to enhance a performance orientation rather than a mastery orientation are a focus on absolute correctness and comparison with the achievement of others (Ames, 1984; Brophy, 1983a, 1983b). Rather than being motivated to succeed, some students respond to these conditions by developing an urge to avoid failure. This motivation leads to behaviors such as refusal to participate and lack of engagement. A focus on self-improvement (in contrast to comparing oneself with others) is more likely to lead to increased effort and a preference for challenge.

Failure affects children's subsequent task persistence (Lyman, Prentice-Dunn, Wilson, & Bonfilio, 1984). This relationship is a reciprocal, interactional one so that children who do not persist will inevitably fail and those who fail are likely not to persist (Yarrow et al., 1983). Students who believe they can succeed will transcend failure experiences and keep trying (Bandura, 1986; Schunk, 1989).

There is some evidence that children with Down syndrome will "switch off" tasks that are at or near their ability level (Wishart & Duffy, 1990), rather than being challenged to persist. However, Duffy and Wishart (1987) demonstrated that errorless learning enhanced the children's willingness to persist with a task in which error was the usual experience. It is possible that this strategy is useful initially, since it counteracts the children's past experiences with error and acts to increase motivation as their involvement is reinforced through success. As an invariant strategy, however, errorless learning may undermine children's capacity to withstand failure, and Duffy and Wishart (1994) were disappointed to find that skills learned in this way did not transfer readily to a second task, despite similar task requirements. They concluded that errorless teaching strategies may be most effective when used in conjunction with conventional trial-and-error methods.

Wishart (1996) suggested that poor task persistence may be due to a fear of failure and low expectancies of success.

> In comparison to children who are developing at the usual rate, most skills will take much longer to learn, and inevitably a greater degree of failure is experienced over a longer period of time before success is finally achieved. This can hardly help the child with DS [Down syndrome] to establish any great faith in his or her own learning ability. (p. 198)

Although Wishart (1996) was describing performance on cognitive tasks, these observations have direct relevance to the learning of tasks that develop social rather than cognitive competence. The rules and rituals of social behavior are important aspects of the behavioral repertoire of children and adolescents with Down syndrome. Fear of failure in social situations is detrimental for personal development just as fear of failure in cognitive tasks affects cognitive development. If we have not encouraged young people with Down syndrome to have confidence in their own abilities, if they believe they will always fail or that they can succeed with only a limited set of routines, they will be inflexible (obstinate) and unwilling to try new activities.

In addition, we need to examine teaching strategies and their effect on learning. Strategies that are effective in the short term may be detrimental to later learning. For example, very structured learning situations may have the unintended result of producing children who either refuse to engage in one-to-one teaching situations or who cannot adapt to group-oriented instruction. A history of adult direction of activity may exacerbate intellectual deficits (Hupp & Abbeduto, 1991). Adults (at home and school) may teach children to be good respondents but ineffective initiators. If we want young people with Down syndrome to be motivated toward their own self-improvement, we may need to consider further the development of their self-regulatory behaviors.

CONCLUSIONS

Based on the studies discussed in this chapter, our overall conclusion is that the majority of adolescents with Down syndrome present few problems of behavior management. Like other adolescents, however, their behaviors depend on both experiences over time and the opportunities currently available. As Reid (1982) concluded, "boredom, inactivity, and lack of purpose are potent causes of behavior problems" (p. 35). It is important that we do not limit opportunities for adolescents with Down syndrome to engage in stimulating work, further education, or recreational activities. Chicione et al.'s (1994) description of loneliness, withdrawal, and depression as a response to adult life should serve as a warning of the deleterious effects of failing to provide opportunities during the transitional stage from adolescence to adulthood. At the same time, however, if adolescents are to gain from these opportunities and make viable choices, they need to be prepared for lifelong learning through the self-management of their own behaviors.

REFERENCES

Agran, M., Fodor-Davis, J., Moore, S., & Deer, M. (1989). The application of a self-management program on instruction following skills. *Journal of The Association for Persons with Severe Handicaps, 14,* 147–154.

Agran, M., & Martella, R.C. (1991). Teaching self-instructional skills to persons with mental retardation: A descriptive and experimental analysis. *Progress in Behavior Modification, 27,* 36–55.

American Psychiatric Association. (1994). *Diagnostic and statistical manual of mental disorders* (4th ed.). Washington, DC: Author.

Ames, C. (1984). Achievement attributions and self-instructions under competitive and individualistic goal structures. *Journal of Educational Psychology, 76,* 478–487.

Ames, C. (1992). Classrooms: Goals, structures, and student motivation. *Journal of Educational Psychology, 84,* 261–271.

Ames, C., & Archer, J. (1988). Achievement goals in the classroom: Students' learning strategies and motivation processes. *Journal of Educational Psychology, 80,* 260–267.

Bandura, A. (1986). *Social foundations of thought and action: A social cognitive theory.* Englewood Cliffs, NJ: Prentice Hall.

Barker, G., & Graham, S. (1987). Developmental study of praise and blame as attributional cues. *Journal of Educational Psychology, 79,* 62–66.

Block, J.H., Block, J., & Morrison, A. (1981). Parental agreement-disagreement on child-rearing orientations and gender-related personality correlates in children. *Child Development, 52,* 965–974.

Brockman, L.M., Morgan, G.A., & Harmon, R.J. (1988). Mastery motivation and developmental delay. In T.D. Wachs & R. Sheehan (Eds.), *Assessment of young developmentally disabled children* (pp. 267–284). New York: Plenum.

Brophy, J.E. (1983a). Conceptualizing student motivation. *Educational Psychologist, 18,* 200–215.

Brophy, J.E. (1983b). Fostering student learning and motivation in the elementary school classroom. In S. Paris, G. Olson, & H. Stevenson (Eds.), *Learning and motivation in the classroom* (pp. 283–305). Hillsdale, NJ: Lawrence Erlbaum Associates.

Brophy, J.E. (1987). Synthesis of research on strategies for motivating students to learn. *Educational Leadership, 44,* 40–48.

Buckley, S., & Sacks, B. (1987). *The adolescent with Down's syndrome.* Portsmouth, England: Portsmouth Down's Syndrome Trust.

Butler, R. (1989). Interest in the task and interest in peers' work in competitive and noncompetitive conditions: A developmental study. *Child Development, 60,* 562–570.

Butterfield, N., Arthur, M., & Sigafoos, J. (1995). *Partners in everyday communicative exchanges.* Sydney, Australia: MacLennan & Petty.

Carr, J. (1988). Six weeks to twenty-one years old: A longitudinal study of children with Down's syndrome and their families. *Journal of Child Psychology and Psychiatry and Applied Disciplines, 29,* 407–431.

Carr, J. (1992). Longitudinal research in Down syndrome. *International Review of Research in Mental Retardation, 18,* 197–223.

Carr, J., & Collins, S. (1992). *Working towards independence: A practical guide to teaching people with learning disabilities.* London: Jessica Kingsley.

Chicione, B., McGuire, D., Hebein, S., & Gilly, D. (1994). Development of a clinic for adults with Down syndrome. *Mental Retardation, 32,* 100–106.

Cuskelly, M., & Dadds, M. (1992). Behavioural problems in children with Down's syndrome and their siblings. *Journal of Child Psychology and Psychiatry and Applied Disciplines, 33,* 749–761.

Cuskelly, M., & Gunn, P. (1991). Behaviour problems in adolescents with Down syndrome. In C.J. Denholm (Ed.), *Adolescents with Down syndrome: International perspectives on research and programme development* (pp. 53–61). Victoria, British Columbia, Canada: University of Victoria.

Down, J.L.H. (1887). *Mental affections of childhood and youth.* Lettsomian lectures. London: Medical Society of London.

Duffy, L., & Wishart, J.G. (1987). A comparison of two procedures for teaching discrimination skills to Down's syndrome and non-handicapped children. *British Journal of Educational Psychology, 57,* 265–278.

Duffy, L., & Wishart, J.G. (1994). The stability and transferability of errorless learning in children with Down's syndrome. *Down's Syndrome: Research & Practice, 2,* 51–58.

Dweck, C. (1986). Motivational processes affecting learning. *American Psychologist, 41,* 1040–1048.

Fegan, L., Rauch, A., & McCarthy, W. (1993). *Sexuality and people with intellectual disability* (2nd ed.). Sydney, Australia: MacLennan & Petty.

Floyd, F.J., & Zmich, D.E. (1991). Marriage and parenting partnership: Perceptions and interactions of parents with mentally retarded and typically developing children. *Child Development, 62,* 1434–1448.

Gath, A., & Gumley, D. (1986a). Behaviour problems in retarded children with special reference to Down's syndrome. *British Journal of Psychiatry, 149,* 156–161.

Gath, A., & Gumley, D. (1986b). Family background of children with Down's syndrome and of children with a similar degree of mental retardation. *British Journal of Psychiatry, 149,* 161–171.

Gath, A., & Gumley, D. (1987). Retarded children and their siblings. *Journal of Child Psychology and Psychiatry and Applied Disciplines, 28,* 715–730.

Gath, A., & McCarthy, J. (1996). Families and siblings: A response to recent research. In B. Stratford & P. Gunn (Eds.), *New approaches to Down syndrome* (pp. 361–368). London: Cassell.

Gibson, D. (1978). *Down's syndrome: The psychology of mongolism.* Cambridge, England: Cambridge University Press.

Goodman, J.F. (1981). *The Goodman Lock Box.* Chicago: Stoelting.

Goodman, J.F. (1992). *When slow is fast enough.* New York: Guilford Press.

Gunn, P. (1982). Play and the handicapped child. In B.H. Watts, J. Elkins, L.M. Conrad, R.J. Andrews, W.C. Apelt, A. Hayes, J. Calder, A.J. Coulsoton, & M. Willis (Eds.), *Early intervention programs for young handicapped children in Australia, 1979–1980* (pp. 147–155). Canberra: Australian Government Publishing Service.

Gunn, P., & Berry, P. (1985). Down's syndrome temperament and maternal response to descriptions of child behavior. *Developmental Psychology, 21,* 842–847.

Gunn, P., & Cuskelly, M. (1991). Down syndrome temperament: The stereotype at middle childhood and adolescence. *International Journal of Disability, Development, and Education, 38,* 59–70.

Harter, S. (1981). A model of mastery motivation in children: Individual differences and developmental change. In W.A. Collins (Ed.), *Aspects of the development of competence: The Minnesota Symposia on Child Psychology* (Vol. 14, pp. 215–255). Hillsdale, NJ: Lawrence Erlbaum Associates.

Hildebrand, R.G., Martin, G.L., Furer, P., & Hazen, A. (1990). A recruitment-of-praise package to increase productivity levels of developmentally handicapped workers. *Behavior Modification, 14,* 97–113.

Hupp, S.C., & Abbeduto, L. (1991). Persistence as an indicator of mastery motivation in young children with cognitive delays. *Journal of Early Intervention, 15,* 219–225.

Kendall, P.C. (1990). Challenges for cognitive strategy training: The case of mental retardation. *American Journal on Mental Retardation, 94,* 365–367.

Kennedy, C.H. (1994). Manipulating antecedent conditions to alter the stimulus control of problem behavior. *Journal of Applied Behavior Analysis, 27,* 161–170.

Kinzie, M.B. (1990). Requirements and benefits of effective interactive instruction: Learner control, self-regulation, and continuing motivation. *Educational Technology Research and Development, 38,* 5–13.

Kopp, C. (1982). Antecedents of self-regulation: A developmental perspective. *Developmental Psychology, 18,* 199–214.

Lamborn, S., Mounts, N.S., Steinberg, L., & Dornbusch, S.M. (1991). Patterns of competence and adjustment among adolescents from authoritative, authoritarian, indulgent, and neglectful families. *Child Development, 62,* 1049–1065.

Lepper, M.R., & Hodell, M. (1989). Intrinsic motivation in the classroom. In C. Ames & R. Ames (Eds.), *Research on motivation in education: Goals and cognition* (Vol. 3, pp. 73–105). San Diego, CA: Academic Press.

Lyman, R.D., Prentice-Dunn, S., Wilson, D.R., & Bonfilio, S.A. (1984). The effect of success or failure on self-efficacy and task persistence of conduct-disordered children. *Psychology in the Schools, 21,* 516–519.

Malone, T.W., & Lepper, M.R. (1987). Making learning fun: A taxonomy of intrinsic motivation for learning. In R.E. Snow & M.J. Farr (Eds.), *Aptitude, learning, and instruction: Cognitive and affective process analyses* (Vol. 3). Hillsdale, NJ: Lawrence Erlbaum Associates.

Marshall, H.H., & Weistan, R.S. (1984). Classroom factors affecting students' self-evaluations: An interactional model. *Review of Educational Research, 54,* 301–325.

Miller, A., & Hom, H.L., Jr. (1990). Influence of extrinsic and ego incentive value on persistence after failure and continuing motivation. *Journal of Educational Psychology, 82,* 539–545.

Moody, P., & Moody, R. (1986). *Half left.* Oslo, Norway: Dreyers Forlag.

Myers, B.A. (1992). Psychiatric disorders. In S.M. Pueschel & J.K. Pueschel (Eds.), *Biomedical concerns in persons with Down syndrome* (pp. 197–207). Baltimore: Paul H. Brookes Publishing Co.

Pintrich, P.R., & de Groot, E.V. (1990). Motivational and self-regulated learning components of classroom academic performance. *Journal of Educational Psychology, 82,* 33–40.

Pitcairn, T.K., & Wishart, J.G. (1994). Reactions of young children with Down's syndrome to an impossible task. *British Journal of Developmental Psychology, 12,* 485–489.

Prasher, V.P., & Krishnan, V.H.R. (1993). Mental disorders and adaptive behavior in people with Down's syndrome [Letter]. *British Journal of Psychiatry, 162,* 848–849.

Pressley, M. (1990). Four more considerations about self-regulation among mentally retarded persons. *American Journal on Mental Retardation, 94,* 369–370.

Quay, H.C., & Peterson, D.R. (1983). *Interim manual for the Revised Behavior Checklist.* Highland Park, NJ: Authors.

Reid, A.H. (1982). *The psychiatry of mental handicap.* Oxford, England: Blackwell Scientific Publications.

Schunk, D.H. (1989). Self-efficacy and cognitive skill learning. In C. Ames & R. Ames (Eds.), *Goals and cognitions: Vol. 3. Research on motivation in education* (pp. 13–44). San Diego, CA: Academic Press.

Shepperdson, D. (1984, February). Care of Down's syndrome teenagers. *Update,* 370–372.

Shepperdson, D. (1988). *Growing up with Down's syndrome.* London: Cassell.

Sigafoos, J., & Meilke, E. (1996). Functional communication training for treatment of multiply determined challenging behavior in two boys with autism. *Behavior Modification, 20,* 60–84.

Steege, M.W., Wacker, D.P., Berg, W.K., Cigrand, K.K., & Cooper, L.J. (1989). The use of behavioral assessment to prescribe and evaluate treatments for severely handicapped children. *Journal of Applied Behavior Analysis, 22,* 331–343.

Stipek, D., & MacIver, D. (1989). Developmental change in children's assessment of intelligence. *Child Development, 60,* 521–538.

Thomas, A., Chess, S., & Birch, H. (1963). *Temperament and behavior disorders in children.* New York: Brunner/Mazel.

Weiner, B. (1986). *An attributional theory of motivation and emotion.* New York: Springer-Verlag.

Weiner, B. (1990). History of motivational research in education. *Journal of Educational Psychology, 82,* 616–622.

White, R.W. (1959). Motivation reconsidered: The concept of competence. *Psychological Review, 66,* 297–333.

Whitman, T.L. (1990). Self-regulation and mental retardation. *American Journal on Mental Retardation, 94,* 347–362.

Wishart, J.G. (1996). Avoidant learning styles and cognitive development in young children. In B. Stratford & P. Gunn (Eds.), *New approaches to Down syndrome* (pp. 173–205). London: Cassell.

Wishart, J.G., & Duffy, L. (1990). Instability of performance on cognitive tests in infants and young children with Down's syndrome. *British Journal of Educational Psychology, 59,* 10–22.

Yarrow, L.J., McQuiston, S., MacTurk, R.H., McCarthy, M.E., Klein, R.P., & Vietze, P. (1983). Assessment of mastery motivation during the first year of life: Contemporaneous and cross-age relationships. *Developmental Psychology, 19,* 159–171.

Zelazo, P.D., & Reznick, J.S. (1991). Age-related asynchrony of knowledge and action. *Child Development, 62,* 719–735.

12

Psychiatric Disorders

Beverly A. Myers

Psychiatric disorders in young people with Down syndrome encompass various disturbances of mood, thought, and behavior that stem from different causes and have varying relationships to Down syndrome. Biologic and psychologic influences must be considered. Possible biologic factors include

1. The disorder may be distinctively associated with and apparently caused by the excess chromosomal/genetic material present in people with Down syndrome (e.g., Alzheimer's dementia).
2. The psychiatric disorder may be one that is completely separate and independent of Down syndrome (e.g., schizophrenia).
3. The disorder may not be related to Down syndrome, but may be related to mental retardation, which occurs in the majority of individuals with Down syndrome (e.g., infantile autism).
4. The hormonal changes associated with puberty not only bring on normal changes in heterosexual interests but also increase the risks for behaviors such as aggression.

Psychosocial stressors and other environmental influences may be significant factors leading to psychiatric disorders in young people with Down syndrome. Conflicts, losses, life changes, and the individual's increasing awareness of his or her disabilities are but a few examples of the many stressors that may occur in the lives of these adolescents. Both biologic *and* psychosocial factors may be important (e.g., major depressive disorder). In examining psychiatric disorders in young people with Down syndrome 10–30 years of age, all these etiologic possibilities must be considered.

EPIDEMIOLOGY

To understand the occurrence of and possible causes of psychiatric disorders in young people with Down syndrome, one must compare the distribution of psychiatric disorders in individuals with Down syndrome to the frequencies of psychiatric disorders both in the population of those with mental retardation from other causes, as well as in the general population. Young people with Down syndrome may be at lower risk for psychiatric disorders than those with mental retardation from other causes.

In one epidemiologic survey of the overall psychopathology of people with Down syndrome, the prevalence of psychiatric disorders in these people was found to be lower than in those with mental retardation of other causes (Collacott, Cooper, & McGrother, 1992). This survey compared all individuals with Down syndrome (including those in institutions) in a region in England to an equal number of individuals with mental retardation of other causes. The authors found psychiatric disorders in 25.9% of 371 individuals with Down syndrome, compared to 37.7% of 371 people with mental retardation of other causes ($p < 0.001$).

Since the mid-1980s, three noteworthy epidemiologic studies of young people with Down syndrome and mental retardation have been conducted. A controlled study by Gath and Gumley (1986) revealed that 38% of 193 children and adolescents with Down syndrome from the community had psychiatric disorders, compared with 49% of 154 age-, sex-, physical-, and mental-disability–matched controls with mental retardation and 4% of sibling controls with no mental retardation. Another epidemiologic study of teenagers with mental retardation (including Down syndrome) from a city in Sweden found that 35% of 20 teenagers with Down syndrome had psychiatric disorders, whereas 61% of the 129 with mental retardation of other causes had psychiatric disorders ($p < 0.02$) (Gillberg, Persson, Grafman, & Themner, 1986). Myers and Pueschel (1991), in a survey of 425 outpatient children, adolescents, and adults with Down syndrome, reported that 13% of children under age 10 revealed psychiatric disorders; 20% of those between ages 10 and 20 had such disorders; and 25% of outpatient adults (over age 20, but with a mean age of 26) had such disorders. No control populations were included.

This chapter focuses on psychiatric disorders in young people with Down syndrome ages 10–30 years, because these disorders tend to be ongoing. Some begin in early childhood and persist into adolescence and young adulthood. The age range of this review extends from adolescence into young adulthood because the psychiatric disorders beginning in adolescence and young adulthood are similar. This discussion, therefore, examines those disorders that begin in infancy or early childhood and persist into adulthood separately from those appearing during adolescence and young adulthood.

PSYCHIATRIC DISORDERS BEGINNING IN CHILDHOOD

Disruptive Behavior Disorders

Disruptive behavior disorders (i.e., attention-deficit/hyperactivity disorder [ADHD], conduct disorder, oppositional disorder) are the most common psychiatric disorders in children with Down syndrome (Myers & Pueschel, 1991), as well as in children in the general population. Whereas some of these disruptive behavior disorders are observed only during childhood, many continue into adolescence, presenting significant problems in the young adult.

Attention-Deficit/Hyperactivity Disorder   The relationship between ADHD and Down syndrome is unknown. Pueschel, Bernier, and Pezzullo (1991) noted in 40 children with Down syndrome ages 4–16 years a significantly increased frequency of hyperactive behavior on the Achenbach Child Behavior Checklist when compared with 40 sibling controls. Short attention span and impulsivity were specifically increased, but other items of the full syndrome of ADHD, including fidgetiness, out-of-seat behavior, distractibility, speaking out of turn, incompletion of activities, poor following of instruction, excessive talking, rowdy play, poor listening, frequent loss of things, and poor regard of danger, were not studied.

In their review of a sample group of young people with Down syndrome under age 20, Myers and Pueschel (1991) noted attentional disorders in 6.1% of 264 such individuals. This prevalence figure does not differ appreciably from that found in children in the general population: 3%–5% (Brunstetter & Silver, 1985) or 6.9% (Burd et al., 1988). Gath and Gumley (1986) found ADHD in 1% of 193 youngsters with Down syndrome (plus 7.5% with hyperkinetic conduct disorder), compared to 6% in 154 controls with mental retardation (plus 1.3% with hyperkinetic conduct disorder). These findings are difficult to interpret, however, since diagnostic categories in England differ from those in the American Psychiatric Association's *Diagnostic and Statistical Manual of Mental Disorders* (3rd ed., DSM-III, 1980)—the latest edition at the time of Gath and Gumley's study. To establish the relationship between ADHD, which itself has a known genetic inheritance (Biederman et al., 1992), and Down syndrome, further studies are required.

The following is a case example of an adolescent with Down syndrome and ADHD:

Case Study A

A is a 13-year-old boy with Down syndrome and mental retardation requiring moderate supports who came to the Child Development

Center (at Rhode Island Hospital, Providence) at age 8 years with behavior problems consisting of tantrums, oppositional behaviors, and a short attention span. These behaviors were interfering with his ability to be educationally mainstreamed. At that time, he was in a structured, self-contained, special education class, and his mother was eager for him to be included as much as possible into the general school population. Behavior modification approaches using time-out and withdrawal of privileges had helped his mother in handling him more firmly at home, but additional measures were needed for school. A has been hyperactive, impulsive, and inattentive since early childhood but is very friendly and sociable. His performance on the Conner's Rating Scale was strongly positive. ADHD was diagnosed, and he was placed on Dexedrine Spansule, increasing to 10 mg/day on school days. This has enabled him to work more independently and to be mainstreamed for significant portions of time. He has friends and participates in many recreational activities.

Conduct and Oppositional Disorders   Conduct disorders (e.g., fighting, temper tantrums, destructiveness, stealing, running away, fire setting) and oppositional disorder (e.g., uncooperative behavior within the family) are probably no more frequent in children and adolescents with Down syndrome than in those with mental retardation of other causes. Gath and Gumley (1986) noted conduct disorders in 20% of 193 children and adolescents with Down syndrome and also in 20% of 153 children and adolescents with mental retardation. Myers and Pueschel (1991) noted that 12% of 264 young people with Down syndrome under age 20 had conduct, oppositional, or aggressive behaviors. Pueschel et al. (1991), using the Achenbach Child Behavior Checklist, found children with Down syndrome to disobey more frequently than sibling controls and were reportedly more stubborn, sullen, and irritable. The extent to which these behavioral disturbances persist into adulthood is not clear (see also Chapter 11).

Infantile Autism and Pervasive Developmental Disorders
Infantile autism is defined as a disorder that appears under the age of 30 months, with severe deficits in language (poor use of speech to communicate), marked social withdrawal, and various repetitive behaviors. Although the symptoms improve with time with behavioral interventions, the disorder is generally lifelong. Thus, a small percentage of adolescents with Down syndrome will be noted to have infantile autism in combination with mental retardation, which has begun in early childhood.

Although the relationship of infantile autism to Down syndrome is unclear, the two disorders are probably not specifically related to each other. Five case reports of infantile autism and Down syndrome have been published in the literature (Bregman & Volkmar, 1988; Ghaziuddin, Tsai,

& Ghaziuddin, 1992; Wakabayashi, 1979). In children, Gath and Gumley (1986) found no difference in the frequency of children with Down syndrome and infantile autism (1%) when compared to controls with mental retardation (2%). Gillberg et al. (1986) noted 1 in 20 teenagers with infantile autism and Down syndrome and 7.2% of 129 controls with mental retardation. In their study of 425 people with Down syndrome, Myers and Pueschel (1991) noted that 1.1% of 261 young people under 20 years of age and 1.2% of 164 adults had infantile autism and Down syndrome. Collacott et al. (1992), in a controlled lifelong survey of Down syndrome and psychiatric disorders, noted infantile autism in 2.2% of 371 people with Down syndrome but noted infantile autism in 4.3% of 371 people with mental retardation of other causes ($p > 0.5$).

The following is a case example of an adolescent with Down syndrome and infantile autism:

Case Study B

B is a 15-year-old with Down syndrome who developed slowly after birth, not walking until age 32 months. He was fairly sociable despite severe language delay and related warmly to his brother, who was born when he was 2 years old. When *B* was 4 years old, the two brothers appeared to be like twins, playing affectionately with each other. With the birth of his second brother when *B* was 5, *B* regressed and became less socially responsive to others. He also stopped being able to play imaginatively with cars. Psychologic testing of *B* at age 9 years revealed an unresponsive boy in diapers with no social responses, unintelligible jabber and grunting, short attention span, rocking, and hair flicking, who eventually became noncompliant and kicked the examiner. The Vineland Adaptive Behavior Scales rated *B* at the 2½- to 3½-year level, with intellectual functioning in the range of mental retardation requiring extensive supports. *B* has continued to be extremely aloof to the present, with persistent, repetitive behaviors and little verbal communication.

Tourette Syndrome and Tics

Tics and Tourette syndrome, with multiple motor and vocal tics, usually begin in childhood. As with infantile autism, the relationship of Tourette syndrome to Down syndrome is unclear. Ten individuals with Tourette syndrome and Down syndrome have been reported in the literature (Barabas, Wardell, Sapiro, & Matthews, 1986; Collacott & Ismail, 1988; Karlinsky, Sandor, Berg, Muldofsky, & Crawford, 1986; Myers & Pueschel, 1994; Sacks, 1982). Of these 10 people, 7 were noted to have an onset of tics beyond the age of 21 years, none had a positive family history, 6 were exposed to phenothiazines as children and adolescents, and 1 child received psychostimulants, suggesting an atypical or tardive Tourette disorder. The 5 individuals with Down syndrome and Tourette disorder reported by Myers and Pueschel (1994) were observed out of a total of 425 (1.2%) individuals with Down syndrome. With a prevalence rate of 0.03%–1.6% in the general population (Kurlan, 1989), there appears to be no increased prevalence of Tourette syndrome in Down syndrome, and thus there is no relationship between the two disabilities.

The following is a case example of an adolescent with Down syndrome and Tourette syndrome:

Case Study C

C is an 11-year-old boy with Down syndrome (14/21 chromosomal translocation, a variant of Down syndrome) who has displayed increasing aggressiveness, tantrums, noncompliance, and fire-setting behavior (including setting fire to his own home). He has also developed motor and vocal tics, which include eye blinks, facial grimaces, grunts, and cattle noises. He had been treated with methylphenidate and diazepam, which did not decrease his impulsive acting-out behavior. Down syndrome was known to occur in his father's family. C was admitted and treated at a child psychiatry hospital, and a psychiatrist was consulted on his care. He has mild motor delay, severe language developmental delay, and a severe articulation disorder. Psychologic testing revealed that he has mental retardation requiring extensive supports, including adaptive levels. Clonidine was ineffective for the tics, whereas haloperidol was effective, but the latter medication had to be discontinued because of bradycardia (i.e., slow heart rate).

Stereotypic Behavior

Repetitive, nonfunctional, self-stimulatory behaviors are primarily observed in severe to profound mental retardation with a need for pervasive supports and in association with autistic symptoms, particularly in those with failure to use verbal communication and with social unrelatedness. Stereotypic behavior is likely to begin in childhood. The frequency of such behavior appears to be low in people with Down syndrome. Myers and Pueschel (1991) noted that 2.7% of 264 people with Down syndrome under 20 years of age and 4.3% of 164 adults with Down syndrome treated in the outpatient clinic displayed stereotypic behavior.

Encopresis and Enuresis

Although control of bowel and bladder functions usually is delayed in individuals with impaired cognitive development, encopresis or bowel incontinence may have other causes and is often associated with environmental and psychosocial stressors. It is an ongoing disorder. The prevalence of encopresis in the general population is estimated to be about 1.3% in boys age 10–12 years (Rutter, Graham, & Yule, 1970). In the only study to note encopresis in people with Down syndrome, Myers and Pueschel (1991) reported encopresis in 5 out of 425 outpatients with Down syndrome, 4 of whom were under 20 years of age; 4 of the 5 also had associated conduct disorders.

PSYCHIATRIC DISORDERS APPEARING IN ADOLESCENCE AND YOUNG ADULTHOOD

Affective Disorders

Major Depression, Dysthymic Disorder, and Unipolar Disorder It is possible to identify major depressive disorder even in people with mental retardation requiring limited to pervasive supports (Myers & Pueschel, 1995). Although it may be difficult for such individuals to verbalize complaints of depression, self-deprecation, guilt, suicidal thoughts, or fatigue, specific behaviors such as crying, loss of interest or pleasure, poor appetite and weight loss, insomnia, psychomotor agitation or retardation, and poor concentration can be observed to support a diagnosis of major depressive disorder.

Although there is no evidence for the occurrence of depressive disorders in children with Down syndrome, several case reports of major depressive disorder in adults with Down syndrome have been published since 1960 (Jakab, 1978; Keegan, Pettigrew, & Parker, 1974; Myers & Pueschel, 1995; Roith, 1961; Storm, 1990; Szymanski & Biederman, 1984; Warren, Holroyd, & Folstein, 1990). Myers and Pueschel (1995) noted a frequency of major depression in 5.5% of 164 young adults with Down syndrome in a 10-year review. Collacott et al. (1992) noted a lifetime frequency of all levels of severity of depression in 11.3% of 371 people with Down syndrome, compared to 4.3% in a control group of 371 with mental retardation of other causes ($p < 0.001$). This greater prevalence of depression in Down syndrome than in other causes of mental retardation suggests the possibility of a specific relationship between Down syndrome and depression. To determine whether there is a significant increase in the risk for depressive disorders in young adults with Down syndrome or whether the risk is no greater than in the general population (point prevalence of major depression of 1.8%–2.6%; lifetime prevalence, 14%–19% [Regier & Burke, 1985]) will require careful epidemiologic studies of affective disorders in Down syndrome.

The major depression noted by Myers and Pueschel (1995) appeared to be intense, prolonged, and sometimes difficult to treat. People with Down syndrome and depression were also found to have lower adaptive skills after recovery from the depression than occurred in matched controls (Cooper & Collacott, 1993), a decline that has been suggested to reflect a loss of confidence that persists after the depression. A marked deterioration in mental and social abilities in a young person with Down syndrome may suggest Alzheimer's disease, but is more likely to be a major depression, even though the two disorders can occur together (Warren et al., 1990). Persistent efforts with antidepressants (and sometimes also antipsychotics) are indicated to treat such a young person, since major depression in those with Down syndrome may be unresponsive to treatment. Depression may be more likely to respond to serotonergic antidepressants. Low levels of serotonin and norepinephrine in the brains of those with Down syndrome may have a relationship to depression (Collacott et al., 1992).

The following is a case example of a young person with Down syndrome and major depression with psychosis:

Case Study D

D is a 21-year-old woman with Down syndrome and mental retardation requiring moderate supports who had been outgoing and active until age 18. After two family members and a friend died, she became depressed, inactive, anxious, insomnious, anorexic, and tearful. She had auditory hallucinations and stopped talking. Unsuccessful treatment included haloperidol, nortriptyline, desipramine, trazodone, clonazepam, and carbamazepine. D was then placed on fluoxetine (i.e., Prozac), 20 mg per day. Her mother felt that D was significantly better after the introduction of fluoxetine.

Bipolar Disorder (Manic-Depressive Disorder)   The prevalence of bipolar (manic depression) and unipolar (depression) disorders have been difficult to ascertain in people with mental retardation because, prior to 1980, bipolar and unipolar disorders were combined and identified as major affective disorders. The prevalence of bipolar disorder in the general population is 0.6%–0.9% (Regier & Burke, 1985).

Since 1985, several cases of mania in Down syndrome have been reported (Collacott et al., 1992; Cook & Leventhal, 1987; Cooper & Collacott, 1991, 1993; McLaughlin, 1987; Singh & Zolese, 1986; Sovner, 1991). Collacott et al.'s (1992) survey found bipolar disorder in 0.5% of 371 individuals with Down syndrome, compared to 1.4% in 371 controls with mental retardation ($p = .624$). Cooper and Collacott (1993) reviewed all the preceding cases and suggested that both a predisposition to depression and a relative protection from mania occurs in young people with Down syndrome as a possible result of reduced serotonergic and noradrenergic function in the central nervous system.

Schizophrenia

Schizophrenia is a mental disorder that usually is manifested in adolescence and young adulthood, with a general prevalence of 0.5%–0.8% (Regier & Burke, 1985). Myers and Pueschel (1991) initially did not identify anyone with schizophrenia in their study population of 164 adults with Down syndrome. Later one of these adults developed schizophrenia (Myers & Pueschel, 1993). In their controlled study, Collacott et al. (1992) observed a 1.6% prevalence rate in 371 people with Down syndrome, in contrast to a 5.4% rate in 371 people with mental retardation of other causes ($p < 0.011$). Therefore, it is unlikely that there is a specifically increased risk for schizophrenia in Down syndrome. Moreover, if any increased risk for schizophrenia were to be identified in Down syndrome, it would likely be related to the increased risk for schizophrenia in the population with mental retardation in general, rather than being specific to Down syndrome.

Dementia

The occurrence of Alzheimer's disease (dementia) in people with Down syndrome under the age of 30 is rare. The average age of clinical onset of Alzheimer's disease in prospective studies of the disease in Down syndrome is ages 51–54 years, with 8% appearing in those by 35–49 years of age, 55% in those by 50–59 years of age, and 75% in those over 60 years of age (Lai & Williams, 1989). Those with dementia in Collacott et al.'s (1992) study had a mean age of 54, whereas those with depression had a mean age of 29 ($p < .001$).

Thus, the cause of a mental and social decline in a young person with Down syndrome from ages 10–30 is unlikely to be Alzheimer's disease. Cognitive and social decline in a person under the age of 35 should be investigated for other causes of dementia or pseudodementia. Such treatable causes include depression, hypothyroidism, folate or B_{12} deficiencies, or hydrocephalus, with depression being the most likely. Treating depression may entail courses of several antidepressants (and sometimes, additionally, antipsychotics).

Eating Disorders and Anorexia Nervosa

In the general population, anorexia nervosa, with intentional weight loss and a recurrent feeling of being fat, develops mostly in girls and women during ages 10–30 years. Four young people with Down syndrome have been reported to have anorexia nervosa (Cottrell & Crisp, 1984; Fox, Karan, & Rotatori, 1981; Hurley & Sovner, 1979; Szymanski & Biederman, 1984). Their symptoms included weight loss, decreased food intake, amenorrhea, depression, withdrawal, and behavioral regression. Two of these young people showed an intense and irrational fear of becoming obese, whereas the other two showed a more prominent depression, decreased food intake, and self-induced vomiting without obsession with weight. Although it may be difficult to identify the thoughts of a person with Down syndrome and mental retardation, poor food intake and weight loss is more likely to be a symptom of depression, a condition of significant risk in Down syndrome. Myers and Pueschel (1991) identified three young adults with problems of intake, one of whom had intentional vomiting but apparently no fear of fatness and later developed major depression. The following case example relates the story of this young person:

Case Study E

E is a 22-year-old man with Down syndrome and mental retardation requiring moderate supports who lived alone with his mother after his mother's breast cancer surgery and his father's sudden death 2 years before. For more than a year, he continued to be sociable and was able to work part-time in a restaurant. Three months before this evaluation, his brother, who is messy, returned home to share a room with *E*, who is neat and orderly. *E* began to vomit intentionally and in a short time lost 20 pounds. A mental status examination of *E* revealed a thin, active man who appeared animated. He denied sadness about his father's death, but he openly displayed anger toward his brother. Behavior modification therapy led to complete cessation of vomiting in 2 months. Four months later, however, *E* became depressed, with crying, agitation, insomnia, preoccupation about his father's death, self-deprecatory thoughts, self-abusive behavior (i.e., biting his arm), and paranoid thinking. Desipramine up to 150 mg for 6 weeks was unsuccessful, but clomipramine (a serotonergic antidepressant) up to 150 mg led to complete recovery from depression. *E's* mother died 3 years after her surgery. Since then, he has lived with his sister and remains well on 100 mg of clomipramine to prevent a recurrence of depression.

Anxiety Disorders

Anxiety disorders include panic disorder with or without agoraphobia, specific phobias, social phobia, posttraumatic stress disorder, generalized anxiety disorder, and obsessive-compulsive disorder. Surveys of Down syndrome earlier than 1980 noted emotional problems that may have represented anxiety disorders but were not identifiable in the terms used in DSM-III (American Psychiatric Association, 1980). Gath and Gumley (1986) found 3% of 194 children with Down syndrome exhibited anxiety and fearfulness, compared to 2.6% of 153 controls with mental retardation of other causes. Myers and Pueschel (1991) noted specific phobias in 1.5% of 261 individuals with Down syndrome under 20 years of age, and in

0.6% of 164 people with Down syndrome over 20 years of age. Collacott et al. (1992) identified neurotic disorders excluding depression in 0.3% of 371 people with Down syndrome as compared to in 2.4% of 371 people with mental retardation of other causes ($p = 0.011$).

Obsessive-compulsive disorder (in which a person exhibits persistent obsessions or repetitive thoughts and compulsions or recurrent unusual behaviors) can be recognized in people with mental retardation (Vitiello, Spreat, & Behar, 1989). Two individuals with obsessive-compulsive disorder and Down syndrome have been reported by O'Dwyer, Holmes, and Collacott (1990). Obsessive-compulsive disorder occurs in 1.2%–2.4% of the general population (Lewis, 1991). Myers and Pueschel (1991) identified 1 young person with obsessive-compulsive disorder and Down syndrome out of 164 (0.6%) adults with Down syndrome. The following case example relates this young person's story:

Case Study F

F is a 22-year-old male with Down syndrome who lives at home with his parents and who developed rituals and compulsive behavior as a 15-year-old. He dresses, cleans, and bathes himself meticulously. He folds his clothing neatly and keeps his room tidy. His rituals include greeting his toys one-by-one in the morning and evening. He resists distraction, frequently gets stuck in the rituals, and repeats them, so that he is often late for meals and for his workshop. Pressuring has led to many conflicts with his parents. Mental status examination revealed a cheerful young man with features of Down syndrome who perseverated on his jacket being in the waiting room until he was allowed to retrieve it. Clomipramine up to 125 mg/day led to moderate improvement, but side effects of falling episodes, constipation, and abdominal pain led to discontinuation. Fluoxetine up to 40 mg/day was partially effective, but sertraline 25 mg/day has been optimal. Parental avoidance of confrontations has also helped. F now has a more active day program, rather than benchwork.

Self-Injurious Behavior

Although self-injurious behavior may appear in children with mental retardation, particularly concomitant with self-stimulatory and autistic behaviors, it more frequently becomes a problem as the person with mental retardation moves into adulthood. Self-injurious behavior occurs in 3% of adults with mental retardation living in the community, but in 8%–15% of those living in institutions (Oliver, Murphy, & Corbett, 1987). It appears to be less frequent in those with Down syndrome. In Myers and Pueschel's (1991) Down syndrome study, self-injurious behavior was observed in

0.8% of 261 children and 1.2% of 164 outpatient adults. Self-injurious behavior has also been observed in association with depression in adults with mental retardation of other causes and has responded to anti-depressants.

Aggression and Intermittent Explosive Disorder

The sudden appearance of conduct disorders, particularly of aggressive behavior, in adolescents and young adults with Down syndrome deserves careful diagnostic study (see also subsection on "Conduct and Oppositional Disorders"). Although some conduct disturbances represent a clear reaction to changes or stressful events in the environment, they may sometimes be a manifestation of such mental disorders as mania, major depressive disorder, or schizophrenia. Specific psychoactive medications are indicated in each disorder in addition to behavioral interventions, psychotherapy, or both (see also Chapter 11).

CONCLUSIONS

More than 75% of adolescents and young adults with Down syndrome develop normally through adolescence without the appearance of psychiatric disorders (disturbances of mood, thought, or behavior). Conduct and attentional disorders are the most frequent psychiatric disorders occurring in these young people but are no more frequent than in young people with mental retardation of other causes. Major depression may be a disorder that occurs significantly more frequently in young people with Down syndrome than in young people with mental retardation of other causes. Other psychiatric disorders occur in young people with Down syndrome no more often than in people with mental retardation of other causes or in the general population. Self-injurious behavior may be distinctively lower in people with Down syndrome than in people with mental retardation of other causes. Treatments for psychiatric disorders occurring in young people with Down syndrome are the same as for each psychiatric disorder occurring in the general population, including specific psychotropic medications, behavioral modification, psychotherapy, parental counseling, and education.

REFERENCES

American Psychiatric Association. (1980). *Diagnostic and statistical manual of mental disorders* (3rd ed.). Washington, DC: Author.

Barabas, G., Wardell, B., Sapiro, M., & Matthews, W.S. (1986). Coincident Down's and Tourette syndromes: Three case reports. *Journal of Clinical Neurology, 1,* 358–360.

Biederman, J., Farnone, S.V., Keenan, K., Benjamin, J., Krifcher, V., Moore, C., Sprich-Buckminster, S., Vgaglia, K., Jellinek, Steingard, R., et al. (1992). Further evidence for family-genetic risk factors in attention deficit hyperactivity disorder:

Patterns of comorbidity in probands and relatives in psychiatrically and pediatrically referred samples. *Archives of General Psychiatry, 49,* 728–738.

Bregman, J.D., & Volkmar, F.R. (1988). Autistic social dysfunction and Down syndrome. *American Academy of Child and Adolescent Psychiatry, 27,* 440–441.

Brunstetter, R.W., & Silver, L.B. (1985). Attention deficit disorder. In H.I. Kaplan & B.J. Sadock (Eds.), *Comprehensive textbook of psychiatry* (pp. 1684–1690). Baltimore: Williams & Wilkins.

Burd, H.R., Camino, G., Rubio-Stipic, M., Gould, M.S., Ribera, J., Sesmand, M., Woodbury, M., Huertes-Goldman, S., Pagan, A., Sanchez-Lacay, A., et al. (1988). Estimates of the prevalence of childhood maladjustment in a community survey in Puerto Rico. *Archives of General Psychiatry, 45,* 1120–1126.

Collacott, R.A., Cooper, S., & McGrother, C. (1992). Differential rates of psychiatric disorders in adults with Down's syndrome compared to other mentally handicapped adults. *British Journal of Psychiatry, 161,* 671–674.

Collacott, R.A., & Ismail, I.A. (1988). Tourettism in a patient with Down's syndrome. *Journal of Mental Deficiency Research, 32,* 163–166.

Cook, E.H., & Leventhal, B.L. (1987). Down's syndrome with mania. *British Journal of Psychiatry, 150,* 249–250.

Cooper, S., & Collacott, R.A. (1991). Manic episodes in Down's syndrome. *Journal of Nervous and Mental Disease, 179,* 635–636.

Cooper, S., & Collacott, R.A. (1993). Mania and Down's syndrome. *British Journal of Psychiatry, 162,* 739–743.

Cottrell, D.J., & Crisp, A. H. (1984). Anorexia nervosa in Down's syndrome—A case report. *British Journal of Psychiatry, 145,* 195–196.

Fox, R., Karan, O.C., & Rotatori, A.F. (1981). Regression including anorexia nervosa in a Down's syndrome adult: A seven-year follow-up. *Journal of Behavior Therapy and Experimental Psychiatry, 12,* 351–354.

Gath, A., & Gumley, D. (1986). Behaviour problems in retarded children with special reference to Down's syndrome. *British Journal of Psychiatry, 149,* 156–161.

Ghaziuddin, M., Tsai, L.Y., & Ghaziuddin, N. (1992). Autism in Down's syndrome: Presentation and diagnosis. *Journal of Intellectual Disability Research, 36,* 449–456.

Gillberg, C., Persson, E., Grafman, M., & Themner, U. (1986). Psychiatric disorders in mildly and severely mentally retarded urban children and adolescents: Epidemiological aspects. *British Journal of Psychiatry, 149,* 68–74.

Hurley, A.D., & Sovner, R. (1979). Anorexia nervosa and mental retardation: A case report. *Journal of Clinical Psychiatry, 40,* 480–482.

Jakab, I. (1978). Basal ganglia calcification and psychosis in mongolism. *European Neurology, 17,* 300–314.

Karlinsky, H., Sandor, P., Berg, J.M., Muldofsky, H., & Crawford, E. (1986). Gilles de la Tourette's syndrome in Down's syndrome: A case report. *British Journal of Psychiatry, 148,* 601–604.

Keegan, D.L., Pettigrew, A., & Parker, Z. (1974). Psychosis in Down's syndrome treated with amitriptyline. *Canadian Medical Association Journal, 110,* 1128–1133.

Kurlan, R. (1989). Tourette's syndrome: Current concepts. *Neurology, 39,* 1625–1630.

Lai, F., & Williams, R. (1989). A prospective study of Alzheimer disease in Down syndrome. *Archives of Neurology, 46,* 849–853.

Lewis, M. (1991). *Child and adolescent psychiatry.* Baltimore: Williams & Wilkins.

McLaughlin, M. (1987). Bipolar affective disorder in Down's syndrome. *British Journal of Psychiatry, 151,* 116–117.

Myers, B.A., & Pueschel, S.M. (1991). Psychiatric disorders in population with Down syndrome. *Journal of Nervous and Mental Disease, 179,* 609–613.

Myers, B.A., & Pueschel, S.M. (1993). Brief report: A case of schizophrenia in a population of Down syndrome. *Journal of Autism and Developmental Disorders, 24,* 95–98.

Myers, B.A., & Pueschel, S.M. (1994). Tardive or atypical Tourette syndrome in a large population with Down syndrome? *Research in Developmental Disabilities, 16,* 1–9.

Myers, B.A., & Pueschel, S.M. (1995). Major depressive disorder in a small group with Down syndrome. *Research in Developmental Disabilities, 16,* 285–289.

O'Dwyer, J., Holmes, J., & Collacott, R.A. (1990). Two cases of obsessive-compulsive disorder in individuals with Down's syndrome. *Journal of Nervous and Mental Disease, 9,* 603–604.

Oliver, C., Murphy, G.H., & Corbett, J.A. (1987). Self-injurious behaviour in people with mental handicap: A total population study. *Journal of Mental Deficiency Research, 31,* 147–162.

Pueschel, S.M., Bernier, J.C., & Pezzullo, J.C. (1991). Behavioural observations in children with Down's syndrome. *Journal of Mental Deficiency Research, 35,* 502–511.

Regier, D.A., & Burke, J.D. (1985). Epidemiology. In H.I. Kaplan & B.J. Sadock (Eds.), *Comprehensive textbook of psychiatry* (4th ed., pp. 295–311). Baltimore: Williams & Wilkins.

Roith, A.I. (1961). Psychotic depression in a mongol. *Journal of Mental Subnormality, 7,* 45–47.

Rutter, M., Graham, P., & Yule W. (1970). *Clinics in developmental medicine.* London: SIMP/Heinemann Medical.

Sacks, O.W. (1982). Acquired Tourettism in adult life. In A.J. Friedhiff & T.N. Chase (Eds.), *Gilles de la Tourette syndrome.* New York: Raven Press.

Singh, I., & Zolese, G. (1986). Is mania really incompatible with Down's syndrome? *British Journal of Psychiatry, 148,* 613–614.

Sovner, R. (1991). Divalproex-responsive rapid bipolar disorder in a patient with Down's syndrome; Implications for the Down's syndrome hypothesis. *Journal of Mental Deficiency Research, 35,* 171–173.

Storm, W. (1990). Differential diagnosis and treatment of depressive features in Down's syndrome: A case illustration. *Research in Developmental Disabilities, 11,* 131–137.

Szymanski, L.S., & Biederman, J. (1984). Depression and anorexia nervosa of persons with Down syndrome. *American Journal of Mental Deficiency, 89,* 246–251.

Vitiello, B., Spreat, S., & Behar, D. (1989). Obsessive-compulsive disorder in mentally retarded patients. *Journal of Nervous and Mental Disorders, 177,* 232–236.

Wakabayashi, S. (1979). A case of infantile autism associated with Down's syndrome. *Journal of Autism and Developmental Disorders, 9,* 31–36.

Warren, A.C., Holroyd, S., & Folstein, M.P. (1990). Major depression in Down's syndrome. *British Journal of Psychiatry, 155,* 202–205.

III

EDUCATION

13

Inclusive Educational Schooling

Mary A. Falvey
Richard L. Rosenberg
Eileen M. Falvey

A growing number of adolescents with Down syndrome are enrolled in general education classes in secondary schools within their communities while receiving supports from both special and general education personnel as well as classmates. This service delivery model, although gaining in popularity, has not always been available for students with Down syndrome.

Prior to the 1950s, services and programs for children and adolescents with Down syndrome were largely nonexistent. In the early 1950s, parents organized the Association for Retarded Children of the United States (now named The Arc: A National Organization on Mental Retardation). Efforts of such parent organizations and others led in the 1950s and 1960s to the development and delivery of school services and other programs for children and adults with disabilities. These early programs were designed to give parents respite from the care of their children and to provide sons and daughters with education and training, because the public schools had denied them access. The settings were typically segregated; often children and adults attended school together in rented church basements or vacant old schools. In the 1960s and 1970s, local school districts began to assume responsibility for providing public school education for children with disabilities at no cost to individual families. These public school programs were often located at segregated school campuses or in a wing of a general education school campus. With a push toward "integrating" children with disabilities in the late 1970s, groups of students were placed on general education campuses, where they sometimes participated in "nonacademic" events and activities with peers without disabilities, while receiving the majority of their education in segregated special education classes. During the late 1970s and early 1980s, some students were selected to be in the mainstream of these general education settings, which often resulted in their being dumped into general education classrooms without the necessary ongoing supports. The assumption, at that time, was that special education services could be delivered only within a special education classroom or school.

Since the mid-1980s, increasing numbers of schools and school districts have developed and implemented inclusive educational service delivery models, according to which students with disabilities attend the same school they would attend if they did not have a disability. Individualized supports that are needed are identified by the student's family, friends, and teachers. Those supports are provided for students to effectively participate within general education classes (Falvey, 1995).

Inclusive education for students with disabilities, including those students with Down syndrome, has gained in popularity for several reasons. First, research studies conducted since the mid-1980s have demonstrated that students with disabilities who are included in typical classrooms fare better academically (Cole & Meyer, 1991) and socially (Strain, 1983; Straub & Peck, 1994), are more likely to form friendships with peers without disabilities, and are more likely to be successful in employment and continuing education (Ferguson & Asch, 1989). In addition, students without disabilities not only did not demonstrate detrimental effects as a result of inclusion but also gained academically, socially, and emotionally (Costello, 1991; Hollowood, Salisbury, Rainforth, & Palombaro, 1995; Kaskinen-Chapman, 1992).

As a brief case example, consider Jace, a first-grader with Down syndrome. He has often been described by his classmates without disabilities and their parents as one of the most important children in their class. Following his kindergarten graduation, the principal of the school he was attending told Jace's mother that every year he receives numerous requests from parents regarding the teacher they want their child to be assigned to the following year. However, at the end of Jace's kindergarten year, the principal had received many more requests from parents that their child be assigned to Jace's class, regardless of the teacher. These parents recognized the important gifts Jace had given them just by being their child's classmate and friend. Although not yet adolescents, all of these children are learning, by experience, important lessons about valuing diversity that will undoubtedly assist them as they grow into adulthood. This and similar experiences are occurring throughout the United States, Canada, and other countries as schools welcome all of their children.

A second reason for the rising popularity of inclusive education is the precedence established by both legislation and litigation representing a compelling argument in favor of inclusive educational practices. In 1954, the U.S. Supreme Court, in a unanimous decision in *Brown v. Board of Education,* ruled that school segregation was immoral and that it would retard the educational and moral development of those being segregated. This landmark ruling is often cited in cases involving protecting the rights of children with disabilities when segregation has been imposed on them. In 1975, the Education for All Handicapped Children Act (now reauthorized as the Individuals with Disabilities Education Act [IDEA] of 1990), PL 94-142, was passed. The act guarantees to all students with disabilities a free appropriate public education in the least restrictive environment. Since PL 94-142 was first passed, *least restrictive environment* has been defined as:

> To the maximum extent appropriate, handicapped children, including those children in public and private institutions or other care facilities, are educated with children who are not handicapped, and that special classes, separate schooling, or other removal of handicapped children from the regular educational environment occurs only when the nature or severity of the handicap is such that education in regular classes with the use of supplementary aids and services cannot be achieved satisfactorily. (20 U.S.C. § 1412[5][b])

PL 94-142 established the legal framework for the provision of inclusive education. In 1975, the overwhelming majority of children and adolescents with Down syndrome were educated in segregated environments, that is, in special schools or special classes. However, as schools and school districts began creating inclusive educational opportunities and publishing and sharing their results, the professional knowledge base began to grow in terms of the supplementary aids and services that are necessary to effectively educate students with Down syndrome in inclusive educational settings. In the early 1990s, two sets of parents, one with a child with developmental disabilities (*Sacramento City Unified School District v. Rachel H.,* 1994) and the other with a child with Down syndrome (*Oberti v. Board of Education of the Borough of Clementon School District,* 1993), filed for due process in their effort to educate their children within inclusive educational settings, after their school districts had refused their children access to inclusive education. The administrative law judges in both cases ruled in their favor, and each of the defending school districts appealed the decision to federal courts. Once the families' requests for inclusive education for their children were upheld, the school districts in both cases once again appealed the decisions to their respective federal circuit courts of appeals. The justices in both circuit courts ruled in favor of the families' requests. In the *Rachel H.* case, the school district appealed the decision to the U.S. Supreme Court, which refused to review the case, ruling that the Ninth Circuit Court of Appeals finding was the final decision in this case. These cases are important in that the courts, citing the growing knowledge base in the education of students with disabilities, ruled in favor of inclusive educational options.

A third reason for the growing trend toward inclusion is that it is becoming recognized that children and adolescents are more likely to form friendships with their peers if they are within close physical proximity and have frequent opportunities to be together (Lewis & Rosenblaum, 1975). When children with Down syndrome are sent outside their neighborhood to go to school to receive specialized services, it is more difficult for them to form relationships and friendships with their peers who live close to them.

A fourth reason for the growth of inclusion is that schools are seen as a microcosm of society and offer students opportunities to learn about how society is organized and about what is and is not tolerated. When isolation and rejection are perpetuated, owing to the existence of segregated classes and schools for students with disabilities, a message is sent to students without disabilities that it is okay to exclude people with disabilities because the adults in charge of the school are doing it. This can have a powerful and lasting effect on students without disabilities, making it difficult and uncomfortable for them to relate to people with disabilities throughout their lives. This is particularly problematic for siblings, cousins, and family friends of children and adolescents with disabilities, because, on the one hand, they have a personal relationship outside of school; but, on the other hand, the school's structure and outlook discourages such relationships.

CHARACTERISTICS OF INCLUSIVE SCHOOLS

For several years, researchers, educators, and advocates have been studying the characteristics of schools that have effectively included students with disabilities, including those with Down syndrome (Biklen, Ferguson, & Ford, 1989; Falvey, 1995; Lipsky & Gartner, 1989; Stainback & Stainback, 1990; Stainback, Stainback, & Forest, 1989; Thousand, Villa, & Nevin, 1994; Villa & Thousand, 1995). This section discusses a number of the most prominent characteristics displayed by such schools. Although not every school that successfully includes students with disabilities reflects each of the characteristics described here to the same extent, they are present within a majority of schools where inclusive education is occurring.

Diversity, multiculturalism, and social inclusion are valued through the creation of a strong sense of democratic communities. For the past several decades in many communities, particularly those with populations that are ethnically diverse, educators, parents, students, and community members have discussed and created curricula that reflect a sense of multiculturalism. When students with disabilities began attending these same schools, it became necessary to broaden the definition of *diversity* to include these students.

Social inclusion is another major aspect of democratic school communities. Both students with disabilities and those without disabilities at times require direct encouragement, strategies, and support to develop friendships. Schools that have successfully included students with disabilities have intentionally designed a strong sense of community and have fostered mutual respect and genuine friendships among staff, parents, students, and the community. These schools also offer access for all students to the total campus and classrooms, including co-curricular and extracurricular activities that are free from prejudice or from physical or psychological barriers.

A sensible and comprehensive professional development process is in place. Teachers, both special and general educators, paraprofessionals, principals, parents, support staff, and students have had little or no prior experience with inclusive educational practices and are in need of strengthening their expertise. In inclusive schools, professional development activities are presented in meaningful ways for specific audiences and include numerous opportunities for staff, parents, and students to participate in creative problem-solving strategies (Thousand et al., 1994; Villa, Thousand, & Rosenberg, 1995). Time and energy are spent examining attitudes, beliefs, and school–community collaboration, as well as specific strategies for accommodating students' needs so that learning is accessible to all. Staff development activities foster team development and skills around a student and his or her needs and community.

There are high expectations for every student, and each student is uniquely important. When schools are adequately prepared to effectively teach all students, including those requiring diverse learning strategies, a rigorous individualized curriculum is generally the outcome. When educators and parents believe in students' potential to acquire and perform numerous skills, generally students rise to the occasion. This notion is referred to as the self-fulfilling prophecy and can have a profound effect on one's performance and motivation. Schools either open doors for students in terms of learning and opportunities or shut them out, reducing or eliminating their opportunities to learn and grow.

Assessment is unbiased, curriculum is meaningful to every student, and instruction is designed to make learning accessible for every student. Classrooms and schools that use a rich and multifaceted curriculum with creative and dynamic instructional strategies are more successful at implementing inclusive educational practices. Focusing on what students can do and how they learn provides essential information about what is needed to make learning accessible to every student. A curriculum that is age-appropriate and reflects students' cultural backgrounds and personal interests is more likely to motivate them as learners. In addition, instructional strategies that reflect students' learning needs and provide them with opportunities to be active participants in the learning process—that is, learning by doing, not by lecturing and having students do meaningless worksheets—are important components of successful inclusion for students.

A broad range of collaborative supports and services is offered. The supports needed for all students to reach their full potential can best be provided in a collaborative system where general and special educators, other specialists, parents, students, and friends each bring specific areas of expertise and experience to the process of defining needs and arranging supports to meet those needs. School personnel must make significant efforts to facilitate meaningful parent and family involvement by acknowledging parents' expertise and experience regarding the needs and abilities of their children, by allowing for variety in the types and amount of family involvement expected, and by being sensitive to the multiple demands that families must balance as they organize their daily routines.

These characteristics are not only reflective of successful inclusion strategies; they are also considered characteristics of good schools for all students. Invariably, too, these schools are in demand as popular educational settings by teachers, principals, parents, and, most important, students.

SECONDARY EDUCATION RESTRUCTURING

Inclusion is not merely dumping students with disabilities into ineffective general education classes where the instruction is didactic and students are expected to, for example, take notes, follow teacher directions, and demonstrate their knowledge base through multiple-choice examinations. In the 1980s, secondary schools have undergone extensive scrutiny, criticism, and efforts at reform as a result of declining academic standards, increased dropout rates, and deteriorating social values. The paragraphs following describe some components of this reform.

Block Scheduling and Creating Smaller Teacher–Student Units

Many secondary schools have divided their daily schedules into time blocks. Instead of teachers teaching five or six periods each day, they might, for example, teach two blocked periods within a team and one class outside of their team. Through block scheduling of core curriculum classes, the teacher-to-student ratio is reduced, in some instances by more than 50% (Sizer, 1992). Block scheduling has also increased opportunities and time for more personalized learning. The teachers, collaborating in teams, use an integrated approach to the curriculum.

Heterogeneous Grouping of Students

Secondary schools are also recognizing the need to group students heterogeneously, in order to encourage all students to focus on higher academic goals, to be prepared for postsecondary education, and to offer all students a solid and comprehensive curriculum. The all-too-frequent method of organizing students in secondary programs, referred to as *tracking*, has not been substantiated in the research as beneficial; on the contrary, many students have suffered negative effects when grouped homogeneously (Oakes, 1985; Sapon-Shevin, 1994). To create a community of learners that reflects the characteristics of the larger community in which they live, students should be taught in groups reflecting the range of abilities, ethnicities, languages spoken, economic status, and other factors within the entire community.

Active Learning Strategies

One of the most distinctive aspects in the secondary school reform movement has been an increased use of cooperative groups for teaching, demonstrating knowledge, and problem solving. Although use of cooperative groups has received substantial attention in the literature, much of the study has focused on the benefits of such an approach for elementary-age students (Johnson & Johnson, 1989; Putnam, 1993). Yet, the benefits for older students are just as pronounced (MacIver & Epstein, 1991). Cooperative groups are designed to teach students the skills of collaborating with others and of reaching common goals, which have been identified by employers as critical skills that workers need. Research has demonstrated that cooperative groups promote high academic achievement, improve self-esteem, promote active learning and social skill development, and influence peer acceptance and friendships (e.g., Johnson & Johnson, 1989; Slavin, 1990). In addition to using cooperative groups, many teachers have adopted a new view on intelligence that has enhanced their efforts to personalize instruction so that it is more meaningful to students, involving them in a variety of multiple intelligence strategies (Armstrong, 1987, 1994; Gardner, 1983). As teachers become more comfortable using a variety of active learning strategies, they also become more comfortable with students working on different levels, referred to as multilevel instruction. The concept is based on the premise that students do not learn the same way, at the same time, using the same materials (Falvey, 1995). Once teachers adopt this concept, strategies for responding to the multiple levels and needs of students can be established.

Authentic Assessment Based on Student Outcomes

A critical issue related to inclusion of students with diverse learning needs and abilities is that of assessment and grading. When students and teachers work closely together as a team using meaningful curriculum and instruction, a more in-depth and comprehensive knowledge of students' strengths, learning, and needs occurs. As a result, teachers are less likely to use standardized methods to assess student performance; instead, they assess skills in more authentic and ongoing ways. Assessment should not be designed to teach students how to take a test for the purpose of passing; rather, it should determine students' knowledge, understanding, and application of course objectives, in addition to determining students' future instructional needs. Authentic assessment, especially the use of multiple examples of exhibitions, is gaining in popularity and acceptability among educators, parents, and students (Darling-Hammond, 1991).

STRATEGIES FOR CREATING INCLUSION IN SECONDARY SCHOOLS

The restructuring efforts at the secondary school level just described can positively influence increased opportunities for inclusive education. In addition, educators, parents, and students have developed a number of strategies that have been used specifically to facilitate the inclusion of students with disabilities, particularly at the secondary level. A description of these specific strategies follows.

Determining Students' Needs Through Making Action Plans (MAPs)

Making action plans (MAPs) are discussion tools designed to help individuals, organizations, and families develop methods for moving into the future effectively and creatively (Falvey, Forest, Pearpoint, & Rosenberg, 1994; Falvey & Rosenberg, 1995). This process brings together the student, his or her friends and family, and other significant members of the student's circle. The participants are asked to collectively contribute to developing a plan to support the student in achieving his or her goals and dreams. A MAPs process can be a useful strategy at the beginning of each school year as new challenges and opportunities arise. The process focuses on the gifts and strengths of the individual student, while listening to and helping him or her to articulate hopes (and fears) for the future. Assumptions of a MAPs process should be that inclusive and heterogeneous communities are based on the premise that each person belongs, that each person can learn, and that in living we discover the truth and dignity of each individual student. Eight key questions are used in the MAPs process, and although all the questions must be asked, the order may be flexible based on group dynamics and contributions. The following are the six MAPs questions.

What is the student's history?
What are your dreams for this student?
What are your nightmares for this student?
What are the student's strengths, gifts, and abilities?

What are the student's needs?

What is the plan of action for the student to reach the dreams and avoid the nightmares?

MAPs have been held in classrooms, living rooms, school cafeterias, corporate board rooms, small offices, and so forth. A MAPs process is not a case conference or a traditional individualized education program (IEP) in which the student is the guest and the professionals are in control. The student, who has the most to gain or lose, is the focus person, and those who are significant to and have the most experience with that student come, participate, and contribute. These might include family members, friends, neighbors, and professionals who have a significant relationship with the focus student. The process leads to a plan of action to assist people to reach their dreams and avoid their nightmares. Such a plan is most likely to lead to positive changes when the student and his or her peers play an active role in planning.

Strategies for Making Learning Accessible

Systematic and organized teaching experiences that utilize multiple strategies to actively involve students are those most likely to succeed in teaching all students, including those with disabilities. In addition, providing learning opportunities in areas in which students do not have strengths will assist the student to broaden his or her learning and strategies for learning. Howard Gardner's book, *Frames of Mind* (1983), provides a theoretical framework for identifying multiple teaching practices based on individual students' learning strategies. The theory identifies seven areas of intelligence: spatial, musical, linguistic, logical or mathematical, bodily or kinesthetic, interpersonal, and intrapersonal. Traditional schools and classrooms have often valued only linguistic and logical or mathematical intelligence, ignoring students' strengths in others areas or relegating those strengths to art classes, music classes, or physical education classes. The focus should not be on how smart one is but, rather, on how one is smart; indeed, the multiple intelligence theory assumes that everyone is smart, but in different ways (Armstrong, 1987, 1994). Table 13.1 lists behaviors that might be looked for when determining a student's personal learning style. Table 13.2 lists suggested instructional approaches that educators can use once they are familiar with their students' personal learning styles.

Some students will need more specific assistance or additional or different supports than multiple instructional strategies can provide in order to learn. Accommodations are individualized supports that provide access to learning for students when multiple strategies are not enough. Accommodations do not result in changing the performance standards that peers without disabilities are expected to demonstrate. Accommodations simply

Table 13.1.   Multiple intelligences/personal learning style characteristics

Linguistic

- Like to write
- Spin tall tales or tell jokes and stories
- Have a good memory for names, places, dates, or trivia
- Enjoy reading books in spare time
- Spell words accurately and easily
- Appreciate nonsense rhymes and tongue twisters
- Like doing crossword puzzles or playing games such as Scrabble or Anagrams

Logical-mathematical

- Compute math problems quickly in their heads
- Enjoy using computers
- Ask questions like, "Where does the universe end?" "What happens after we die?" and "When did life begin?"
- Play chess, checkers, or other strategy games and win
- Reason things out logically and clearly
- Devise experiments to test out things they do not understand
- Spend lots of time working on logic puzzles such as Rubik's cube

Spatial

- Spend free time engaged in art activities
- Report clear visual images when thinking about something
- Easily read maps, charts, and diagrams
- Draw accurate representations of people or things
- Like the use of movies, slides, or photographs in educational context
- Enjoy doing jigsaw puzzles or mazes
- Daydream a lot

Musical

- Play a musical instrument
- Remember melodies of songs
- Tell you when a musical note is off-key
- Say they need to have music on in order to study
- Collect CDs, records, or tapes
- Sing songs to themselves
- Keep time rhythmically to music

Bodily-kinesthetic

- Do well in competitive sports
- Move, twitch, tap, or fidget while sitting in a chair
- Engage in physical activities such as swimming, biking, hiking, or skateboarding
- Need to touch people when they talk to them
- Enjoy scary amusement rides
- Demonstrate skill in a craft such as woodworking, sewing, or carving

Interpersonal

- Have a lot of friends
- Socialize a great deal at school or around the neighborhood
- Seem to be "street-smart"
- Get involved in after-school group activities
- Serve as the "family mediator" when disputes arise
- Enjoy playing group games with other children
- Have a lot of empathy for the feelings of others

Intrapersonal

- Display a sense of independence or a strong will
- React with strong opinions when controversial topics are being discussed

(continued)

Table 13.1.   (*continued*)

- Seem to live in their own world
- Like to be alone to pursue some personal interest, hobby, or project
- Seem to have a deep sense of self-confidence
- March to the beat of a different drummer in their style
- Motivate themselves to do well on independent study projects

From Gage, S.T., & Falvey, M.A. (1995). Assessment strategies to develop appropriate curricula and educational programs. In M.A. Falvey (Ed.), *Inclusive and heterogeneous schooling: Assessment, curriculum, and instruction* (pp. 65–66). Baltimore: Paul H. Brookes Publishing Co.; reprinted by permission.

mean that strategies used for learning or demonstrating skills or knowledge might be different. Accommodations may mean, for instance, *extending the time* for a student to take a test who, because of his or her learning disability, reads at a slower pace than his or her peers. The student may be given a study hall period to complete the test, or perhaps the student will take the work home to complete. *Technological or other adaptive devices* can also be considered accommodations for students with physical or learning disabilities. Adaptive devices range from the highly technical to those using minimal technology and are often portable (e.g., a laptop computer or electronic notetaker, a picture book, or an extended grabber for a student who needs help reaching things, to mention a few).

Accommodations might also involve providing students with additional supports. Personal supports can range from periodic checks on an individual student, continuous support for a specific activity (e.g., assisting with a student's personal care needs in the restroom), or continuous support across all activities. Student transitions (e.g., from one service delivery model to another, moving to a new school in a different community, or moving from elementary school to middle school or from middle school to secondary school) may require additional supports. Personal supports can be provided by same-age or older students, special or general education teachers, related services personnel, instructional or health care assistants, volunteers, or administrators. Peer supports are the most natural supports, often generating ideas for and creating the most effective supports.

Accommodations should be provided to students only when necessary to facilitate their learning. As students' skills become more proficient, the need for accommodations is reduced, and their use should be faded and, if possible, eliminated. Some students, however, will always require specific accommodations, and those should not be faded—only updated and modified as the curriculum and students' ages and needs indicate.

When accommodations are provided, care should be taken to assist both students with and without disabilities to use them in ways that ensure students' physical, social, and emotional inclusion in all activities. This may require teaching students not yet familiar with a particular accommodation about its use and purpose. Giving all students the opportunity to

Table 13.2.   Instructional approaches and strategies for seven areas of intelligence

Linguistic
- Saying, hearing, and seeing what needs to be learned
- Telling or listening to tales and stories
- Using tape recorders, taped stories, typewriters, word processors
- Creating newsletters, journal writing
- Using word problems
- Reciting math problems
- Using crossword puzzles or playing games that use words

Logical-mathematical
- Using concrete objects for teaching
- Using computers
- Allowing for experimentation, exploration of new ideas, and time to answer
- Using strategy games such as chess and checkers
- Enlisting student's involvement in developing a behavior management plan
- Using visual cues to teach, for example, a picture of a snake in the shape of an ''S''

Spatial
- Allowing student to be engaged in art activities, especially drawing and painting
- Teaching through images, pictures, and colors
- Using three-dimensional objects for teaching
- Using jigsaw puzzles or mazes
- Using student's ''daydreaming'' to create stories

Musical
- Teaching to play musical instrument
- Using rhythm and melodies
- Working with music playing in the background
- Using records or tape
- Singing songs, especially ones that have concepts or messages to teach

Bodily-kinesthetic
- Using tactile images and interactions to teach
- Moving, twitching, tapping, or fidgeting while sitting in a chair
- Providing opportunities to engage in physical activities, such as jumping, skipping, crawling, somersaulting
- Using patterns and computers
- Using the outdoors to teach, with students working out math problems or reading

Interpersonal
- Using mutual reading activities
- Reading to others and/or teaching others to read
- Using group problem-solving activities
- Facilitating involvement in after-school group activities
- Mediating when student disputes arise
- Playing group games with other children
- Using community volunteering to teach

Intrapersonal
- Providing opportunity for independent work
- Giving students answer sheets to do self-correcting
- Using high-interest reading materials
- Providing opportunity to be alone to pursue personal interest, hobby, or project

(continued)

Table 13.2. (*continued*)

* Providing cozy and private sections of the room
* Respecting and honoring individual differences and learning approaches
* Allowing for plenty of leisure reading time

From Falvey, M.A., & Grenot-Scheyer, M. (1995). Instructional strategies. In M.A. Falvey (Ed.), *Inclusive and heterogeneous schooling: Assessment, curriculum, and instruction* (p. 144). Baltimore: Paul H. Brookes Publishing Co.; reprinted by permission.

use accommodations in order to reduce any mystique about them can facilitate the social and emotional inclusion of students. For example, students who use communication picture books should be encouraged to share them with their peers, so that they can become more familiar and comfortable with this assistive form of communication.

Occasionally, a student, even given multiple teaching strategies and accommodations, is still unable to gain meaningful access to the curriculum and requires additional supports, referred to as *multilevel instruction. Multilevel instruction* is defined as providing students with individualized supports to facilitate their access to learning, including modifying the performance standards. Multilevel instruction thus provides students opportunities to participate, even if only partially. It can include

* Teaching the same curriculum but at a less complex level
* Teaching the same curriculum but with functional or direct application to daily routines of life
* Teaching the same curriculum but reducing the performance standards
* Teaching the same curriculum but at a slower pace
* Teaching a different or substitute, but related, curriculum

Multilevel instruction should be used in such a way that it involves the least intrusive modification possible. There will be students who have such significant learning needs that certain adaptations or modifications must be made to structure the learning task in order for them to succeed. Such modifications should not be used unless absolutely necessary, and should be faded as soon as possible so as not to limit students' possibilities.

To plan and organize the needs of a student using the strategies described here, a matrix can be used to indicate when students' IEP objectives will be addressed within the context of the general education schedule. In addition, the matrix provides the opportunity to identify which strategies will be used to facilitate the students' access to learning within each subject. Figure 13.1 provides a sample matrix for Carlos, a junior with Down syndrome who is included in his local high school.

CONCLUSIONS

This chapter has described pragmatic tools and strategies to facilitate the learning of diverse students in heterogeneous classrooms and schools. Still,

IEP objectives	Carlos's schedule						
	English	History	Math	Science	Band	Physical education	Lunch
Greet others	X	X	X	X	X	X	X
Read 50 new words	X	X		X			
Add and subtract two-digit numbers without carrying and borrowing		X	X	X			X
Type on a computer, with facilitation, one-page report/summary	X	X		X			
Demonstrate understanding of the value of $1–$5			X				X
Develop relationships and friendships with at least four peers	X	X	X	X	X	X	X
Demonstrate use of personal hygiene skills		X			X	X	X
Develop leisure skills				X	X	X	X

Figure 13.1.   Opportunities for Carlos to work on specific IEP objectives.

there are no easy recipes or formulas (Falvey, 1995). An individualized planning process must occur for each student that is collaborative across staff, students, and family members. Such collaborative planning offers the opportunity to identify, create, and provide students with the supplementary aides, supports, and services necessary for inclusive education to be meaningful and productive for all students.

Every student has the right to learn from his or her peers. In the context of inclusive education, *learning* means the core curriculum that all students have access to, as well as opportunities to develop friendships and relationships. Schools need to develop partners with students, their families, and the community. For example, David, a 16-year-old student with Down syndrome who had always attended a segregated school for other children with disabilities, moved to a community where inclusive educational practices were used at the local high school. Reluctantly, his mother agreed to enroll him, but she requested that after 3 months an IEP team meeting be held to evaluate his placement. At the 3-month IEP, David's mother tearfully said that, until his enrollment in the local high school, she had not known that David liked science. "How could anyone know if he liked science?" she asked. "He never had science; instead, he had 'special education curriculum,' which often excluded most aspects of the core academic curriculum."

REFERENCES

Armstrong, T. (1987). *In their own way.* Los Angeles: Jeremy P. Tarcher.

Armstrong, T. (1994). *Multiple intelligences in the classroom.* Alexandria, VA: Association for Supervision and Curriculum Development.

Biklen, D., Ferguson, D.L., & Ford, A. (1989). *Schooling and disability: Eighty-eighth yearbook of the National Society for the Study of Education.* Chicago: University of Chicago Press.

Brown v. Board of Education, 347 U.S. 483 (1954).

Cole, D.A., & Meyer, L.H. (1991). Social integration and severe disabilities: A longitudinal analysis of child outcomes. *Journal of Special Education, 25,* 340–351.

Costello, C. (1991). *A comparison of students' cognitive and social achievement for handicapped and regular students who are educated in integrated versus a substantially separate classroom.* Unpublished doctoral dissertation, University of Massachusetts, Amherst.

Darling-Hammond, L. (1991). The implications of testing policy for quality and equality. *Phi Delta Kappan, 73*(3), 220–224.

Education for All Handicapped Children Act of 1975, PL 94-142, 20 U.S.C. §§ 1400 *et seq.*

Falvey, M.A. (Ed.). (1995). *Inclusive and heterogeneous schooling: Assessment, curriculum, and instruction.* Baltimore: Paul H. Brookes Publishing Co.

Falvey, M.A., & Grenot-Scheyer, M. (1995). Instructional strategies. In M.A. Falvey (Ed.), *Inclusive and heterogeneous schooling: Assessment, curriculum, and instruction* (pp. 131–158). Baltimore: Paul H. Brookes Publishing Co.

Falvey, M.A., & Rosenberg, R. (1995). Developing and fostering friendships. In M.A. Falvey (Ed.), *Inclusive and heterogeneous schooling: Assessment, curriculum, and instruction* (pp. 267–283). Baltimore: Paul H. Brookes Publishing Co.

Falvey, M.A., Forest, M., Pearpoint, J., & Rosenberg, R.L. (1994). Building connections. In J.S. Thousand, R.A. Villa, & A.I. Nevin (Eds.), *Creativity and collaborative learning: A practical guide to empowering students and teachers* (pp. 347–368). Baltimore: Paul H. Brookes Publishing Co.

Ferguson, P., & Asch, A. (1989). Lessons from life: Personal and parental perspectives on school, childhood and disability. In D. Biklen, A. Ford, & D. Ferguson (Eds.), *Disability and society* (pp. 108–140). Chicago: National Society for the Study of Education.

Gage, S.T., & Falvey, M.A. (1995). Assessment strategies to develop appropriate curricula and educational programs. In M.A. Falvey (Ed.), *Inclusive and heterogeneous schooling: Assessment, curriculum, and instruction* (pp. 59–110). Baltimore: Paul H. Brookes Publishing Co.

Gardner, H. (1983). *Frames of mind.* New York: Basic Books.

Hollowood, T., Salisbury, C., Rainforth, B., & Palombaro, M. (1995). Use of instructional time in classrooms serving students with and without severe disabilities. *Exceptional Children, 61*(3), 242–253.

Individuals with Disabilities Education Act (IDEA) of 1990, PL 101-476, 20 U.S.C. §§ 1400 *et seq.*

Johnson, D.W., & Johnson, R.T. (1989). *Cooperation and competition: Theory and research.* Edina, MN: Interaction Books.

Kaskinen-Chapman, A. (1992). Saline area schools and inclusive community CONCEPTS (Collaborative organization of networks: Community, educators, parents, the workplace, and students). In R.A. Villa, J.S. Thousand, W. Stainback, & S.

Stainback (Eds.), *Restructuring for caring and effective education: An adminis-trative guide to creating heterogeneous schools* (pp. 169–185). Baltimore: Paul H. Brookes Publishing Co.

Lewis, M., & Rosenblaum, L.A. (1975). *Friendships and peer relations.* New York: John Wiley & Sons.

Lipsky, D.K., & Gartner, A. (1989). *Beyond separate education: Quality education for all.* Baltimore: Paul H. Brookes Publishing Co.

MacIver, D.J., & Epstein, J.L. (1991). Responsive practices in the middle grades: Teacher teams, advisory groups, remedial instruction, and school transition pro-grams. *American Journal of Education, 99,* 587–622.

Oakes, J. (1985). *Keeping track: How schools structure inequality.* New Haven, CT: Yale University Press.

Oberti v. Board of Education of the Borough of Clementon School District, 995 F.2d 1204 (3rd Cir. 1993).

Putnam, J.W. (Ed.). (1993). *Cooperative learning and strategies for inclusion: Cel-ebrating diversity in the classroom.* Baltimore: Paul H. Brookes Publishing Co.

Sacramento City Unified School District v. Rachel H., 14 F.3rd 1398 (9th Cir. 1994).

Sapon-Shevin, M. (1994). *Playing favorites: Gifted education and the disruption of community.* Albany: State University of New York Press.

Sizer, T. (1992). *Horace's school: Redesigning the American high school.* Boston: Houghton Mifflin.

Slavin, R.E. (1990). *Cooperative learning: Theory, research, and practice.* Engle-wood Cliffs, NJ: Prentice Hall.

Stainback, W., & Stainback, S. (Eds.). (1990). *Support networks for inclusive schooling: Interdependent integrated education.* Baltimore: Paul H. Brookes Pub-lishing Co.

Stainback, S., Stainback, W., & Forest, M. (Eds.). (1989). *Educating all students in the mainstream of regular education.* Baltimore: Paul H. Brookes Publishing Co.

Strain, P. (1983). Generalization of autistic children's social behavior change: Ef-fects of developmentally integrated and segregated settings. *Analysis and Inter-vention in Developmental Disabilities, 3*(1), 23–34.

Straub, D., & Peck, C. (1994). What are the outcomes for nondisabled students? *Educational Leadership, 52*(4), 36–40.

Thousand, J.S., Villa, R.A. & Nevin, A.I. (Eds.). (1994). *Creativity and collabo-rative learning: A practical guide to empowering students and teachers.* Balti-more: Paul H. Brookes Publishing Co.

Villa, R.A., & Thousand, J.S. (1995). *Creating an inclusive school.* Alexandria, VA: Association for Supervision and Curriculum Development.

Villa, R.A., Thousand, J.S., & Rosenberg, R.L. (1995). Creating heterogeneous schools: A systems change perspective. In M.A. Falvey (Ed.), *Inclusive and het-erogeneous schooling: Assessment, curriculum, and instruction* (pp. 395–414). Baltimore: Paul H. Brookes Publishing Co.

14

Secondary Education

Planning for the Future

H.D. Bud Fredericks

As the young person with Down syndrome approaches the high school years, the student and his or her parents face a myriad of choices regarding the type of secondary school program that the student prefers, as well as his or her thoughts about the future beyond high school. This chapter examines a number of those potential choices and the implications of each.

Prior to discussion of such choices in this chapter, it is important to define the purpose of the high school educational program. Simply stated, high school should help the student prepare for what lies beyond high school in the adult world. For some students, high school provides the preparation and groundwork necessary for further studies, whether at a 4-year college, a 2-year college, or advanced vocational training. For other students, high school constitutes the end of their academic preparation, and, upon graduation, they expect to enter directly into the world of work. Few students entering high school have a clear vision of what they want their futures to be in terms of school, work, or living situation. Moreover, this vision does not necessarily become clearer as the secondary program progresses. Nevertheless, most students endeavor to make choices that conform to their academic and personal interests and that help pave the way for their future, however dimly envisioned.

FUTURES PLANNING

For adolescents with Down syndrome, planning for the future is vitally important in order to keep their options open (see also Chapter 13). Some techniques have been developed to assist students and their parents to think about the future and to design the high school program accordingly. One of these techniques, futures planning or mapping, tries to help the student conceptualize what he or she wants in the future relative to school, work, living situations, and social relationships. Mapping should be done before the student enters high school. Decisions reached at this stage should then be reexamined yearly and altered, if necessary, as the student acquires new skills or interests. Who participates in this futures planning? Certainly, the student should have the main voice, assisted by his or her parents, teachers, friends, other relatives, case managers or service coordinators, and anyone else closely associated with him or her.

Many communities have individuals trained to facilitate a futures planning meeting, and, if available, they should be used. However, anyone who is sensitive to the person with Down syndrome and is skilled at drawing out information from groups can act as a facilitator. Wall charts on which pictures, words, and diagrams can be placed are useful to help the group move through the process.

The mapping process will vary depending on the facilitator. However, the end result should be similar in all cases—a vision of the future that includes five major areas—education, residential living, work, peer social relationships, and recreation. Numerous questions are pertinent to each area. For instance: Does the student wish to continue his or her education beyond high school? If so, what will be studied? Where? Where would the student like to live—with his or her parents or in his or her own apartment, house, duplex, or group home? With whom would he or she like to live if not with parents? How can this be paid for? Does someone need to investigate alternatives and get back to the group in the future? What kind of work would the student like to do upon graduating from high school? (Unless the student has had some vocational experience, this will be a difficult area to discuss. The student may have formulated some ideas from watching television or talking to adults about their jobs.) The facilitators can assist the student by asking questions such as whether the student likes to work indoors or outdoors (weather conditions of the anticipated geographic area should thus be considered). Also, does the student like to work with people, or would a more solitary type of job be preferable? Does he or she like to move around, or would a sedentary job be preferred? These types of questions will elicit choices. The group then needs to consider who will help the student find a job, who will train the student, and who will monitor the student's progress. Also, how much support will the student need on a job?

The facilitator proceeds to ask similar questions for each major area. No attempt should be made to discourage dreams, but reality checks may be necessary. For instance, Jonathan (not his real name), a student in Oregon, wanted to live in a beach house on the Oregon coast. It was explained to him that such a house would probably cost between $300,000 and $500,000. He should keep his dream, but until sufficient money could be raised, what would be another alternative? The young man now lives in half of a duplex with an apartment mate without disabilities, but he still has his dream and has accepted the fact that the only way he will ever achieve it will be to win the state lottery—so, every week, he buys one chance at the lottery.

The process of futures planning should be carefully and sensitively done. It usually takes about 3 hours. Sometimes, to complete the initial planning, two sessions are necessary. A summary of the proceedings is prepared. Each year while the student is in high school, the process should be repeated in order to review previous decisions and alter the plan based on the student's new interests or new information about resources available to adults in the community where the student chooses to live.

It is often a good idea during the last 2 years of high school to invite adult residential and vocational agencies to send representatives to the futures planning meeting. They can provide valuable information about what services are available and about the possibilities for obtaining those services. Even if they are unable to provide services to the youth when he or she graduates, they may be able to suggest ways in which the student can achieve his or her desires.

When each year's futures plan is completed, the student and his or her parents are ready to choose what they want to happen in the high school experience. If we return to the assumption that high school prepares one for life after high school, then the futures plan should dictate the secondary school program and activities. The five areas considered in the futures planning process are also the five areas around which choices will need to be made in high school. These are academic curriculum, life or functional skills to prepare for residential living, employment/vocational training, recreational activities and extracurricular undertakings, and social relationships with peers. Decisions made in each of these areas will determine the type of high school program developed. These areas are discussed in turn, on the pages following, with additional subsections on the transition years and community college.

Inclusion and Supported Education

In addition to developing a high school curriculum that will meet the needs of the student, choices need to be made as to the degree of inclusion of the child in the general high school program. The high school curriculum and the question of inclusion are not separate issues, but are inextricably bound together, depending on the choices made. Although this author favors the concept of inclusion and insisted on his son with Down syndrome being included in a general education program before the word *inclusion* became part of educational parlance, he believes that the quality of education is the primary consideration and that some instruction can, if necessary, be effectively delivered in a noninclusive setting. This is especially the case in some high schools where there is a shortage of special education aides and resistance by some general education teachers to include students with disabilities in their classrooms.

For a student to be included in general education classes, there must be adequate supports to ensure that the student benefits from such a placement. Some students in some classes will need no supports and will function independently and effectively. Within other classes, students may need one or more of a variety of supports such as a teaching assistant, modified materials, or a peer tutor.

Placement within each class in the high school program needs careful analysis to determine the student's capabilities vis-à-vis the course requirements. This analysis, which should be conducted with both special and general education teachers during the individualized education program (IEP) process, will determine the type and degree of support necessary. As stated, this support will vary depending on the course and the expectations of what the student will learn during the course.

Parents should look askance at any support system that is uniformly prescribed across courses. This can happen when the IEP process has not thoroughly examined the needs of each class. Tailoring the support to each educational class or school environment is now frequently referred to as supported education. Supported education delivers the amount of support necessary for the student to achieve effectively in a given educational endeavor and can vary from modified materials to an individual teaching assistant. The concept of supported education follows logically from the practices of supported employment and supported living. Both of these now widely accepted practices tailor the support needed on the job or in the residence to the individual's competencies.

If during the IEP process the parents, the adolescent, and the rest of the IEP team decide that placement in certain general classes will not provide an appropriate education because of the lack of adequate supports, the parents certainly can insist on the provision of such supports in order to achieve a satisfactory placement in inclusive classes. In some instances, schools may balk at meeting the parents' demands. If so, the parents are then faced with deciding whether to continue efforts to achieve the included placement or to accede to the school's designated placement.

Parents who choose to demand an inclusive setting with appropriate supports despite a school's refusal may have to seek outside assistance such as a federally funded parents' organization, a local or state association for citizens with retardation, or other parents within the school who feel the same way. If these types of intercessions do not change the school's refusal, the parent always has the options of insisting on mediation and possibly taking legal action.

Some parents may accept the school's decision that included opportunities are not available in certain curricular areas for the student. If so, the student may be placed in a special education setting for certain instructional periods of the day. In such a situation, the student may be placed in a resource room or in a separate class for students with disabilities. In either such placement, the parent must ensure through the IEP process that the coursework presented to the student is what the parent and the student desire.

Academic Considerations

The term *academic* can be broadly or narrowly defined. For purposes of this discussion, this author defines it narrowly to refer to traditional coursework such as language arts, social studies, mathematics, and science, in addition to courses such as home economics, music, art, in-school vocational training, and physical education.

To what degree should a secondary student with Down syndrome take academic courses such as language arts, social studies, mathematics, and science? The answer depends on which of these academic subjects are deemed appropriate and desirable for the student. Many parents encourage their child to continue to expand his or her abilities in mathematics, reading, and writing. High school classes in these subjects can accommodate students with disabilities. In rare instances, the student can cope with the curriculum being offered without support. More often, the general education teacher, with the assistance of a special education consultant, can modify the curriculum so that the student can attend the general class but complete coursework more suited to his or her ability level.

It is also possible that a separate curriculum with materials appropriate to the student's abilities can be delivered within a general classroom that is focusing on the same academic area. Some general education teachers have the ability to teach the student with this curriculum without assistance; more often, however, additional classroom help is needed. This can be provided by a teaching assistant or a peer tutor.

For instance, a student's IEP indicates that she is to be provided instruction in reading so that her grade-level proficiency in reading will continue to improve. This curricular objective was chosen because the youth likes to read and does so for recreational purposes. The futures planning group and the IEP team have determined that continued instruction in reading competency is appropriate so that she can enhance her reading ability and thereby take advantage of a wider range of reading materials. The IEP team determines that the instruction could be delivered in a language arts class with a particular teacher who has in the past been effective with students with disabilities. The special education consultant, together with the parents and the student's previous teachers, selects materials appropriate for the student. The general education teacher and the consultant determine when the student can participate fully in the materials being presented to the class, when she can work independently, and when she needs the assistance of a peer tutor (chosen from volunteers within the class who take turns assisting the student). Each volunteer works with the student on an average of once every 3 weeks. As a result of these combined efforts, not only do the student's reading abilities improve but through the system of peer tutors, she widens her social contacts within the school.

It should be noted that the same instruction could have been delivered in a special education class. However, the student might not have felt welcomed as an integral part of the general education program and might not have had an opportunity to increase social contacts within the school.

In academic areas in the high school such as home economics, in-school vocational training, art, music, and physical education, accommodations for the student with disabilities seem to be made more easily than in traditional academic subjects such as mathematics, science, and language arts. For instance, most home economics teachers already have in their collection of materials programs that have been carefully task analyzed and can be used with minimal modification for the student with disabilities. Many vocational training instructors are also willing to forgo the required book learning in their courses to give a student with Down syndrome the opportunity for "hands-on" vocational experience such as in the woodworking or automobile mechanics class.

Functional Curriculum

A functional curriculum can also be referred to as a life skills curriculum. Frequently during the futures planning session, parents begin to realize the large number of skills needed by their adolescent to eventually live in his or her own apartment or in any type of independent or semi-independent living situation. They further realize that much learning will need to occur if the adolescent is to achieve that goal of independence. If parents reflect at any length on the situation, they can easily feel overwhelmed for their son or daughter.

At that point what is needed is a system of inventorying skills for the student. Such a system has been developed by Petersen, Trecker, Egan, Fredericks, and Bunse (1983). This program identifies skills present and skills absent across a number of curricular domains and offers a method for prioritizing the missing competencies. Table 14.1 shows the domains covered within the system, which encompass most of the skills needed to function independently in the community and to live a full life. Table 14.2 lists specific skills contained, for instance, within the domain of food preparation.

If functional skills are deemed important for the student with Down syndrome, parents, together with the adolescent, should undergo the assess-

Table 14.1.   Domains for skill assessment purposes

Communication	Community mobility
Social	Personal information
Sexual awareness	Money management
Personal hygiene	Time management
Dressing	Meal planning, shopping, and storing
Clothing care and selection	Food preparation
Eating	Leisure skills—home based
Home and yard maintenance	Leisure skills—community based
Health and safety	

ment process recommended by Petersen et al. (1983). Those authors have prepared forms for checking off those skills that the student has and those that are needed. Many of the skills can be taught at home, if parents have the time, skill, and inclination to do so. Others can best be taught within the school. For instance, most of the skills for food preparation shown in Table 14.2 can be taught within a home economics class. The opportunity to practice them at home would be ideal.

Table 14.2.   Food preparation

Prepares work area and self for cooking
Cleans food when necessary
Peels and grates food
Dices food with knife
Cleans up spills
Opens and closes various types of containers
Prepares food from recipe
Prepares food from can/box
Sets and cleans table
Scrapes and rinses dishes
Washes dishes by hand so they are clean and sanitary
Dries dishes or stacks in drying rack
Cleans kitchen after use
Operates dishwasher
Stores food left over from meal
Prepares five different nutritionally balanced breakfasts
Prepares five different nutritionally balanced lunches
Prepares sack lunch
Prepares dinner using prepackaged foods
Prepares five main dishes suitable for evening meal
Prepares frozen vegetables
Prepares two different salads
Prepares two side dishes of pasta, potatoes, or rice

Case Study: Jonathan

It was the goal of Jonathan (the student with Down syndrome mentioned earlier in the chapter) and his parent that after graduation he would live in his own apartment with some staff supervision. It was determined that one of the skills Jonathan would need would be to prepare his own meals. In addition, he would have to learn how to shop, budget his money for food, pick out the best food buys, and then store the food appropriately. Through a combination of general education programs, special education resources, and parental participation, Jonathan's instructional goals were realized.

Jonathan participated in a series of home economics classes through which he became proficient at cooking. The teacher already had some materials that were task analyzed, and modifications were made to other materials to meet Jonathan's needs. He also learned about food groups and good nutrition.

Since Jonathan was still living at home, he worked with his mother to determine weekly menus and what food would need to be purchased to prepare the meals; he also developed a shopping list. At school he spent two periods a week in the special education resource room, where he would examine the local newspaper for food specials that matched his shopping list. A special education teaching assistant would then accompany him to the store 1 day a week to make his purchases during the last 2 hours of school, noting carefully price comparison and nutritional content of food items. On the day of shopping, Jonathan's parent would send money with him for the food purchases. Jonathan's parent would meet the student and teaching assistant at the store to pick up the student and groceries. They would return to the parent's house where the student would store the food in the appropriate places.

This program was carefully orchestrated to allow Jonathan to become proficient at cooking, menu planning, budgeting for food purchases, shopping, and food storage. After graduation, Jonathan did move out of his parent's home into his own apartment with some staff supervision and, as mentioned earlier, subsequently moved into a duplex where he lives with an apartment mate without disabilities. He continues to budget, shop, store food, and cook.

Vocational Training

The term *vocational training* typically denotes two different types of options for high school students. The first is that of the traditional vocational education course, which includes such things as woodworking or automotive mechanics. Formerly computer classes might also have been included, but today computer technology is so pervasive that it is no longer considered a vocational course but a necessary life skill.

The other type of vocational training available to students with disabilities is placement in a job in the community with a vocational trainer while the student is still in school. Not all schools offer this curricular option. Among schools that do provide community-based vocational training, the program usually is offered during the last 2 years of school of a 4-year program. (This author recognizes that many youth with disabilities can attend school in most states until they are 21; the options for those additional school years are discussed in a subsequent section of the chapter.)

During the first year in which the student is enrolled in the community-based vocational training program, he or she is placed in a job in the community for about an hour a day. During the second year, and in subsequent years for students who attend school beyond the 4 years of high school, the amount of time spent in a community job is usually increased to 2 hours a day. A vocational trainer accompanies the student to the job, teaches job skills on site, and also teaches associated work skills or social skills. Figure 14.1 is an example of an associated work skills checklist together with an example of the assessment conducted on one student (Fredericks et al., 1987; see also Chapter 19).

While the student is in the vocational program, every effort is made to provide him or her with a series of different employment experiences, some working inside, some working outside, some working with people, some working alone. The purpose, of course, is not only to observe the student's performance in different types of work situations but also to assist the student to ascertain which types of jobs he or she would prefer after graduation. One high school program had more than 50 different community placements that included restaurants, veterinary clinics, banks, plumbing and electrical establishments, the local fire department, a university, and numerous miscellaneous shops and businesses.

The decision to have a student participate in in-school vocational training is not difficult. Students may express an interest in a particular curricular offering, and it can generally be fit into the student's school program fairly easily, becoming, in essence, just another course. The decision to have the student participate in a community-based vocational training program may be more problematic. There are advantages and disadvantages to such participation. Some parents feel that because the program removes the student from school for a period of time each day, valuable experiences will be lost, such as opportunities to socialize with peers or courses that the parent feels are more important for the student. Still others perceive the community-based programs as merely another form of segregated special education, and therefore they do not want their child to participate.

Associated Work Skills Checklist

Student: John Jones _____ Placement: Animal Hospital _____

Date: 2-1-97 _____ Contact Person: Jim Healer _____

	Has skill	Needs training	Location				
			School	Home	Community	Work	Other
Work-Related Behavior							
1. Checks own work	√					√	
2. Corrects mistakes		√					
3. Works alone without disruptions for specified periods with no contact from supervisor / teacher		√				√	
4. Works continuously at a job station for specified amount of time	√					√	
5. Safety a. Uses appropriate safety gear	√					√	
b. Responds appropriately during fire drill	√					√	
c. Follows safety procedures specific to classroom / shop	√					√	
d. Wears safe work clothing	N.A.						
e. Cleans work area		√				√	
f. Identifies and avoids dangerous areas	√					√	
g. Responds appropriately to emergency situation (sickness, injury, etc.)	√					√	
6. Participates in work environment for specified periods of time		√				√	

(continued)

Figure 14.1. Associated work skills checklist and sample student assessment.

Figure 14.1.   *(continued)*

	Has skill	Needs training	Location				
			School	Home	Community	Work	Other
7. Works in group situation without being distracted		√				√	
8. Works faster when asked to do so		√				√	
9. Completes work by specified time when told to do so		√				√	
10. Time management: a. Comes to class/work for designated number of times per week	√					√	
b. Arrives at class/work on time	√					√	
c. Recognizes appropriate time to take break or lunch	N.A.						
d. Recognizes appropriate time to change task		√				√	
e. Returns promptly from: i. Break	N.A.						
ii. Restroom	√					√	
iii. Lunch	N.A.						
f. Uses time clock/clock appropriately	N.A.						
11. Observes classroom/shop rules		√				√	
12. Does not leave workstation without permission	√					√	
Mobility/Transportation 1. Takes appropriate transportation to and from school/work	√		√			√	

(continued)

Figure 14.1. *(continued)*

	Has skill	Needs training	School	Home	Community	Work	Other
			Location				
2. Locates workstation/ desk	✓					✓	
3. Locates bathroom	✓					✓	
4. Locates break/ lunch area	✓					✓	
5. Locates locker or coat area	N.A.						
6. Moves about class/ work environment independently	✓					✓	
Self-Help / Grooming Independently:							
1. Dresses appropri- ately for school/ work	✓			✓		✓	
2. Cleans self before coming to school/ work	✓			✓			
3. Cleans self after us- ing restroom	✓		✓			✓	
4. Cleans self after eating	N.A.						
5. Shaves regularly		✓	✓	✓			
6. Keeps hair combed	✓			✓			
7. Keeps nails clean	✓			✓			
8. Keeps teeth clean	✓			✓			
9. Uses deodorant	✓			✓			
10. Bathes regularly	✓			✓			
11. Cares for menstrual needs	N.A.						
12. Cares for toileting needs	✓		✓	✓		✓	
13. Eats lunch and takes break	N.A.						
14. Washes before eating	N.A.						
15. Brings lunch/snack independently	N.A.						

(continued)

Figure 14.1. *(continued)*

	Has skill	Needs training	Location				
			School	Home	Community	Work	Other
16. Operates vending machine	N.A.						
17. Uses napkin independently	N.A.						
18. Displays appropriate table manners	N.A.						
Social Communication							
1. Communicates basic needs, such as							
a. Thirst	√					√	
b. Hunger	√					√	
c. Sickness	√		√	√		√	
d. Toileting needs	√			√			
2. Does not engage in							
a. Self-stimulatory or self-abusive behavior	√		√				
b. Aggressive/ destructive behavior	√		√				
c. Self-indulgent (attention-getting) behavior	√		√				
3. Engages in relevant, appropriate conversation		√	√			√	
4. Responds calmly to emotional outbursts of others	√		√				
5. Talks about personal problems at appropriate times	√		√	√			
6. Refrains from exhibiting inappropriate emotions at school/ work	√		√			√	
7. Refrains from bringing inappropriate items to school/ work	√		√			√	

(continued)

Figure 14.1. *(continued)*

	Has skill	Needs training	Location				
			School	Home	Community	Work	Other
8. Refrains from tampering with or stealing others' property	✓		✓			✓	
9. Responds appropriately to changes in supervisors/teachers		✓				✓	
10. Interacts with co-workers/students at appropriate times		✓			✓		
11. Responds appropriately to social contacts such as ``hello'' or ``good morning''		✓			✓		
12. Initiates greetings appropriately		✓			✓		
13. Ignores inappropriate behaviors/comments of co-workers/students	✓		✓			✓	
14. Refrains from inappropriate sexual activity at school/work	✓		✓			✓	
15. Laughs, jokes, and teases at appropriate times		✓	✓			✓	
16. Responds appropriately to strangers	✓		✓			✓	
17. Approaches supervisor/teacher appropriately when							
a. Needs more work		✓					✓
b. Makes a mistake he or she cannot correct	✓					✓	
c. Tools or materials are defective	✓					✓	
d. Does not understand task		✓				✓	
e. Task is finished	✓					✓	
f. Disruption has occurred	✓					✓	
g. Sick	✓					✓	

(continued)

Figure 14.1. *(continued)*

	Has skill	Needs training	School	Home	Community	Work	Other
18. Complies with supervisor's/teacher's requests in specified period of time	✓					✓	
19. Responds appropriately to correctional feedback from supervisor/teacher	✓					✓	
20. Responds appropriately to changes in routine		✓				✓	
21. Follows instructions	✓					✓	

The advantages usually cited by both professionals and parents are that the community-based vocational experience is the best preparation for the world of work. Transition to paid employment after graduation is easier if the student has had vocational experience while in high school. In addition, proponents of such training cite the fact that the student who is working in the community acquires new social opportunities with fellow workers. Students who have participated in such a program seem to increase their self-esteem and maturity.

Probably the greatest advantage of community-based training is the opportunity to teach associated work skills to the student in an adult setting. The skills on the associated work skills checklist (Figure 14.1) are considered to be among the most important for the adolescent to acquire and to carry into adulthood, especially those listed under "Social Communication." Although the skills were designed to identify effective interaction with others in the workplace, most of them apply to interactions with others in all environments.

Clearly, community-based vocational training has both advantages and disadvantages for the student. Parents and the student will need to weigh carefully those considerations as they decide whether to participate in such a program.

Socialization

When most people look back on their secondary school years, they remember their friends and the social experiences those years provided. Such opportunities should also be available for the student with Down syndrome. In fact, the participation in social activities and the opportunities to develop friendships should be an integral part of the student's school program and should be reflected in his or her IEP.

Proponents of full inclusion cite opportunities for social interaction as an important aspect of inclusion. Certainly the truth of their claim has been demonstrated repeatedly. However, merely placing a youth in a general education setting will not ensure that social relationships develop. Usually two things must occur in order for social relationships to develop for the student with Down syndrome. First, the students without disabilities must become familiar with the student's disorder and with the limitations that it imposes on the student. Even more important, however, students without disabilities need to learn about the *capabilities* of the student with Down syndrome. They also need to know that students with disabilities have the same emotional and social needs that they do.

The second condition that usually breeds successful social relationships is the formation of a circle of friends (Haring, Breen, Pitts-Conway, Lee, & Gaylord-Ross, 1984; Meyer & Putnam, 1988). In such an arrangement, students without disabilities are recruited to be friends of the student with disabilities. As this group becomes more familiar with the student with disabilities, natural friendships emerge and the student with disabilities becomes included in many of the social activities of his or her new friends.

Parents can help facilitate, maintain, and strengthen social relationships. First, as with all young secondary students, parents become the chauffeur, transporting their child to school events. They also agree to give rides to his or her friends. Second, they can invite their son's or daughter's friends to their home for such things as pizza parties or slumber parties.

Recreational Activities

Whereas socialization activities in the elementary school revolve around the student's classroom, at the middle and secondary school levels socialization also occurs in the halls as students move from class to class; in the lunchroom; in the student lounge; and within all the after-school activities such as clubs, sports, and special school events. For students with Down syndrome to be totally involved in the school and to enhance their opportunities for social relationships, involvement in after-school activities should be strongly encouraged. The activity, of course, needs to be something in which the student is interested.

For instance, one young girl whose parents took her to numerous stage plays and musicals was fascinated with the theater. During the futures planning meeting, she indicated that she wanted to be an actress. The meeting facilitator suggested that she might want to join the drama club at the high school and become involved with the high school productions.

With the help of a school counselor, she did join the club and was active in all the productions, working on costumes, scenery, acting as an usher, and being part of the chorus in a musical. Her social life in school revolved around the drama club, and she became good friends with a number of the club's members.

In another example, a boy with Down syndrome had played Little League baseball when he was young. The coordinator of the Little League program was also the high school baseball coach, and so when the youth entered high school the coach approached him and asked if he would like to be manager of the high school baseball team. He accepted and for 4 years was the team's manager, for which he received a school letter each year. His socialization group during his high school years revolved around the school's athletes, who included him in many of their social activities (see also Chapter 23).

The Transition Years

As indicated previously, many students with disabilities can remain in school until they are 21 years of age, and in some states even longer. Many schools have established transition programs for these years. Included in these programs are such things as vocational training, functional or life skills training, and preparation for residential living (the more sophisticated programs include all three aspects).

For instance, one school district had as part of its holdings a home that had previously housed part of the school administration. They converted these offices back into a traditional home with three bedrooms, a living room, and a dining area. During the day, this home became the center for the transition program. Vocational trainers would pick up students, take them to community jobs, train them on the job, and also teach them associated work skills. Students were rotated across a number of jobs to help them determine which type of work they liked. There was also close coordination with adult vocational agencies in the community and with the local Vocational Rehabilitation Office in an effort to secure paying positions for the students when they left the transition program (see also Chapter 18).

While some students were working, others were receiving instruction in functional living skills, tailored to their needs. These skills included such things as food and clothes shopping, food storage, cooking, home maintenance, and even more basic skills such as grooming and personal hygiene.

In the late afternoon and evening, the center became a home for three students. Students would live in the home for 4 nights, preparing evening meals, deciding on evening entertainment, preparing breakfast, doing laundry, and maintaining the home as their own. These experiences were designed so that the students could practice skills learned, and the staff could assess the students' remaining functional skills needs.

Certainly, such a program is the ideal for preparing a student to leave school and enter the adult world. But even without such an ideal arrangement, these transitional years should be used to help students practice vocational and functional living skills. Many schools have also encouraged students in the 18- to 21-year-old age group to take advantage of courses offered in community college while they continue their high school education.

Community College

Community colleges offer a variety of courses suitable for students with Down syndrome, such as computer classes (many of which are self-paced) or courses in photography, music, theater, physical education, dance, and art. Moreover, most community colleges now have a special education department that assists students with placement in various courses and also provides tutorial assistance for some courses or note takers and readers for students. In addition, many of these special education departments offer courses in functional skills. Community college courses can provide skills to students with Down syndrome not only during the transition years but also throughout their lives (see also Chapter 16).

Role of the Parent

Most secondary school students prefer that their parents do not visit the high school or observe in classes. In fact, most would be utterly embarrassed should such an event occur. Yet, parents who have visited high schools have found the experience worthwhile and beneficial for their children.

For instance, one father visited the school during lunch hour and spied his son sitting alone eating lunch. Because one of the his son's IEP goals was to increase opportunities for socialization with peers, the father mentioned to the principal of this small school that it might be nice if the two of them could arrange for his son to have some company at lunch. The matter was easily handled. The principal knew many students who liked the boy and suggested to them that they invite him to sit with them. On subsequent visits to the school by the father, the boy was sitting with other boys and was actively engaged in conversation.

School administrators usually see parents only when students are in trouble in school. The experience of having parents visit the school (by prior arrangement) to observe or discuss the program is unusual, and most administrators have welcomed the opportunity to better acquaint parents with the high school and help them determine whether their son or daughter is fitting in. Indeed, most high school administrators would welcome close ties with more parents, since they believe that such opportunities for communication benefit the students.

CONCLUSIONS

For the student with Down syndrome to have a successful, enjoyable, and productive secondary school experience, a number of decisions need to be carefully made by the student and his or her parents. A futures plan that focuses on the student's desires in education, residential living, vocation, socialization, and recreation can assist in making these decisions. In fact, the futures plan can guide the entire high school curriculum.

REFERENCES

Fredericks, B., Covey, C., Hendrickson, K., Deane, K., Gallagher, J., Schwindt, A., & Perkins, C. (1987). *Vocational training for students with severe handicaps.* Monmouth, OR: Teaching Research Publications.

Haring, T., Breen, C., Pitts-Conway, V., Lee, M., & Gaylord-Ross, R. (1984). *The effects of peer tutoring and special friends experiences on nonhandicapped adolescents.* Unpublished manuscript, San Francisco State University, San Francisco.

Meyer, L., & Putnam, J. (1988). Social integration. In V. B. Van Hasselt, P. Strain, & M. Herson (Eds.), *Handbook of developmental and physical disabilities* (pp. 107–133). New York: Pergamon.

Petersen, J., Trecker, N., Egan, I., Fredericks, B., & Bunse, C. (1983). *The teaching research curriculum for handicapped adolescents and adults: Assessment procedures.* Monmouth, OR: Teaching Research Publications.

15

The Computer as
a Tool for Learning

Joan Tanenhaus

Computers can be a powerful learning tool throughout the lives of people with Down syndrome. Along with other work and life experiences, the computer has the potential to contribute to lifelong learning in many respects (e.g., reading and mathematical skills): in specific subject areas relating to social studies or science; in general knowledge and vocabulary development; in motor skills; in eye–hand coordination; in memory strategies; and in critical thinking skills, to mention but a few. With the computer, learning can be in a recreational format that is fun while also helping to develop independence and a positive self-image. Computers are highly motivational: They allow individuals to be in control; they build self-confidence and self-esteem; they provide the much-needed opportunity for repeated success; and they allow users to learn at their own rate, competing only with themselves.

One of the reasons computers are such compelling learning tools for youngsters with Down syndrome is that computers are such visual devices. Pueschel (1987) has shown that children with Down syndrome have fewer difficulties with visual-motor and visual-vocal processing than with auditory-motor and auditory-vocal processing. Computers, with their strong visual information and with their ability to accompany auditory information with visual feedback, are an excellent way to teach to the child's preferred learning style and to his or her individual strengths. At the same time, the computer presents strategies for learning to the weaker auditory area with speech, sounds, and verbal information (see Figure 15.1).

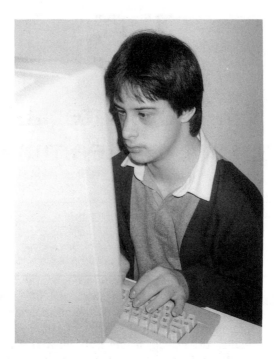

Figure 15.1. Michael, age 15, uses the computer independently for school work and for recreation.

GENERAL PRINCIPLES

The ultimate worth of the computer as an instrument for learning lies in the selection of proper hardware and software; in the effective introduction and modeling of the computer as a learning tool by creative therapists, teachers, and parents; and in its integration with other learning and experiences.

When first introduced, the computer may be used as an interactive tool, with the student and teacher or student and parent working together. The student interacts directly with the computer and the adult is there to guide, to direct, to explain, to model, to question, and most of all, to enhance the experience.

Computer learning is most effective when integrated with other learning. Software should be selected so that language and vocabulary reflect learning in other education settings. It is always important to consider the motor and perceptual skills required to use the particular software. The computer experience can also be enhanced if pictures and other materials are printed out from the software programs and off-computer activities are created. Books and other learning games that deal with the same vocabulary and concepts that are in the software programs will help to generalize the learning. The computer will not replace any other material or techniques; it just adds another tool for learning.

When the student with Down syndrome has acquired basic computer skills (e.g., how to turn on the computer, how to use the mouse, how to open and close a file), he or she will be able to use some programs independently. Parents should also continue to purchase software that needs guided learning at first and can be used independently after a while.

Guided learning stretches students' learning, because students can buy more advanced programs that need to be mastered before independent use. During the period of guided learning, the student and parent can work together to develop strategies, understand computer routines, figure out the program's objectives, learn keyboard shortcuts and input requirements, and so forth. The adult, along with the student, can prepare a guided learning instruction sheet (see Figure 15.2), which gives step-by-step instructions to master the task. Together, the adult and the student can review the sheet to be sure the user can understand and follow the instructions. If the sheet is prepared as a word processing document of a talking word processor, then the learner can call up the document and hear the instructions read aloud.

SELECTING A COMPUTER

When trying to decide what kind of computer to buy, the purchaser must always consider the software that is needed and the adaptive equipment that might be necessary. The first big decision to make when purchasing a computer is whether to select an IBM-compatible or a Macintosh-compatible computer. In general, as of this writing, this decision is becoming less critical. For adolescents, most software and much adaptive equipment are available for both platforms. (Some exceptions to this are discussed in the upcoming section on special access issues.) However, two other factors to consider are cost and complexity of operating the equip-

---

Super Munchers (MECC)
1. Double click the Super Munchers icon on the hard drive.
2. Click Practice to play without score, or click Play for a regular game.
3. Choose a category by clicking once on it. Click OK.
4. Select a level, then click OK.
5. Read the title. That tells you the category you are looking for. If you cannot read the word, click Pause while you look it up in the list you made, or ask someone for help. When you know what the word is, click Continue.
6. Look for all the words that fit into the category. Click once to go to the box; click again to choose it.
7. If you need to get away from a Troggle, go to a box with brackets. Click only once to hide there until the Troggle moves away.
8. To take a break, you can always click the Pause box.
9. To end the game, go to the File menu, click and drag to highlight End Game.

Figure 15.2.   Sample guided learning instruction sheet.

ment. IBM-compatibles, the business standard, are often more reasonably priced; at the same time, they are more complex to use than the Macintosh. Macintosh-compatibles, the educational standard, may be slightly more expensive, but they are easier to use and often have fewer problems with compatibility issues. If purchase of a secondhand computer is being considered, such as the Apple IIGS, the buyer should be aware that obtaining software may be a problem. More important, the software is more of the drill-and-practice type and not the newer, more open-ended, creative-learning software that is available for the IBM-compatible and Macintosh. Speech output is also not as natural sounding, and graphics and animation are less sophisticated. The Apple IIGS is a discontinued computer, and no more software will be published for it. However, sometimes the Apple IIGS is available at minimal cost (under $250) and may be worth considering as a beginning computer if the budget is limited, especially if educational software is included in the price.

If a new multimedia system is being purchased, the following should be included:

1. A family should try to purchase as much RAM (random access memory), hard-drive space (storage space), and speed as they can afford.
2. A CD–ROM drive (i.e., Compact Disk–Read-Only Memory), which is a data storage medium that resembles audio CDs (i.e., compact discs). Its advantages are large memory capacity and durability, in contrast to the more conventional data disks that are magnetic. Quad- to eight-speed CD-ROM drives are now becoming the standard in the industry and should be considered the minimum speed to purchase. Most new software is now appearing on CD-ROM instead of on older floppy data disks.
3. A sound card (necessary only for IBM-compatibles, because the sound capabilities are built into the Macintosh-compatible). This card is placed inside the computer and gives it the capacity for speech output, speech input, and enhanced sound quality.
4. A printer (color, if possible).
5. A modem—optional, but definitely worth considering. A modem is a device that lets the computer communicate and exchange information with other modem-equipped computers over telephone lines (see later section, "Surfin' the 'Net").

Figure 15.3 contains a checklist of questions that can be helpful in determining which computer platform (IBM or Macintosh) is optimal for you and your family.

Potential buyers should visit local computer stores and try out different computers. They can also visit local users' groups to gather more information. If there is a computer resource center, an Alliance for

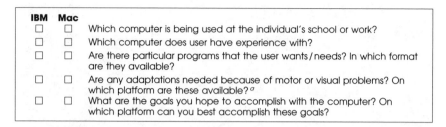

IBM	Mac	
☐	☐	Which computer is being used at the individual's school or work?
☐	☐	Which computer does user have experience with?
☐	☐	Are there particular programs that the user wants/needs? In which format are they available?
☐	☐	Are any adaptations needed because of motor or visual problems? On which platform are these available? [a]
☐	☐	What are the goals you hope to accomplish with the computer? On which platform can you best accomplish these goals?

Figure 15.3.   Choosing a computer platform. ([a] See section in text on "Special Access Issues.")

Technology Access Center, or a United Cerebral Palsy Center in the area that has computers, adaptive equipment, and software on loan or display for individuals with disabilities, these are good resources to contact or visit. Often different computers, programs, and adaptive equipment are available to be tried. Computer magazines, both general and model-specific, may offer good ideas and answer technical questions. Most of all, the buyer should not be pressured to make a fast purchase. Time spent looking always adds to general knowledge and to a more informed decision. Computer novices should consider purchasing their computers from a store that will be able to give ongoing support and assistance when difficulty is experienced. Mail-order prices may be slightly cheaper, but the lack of support makes them more expensive in the long run. A local dealer who can be visited easily and who is willing to spend time with the new user is often the better choice.

SPECIAL ACCESS ISSUES

If the individual with Down syndrome has motor, visual, cognitive, or attention difficulties that prevent the use of the standard keyboard or standard-size monitor, this can often be remedied with special adaptive equipment that is available for both IBM-compatibles and Macintosh-compatible computers (see Figure 15.4). This section briefly discusses some adaptive components.

Single Switches

If a severe motor impairment prevents the young person with Down syndrome from using his or her hands to gain access to the computer, many types of single switches are available to be used with any part of the body that the individual can control. Pressing and releasing these switches signals a response to the computer. Used together with hardware or software interfaces such as Ke:nx (manufactured by Don Johnston Inc.), Cross-Scanner (manufactured by R.J. Cooper), ClickIt! (manufactured by IntelliTools), or WinSCAN (Academic Software), complete computer access is available. CrossScanner, a software option, is available for IBM and

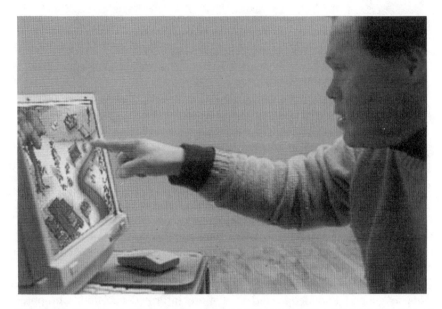

Figure 15.4. Using Touch Window and specialized language-learning software. (Courtesy of Laureate Learning Systems, Winooski, Vermont.)

Macintosh. Ke:nx and ClickIt! are available only for Macintosh-compatible computers, and WinSCAN is for Windows only.

Touch Window

A Touch Window (manufactured by Edmark) (see Figure 15.4) is a touch-sensitive screen that allows users to control the computer by touching the screen rather than using a keyboard. All Macintosh programs and Windows programs for Macintosh- and IBM-compatible computers that use the mouse (a palm-size device for controlling the cursor on the display screen) are 100% compatible with the Touch Window.

IntelliKeys

IntelliKeys (manufactured by IntelliTools) is an expanded keyboard that lets the student use customized keyboards (see Figure 15.5). For example, if a program uses only the four arrow keys and space bar, only those keys will be visible and usable. The icons representing these keys will be larger, spaced farther apart, and, therefore, easier to press. If full keyboard access is necessary, another overlay on IntelliKeys presents all the keys in larger sizes. IntelliKeys is available for both Macintosh and IBM, as is Overlay Maker (IntelliTools), which is used to create and customize one's own keyboard overlays. However, to create overlays for programs that are

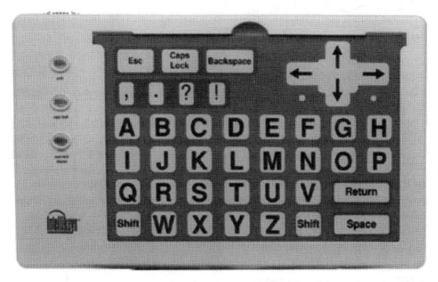

Figure 15.5.   IntelliKeys expanded keyboard with alphabet overlay. (Photo courtesy of Intelli-Tools, Novato, California.)

mouse-driven and have no keyboard equivalents, ClickIt! (IntelliTools) is needed but is available for Macintosh only.

Trackball
Software that uses a mouse places a cursor on the screen. The mouse is used to move the cursor and to select it. It is often more manageable for students to use a trackball rather than a mouse. The trackball is stationary and allows for separate movements to move the cursor and press the mouse button. (The standard mouse moves around the table and then has to be held in the exact position while the click-button is pressed to make the selection.) Trackballs are available for both IBM and Macintosh and are available at all computer stores.

Keyguards
Keyguards (manufactured by Don Johnston Inc.) are designed to fit over the keyboard to isolate the keys, making it easier for people with limited fine motor control to independently make selections without hitting the wrong keys. They are available for both Macintosh and IBM platforms and for different keyboards.

Mouse Emulation
If the user is unable to use the mouse but can use keys on the keyboard, he or she can use the built-in mouse emulation feature of the Macintosh

to move the cursor. This option is also available with IntelliKeys (discussed earlier) for both the IBM and the Macintosh platforms. Windows95 also has mouse emulation.

Screen Enlargement
Macintosh has a built-in screen enlarger, Close View, that may be helpful for people with vision impairment.

Assisted Keyboard
If a computer user is unable to press several keys simultaneously (as when one needs to press Control-Alt-Delete or Control-Command-Reset to restart the computer), the Assisted Keyboard mode allows the user to do this with consecutive key presses. The feature is also helpful for the individual who can use only one hand. Assisted keyboard is available on all Macintoshes, in Windows95, and with IntelliKeys (discussed previously) for both the IBM and the Macintosh.

SEATING AND POSITIONING
Seating and positioning at the computer is an important issue. The user should be seated in a comfortable chair, with his or her feet on the floor with a knee angle that is approximately 90 degrees. If the table height is such that a higher chair is necessary, a foot support of some kind can be used so that the feet rest on it and the knee angle is maintained. The monitor needs to be at eye level, at a comfortable viewing distance. If there is a visual impairment, a CRT Terminal Valet might be considered. This allows the computer monitor to be clamped onto a platform that can be brought closer or farther away, depending on the program's output. Keyboard height should support a comfortable arm position. If there is any unusual positioning (e.g., head tilted all the way up or down, arms elevated), computer placement should be reevaluated. Consultation with an occupational therapist may be helpful. Lighting needs to be bright enough so that the computer screen can be seen easily, but care must be taken to prevent glare on the screen. This needs to be examined during different hours of the day, since daylight and night lighting differ. There should also be adequate light on the keyboard or adaptive equipment. If external speakers are used, one should be placed on each side of the computer so that sound is heard bilaterally.

GENERAL GUIDELINES IN SELECTING COMPUTER SOFTWARE
Software should be appropriate in concepts and vocabulary to the user's age and skill level. Look for clear graphics and easy-to-read text. When educational programs are selected, make sure that rewards for correct responses are interesting and motivating. It is helpful if options such as

speed, sound, varied content, amount of repetition, length of activity, level of difficulty, type of reinforcement, and so forth can be controlled. Look for programs that have authoring capabilities in which the user's own vocabulary, spelling words, mathematics problems, and so on can be entered for individualized work. Look for an instructional manual that also includes suggestions for related, off-computer activities. Always try to review the programs before purchase or try to locate a dealer who will allow returns if the software is not appropriate. Table 15.1 provides a list of questions to ask in reviewing software.

It is easy to see the educational value of programs that provide drill and practice for specific mathematics, reading, and spelling skills. Become aware, also, of the educational and social benefits of some games and of art and music programs. Think about how these software programs might help receptive and expressive language skills, eye–hand coordination, spatial concepts, turn taking, problem solving, sequencing, and so forth. Other areas to consider are development of independence, attention span, and motivation.

When reviewing software, look for the following positive qualities:

1. Open-endedness, which provides an opportunity to explore and think things out
2. Graphics, animation, and sound that provide excitement and motivation and encourage increased attention span and focus
3. Humor

Table 15.1.   Software review questions

---

1. Is the program easy to use and understand? Is it easy to get in or out of an activity at any point? Is the installation procedure straightforward and easy to do? Are there any extra hardware requirements (i.e., a sound card, CD-ROM, etc.)? Are printing routines simple?
2. Does the user have the skills needed to use it?
3. Is it fun, interesting, and motivating?
4. Does the program provide a range of activities so that it can be used over a period of time and still be fun and interesting? Can the user select from a range of difficulty levels?
5. Is the feedback clear? Does it employ meaningful graphic and sound capabilities? Does it reinforce content and guide learning when necessary?
6. Does the program have authoring capabilities (can vocabulary and mathematics levels be entered)?
7. Is the quality of the speech good, and is the vocabulary level appropriate?
8. Is the program free of stereotypes, gender, and ethnic biases? Does it express positive values?
9. Does the program take advantage of the computer's unique abilities? Are random generation techniques employed, so activity is not always the same?
10. What is the overall value—how much does it cost in relation to what it does?

4. Portrayal of positive values
5. A sense of control over the program

There are now specialized collections of public domain software for education and language learning (e.g., Technology for Language and Learning). These are free programs with only a minimal per-disk charge for duplicating, and they offer an excellent and inexpensive way to expand one's computer software collection.

Again, whenever possible, *try before you buy.* Ask for a 30-day review from software companies, request the right to return the software if it is inappropriate to individual needs, or visit a computer resource center or a user's group. Table 15.2 is a resource list of software programs of high quality that may be of interest and value to adolescents with Down syndrome. The companies that produce this software can provide more details as well as their catalogs. This is only a list of suggestions—there are many other programs of great value, with new ones appearing almost daily. At the end of this chapter, the Appendix contains a list of computer resources, including software and hardware references and organizations that can supply information about computer use with adolescents with Down syndrome.

SUGGESTED ACTIVITIES WITH ADOLESCENTS

The following is a brief description of the types of activities that the adolescent with Down syndrome can do with the computer:

1. *Language:* To encourage the development of increased vocabulary skills, a program like Word Attack 3 (published by Davidson) can be used. In this program, the parent or teacher can enter the specific words, definitions, and sentence examples. The program then places those words (both visually and auditorally) into various game and puzzle-type activities, providing opportunities for the learning to be integrated and generalized. Other language-oriented programs include Super Munchers (published by MECC), in which players have to identify all things that belong to a certain category (i.e., sports figures, holidays, presidents, cities) in a PacMan-type game. The faster the players can read and identify the target, the more points they get. This same game format is available for other language and reading skills and vowel identification (i.e., find all the words that have a long *a* sound—in Word Munchers Deluxe [published by MECC]). Story books that are read aloud are also an excellent source of language, reading, and vocabulary development. They are accompanied not only by the spoken and written text but by animations, movie clips, photographs, and so on. Visual and learning materials enhance the reading experience and relate it to other learning—examples include books

Table 15.2. Suggested software to enhance goals

Reading / Language
Alien Tales (Broderbund Software Inc.)
Interactive Movie Books (Sound Source)
GrammarGames (Davidson and Associates)
Laureate Learning Software
Living Books (Broderbund Software Inc.)
Merriam-Webster's Dictionary for Kids (Mindscape)
Reading Maze (Great Wave)
Super Solvers Midnight Rescue (The Learning Company)
Super Solvers Spellbound (The Learning Company)
Treasure Mountain (The Learning Company)
Word Attack 3 (Davidson and Associates)
Word Blaster (Davidson and Associates)
Word City (Sanctuary Woods)
Super Munchers (MECC)
Word Munchers Deluxe (MECC)

Writing
Children's Writing / Publishing Center (The Learning Company)
Co:Writer (Don Johnston Inc.)
Hollywood (Theatrix)
Imagination Express (Edmark)
IntelliTalk (IntelliTools)
Keroppi Day Hopper (Big Top)
Once Upon a Time (Compu-Teach)
Opening Night (MECC)
Spellevator (MECC)
Storybook Weaver (MECC)
Student Writing Center (The Learning Company)
Student Writing & Research Center (The Learning Company)
The Amazing Writing Machine (Broderbund Software Inc.)
Write Out Loud (Don Johnston Inc.)

Mathematics
Logical Journey of the Zoombinis (Broderbund Software Inc.)
Math Blaster Mystery (Davidson and Associates)
Math Munchers Deluxe (MECC)
Math Workshop (Broderbund Software Inc.)
Mighty Math Series (Edmark)
Snootz Math Trek (Theatrix)
Super Solvers Outnumbered (The Learning Company)

Visual-Perceptual Skills
Highlights Puzzlemania (Graphix Zone)
Lost & Found (GTE)

Social Studies
Africa Trail (MECC)
Amazon Trail (MECC)
Carmen Sandiego Series (Broderbund Software Inc.)
Nigel (Lawrence)

Science
Bumptz Science Carnival (Theatrix)
Gizmos & Gadgets (The Learning Company)
Magic School Bus Series (Scholastic)
Ozzie programs (Digital Impact)
The Incredible Machine (Sierra On-Line)
Widget Workshop (Maxis)

(continued)

Table 15.2. *(continued)*

General Information
Compton's Interactive Encyclopedia (Compton's)
Grolier's Encyclopedia (Grolier)
Super Munchers (MECC)
Talking Academic Quiz Kid (Orange Cherry)

Time Management and Organizational Skills
Datebook Pro (After Hours)
In Control (Attain)
What Are You Doing Today, Charlie Brown? (Individual)

Recreaton
KidPix (Broderbund)
Mario's Fundamentals (Interplay)
Print Shop (Broderbund)
Top Secret Decoder (Houghton Mifflin Interactive)

Art and Music
Blocks In Motion (Don Johnston Inc.)
Flying Colors (Davidson)
Origami (Casady & Greene)
Print Shop (Broderbund)
Stationery Store (Davidson)

Sports
Guinness Book of World Records (Grolier)
NFL Math (Sanctuary Woods)
Sports Illustrated for Kids (Creative Multimedia)

Memory
Memory Building Blocks (Sunburst)

Reasoning and Thinking / Problem Solving
Logic Quest (The Learning Company)
Museum Madness (MECC)
Secret Island of Dr. Quandry (MECC)
Sim Town (Maxis)
Strategy Games (Edmark)
Thinkin' Things 1, 2, & 3 (Edmark)

published by Broderbund (e.g., some *Living Books, Alien Tales*), Sound Source (e.g., *Black Beauty, Lassie*), and Disney (e.g., *The Lion King, Pocahontas*).

2. *Articulation and Linguistic Skills:* Meyers (1988) has shown how computer word processing programs with synthesized speech output can give students with Down syndrome opportunities to develop an understanding of the sound patterns of words and sentences and to help them improve their articulation and linguistic skills. Programs such as "IntelliTalk" (published by IntelliTools), "Kid Works" (published by Davidson and Associates), and "Write Out Loud" (published by Don Johnston Inc.) are talking word processors that can be used for this purpose. As the children input to the computer, the letters, words, and sentences appear in written form on the screen and are

spoken aloud. Talking word processors can be used to do homework from school, to write journals, to do reports and school projects, and so forth.

3. *Mathematics:* Drill-and-practice mathematics programs allow the student with Down syndrome to repeatedly practice basic mathematics facts. Rewards are present for correct responses, tutorial help is there for wrong answers, and record-keeping options let the student track progress over time. For word problems and more abstract mathematics activities, programs like the Super Solver series (published by The Learning Company) put the mathematics activities in an adventure game context. Solving the problems allows the player to access special clues, hints, and options that help solve the adventure.

4. *Social Studies:* For help learning about the United States (e.g., cities, states, locations, important facts), the "Carmen Sandiego Series" (published by Broderbund) is invaluable. A thief has stolen a national treasure (i.e., the Statue of Liberty), and the task is to follow the thief around the country until he can be caught. To do this, players learn state locations, important facts, logical thinking skills, sequencing, and so forth, in a totally nonviolent situation. In "Nigel" (published by Lawrence), a similar program, players assume the role of a photographer. They get an assignment to photograph places, landmarks, people, or animals around the world. With each assignment, they have to find new locations. The program begins very simply and increases in difficulty as the player learns.

These are only a few areas and examples of computer-enhanced learning. The possibilities are endless, depending on the child's interest; the skill level; and the academic, cognitive, language, and social areas being addressed. Each new day brings new software programs and new learning challenges.

SURFIN' THE 'NET

One of the new and exciting things that can be done with a computer and a modem is to go online, either on the Internet or on one of the commercial online services and take advantage of the many opportunities and services provided. Parents can read about medical issues, browse through the libraries of many online disability groups, or chat live with other parents.

The easiest way to get onto the Internet is through membership in one of the commercial online services, such as Prodigy (800-PRODIGY), America On-Line (800-827-6364), and CompuServe (800-848-8199). The following sections may give the reader an idea of some of the features of the Internet.

E-mail

E-mail is electronic mail. It can be used to send messages; ask questions; contact and correspond with pen pals; share information and opinions with users around the world through mailing lists; communicate with television stations, local radio stations, and magazines; and so on. An e-mail address is obtained by joining a commercial online service or getting an Internet provider. The following are some of the special mailing lists and e-mail addresses of interest:

- National Down Syndrome Congress: ndsc@charitiesusa.com
- DOWN-SYN@vm1.nodak.edu (discussion group on Down syndrome)
- The Arc: thearc@metro.com (formerly, Association for Retarded Citizens of the United States)
- Apple Computer information: webmaster@apple.com
- listserv@bitnic.educom.edu (contact them for a mailing list of mailing lists)
- Alliance for Technology Access: atafta@aol.com
- Technology for Language and Learning: ForTLL@AOL.com (contact them for information about public domain software and shareware for special needs)

Bulletin Boards

To connect with a bulletin board service (BBS), all that is needed is a modem, a telephone line, and software that comes with the modem. Internet access or commercial online services are not necessary for these numbers. Just follow the modem's program instructions and type in the BBS numbers as follows:

- Able Inform (301-589-3563)—databases, bulletins, files, and information from Abledata, resources for people with disabilities
- Disability Works (303-989-6156)—bulletins geared to advocacy

Chat Rooms

Chat rooms give people sitting at their computers the amazing capacity to type messages that other users see on their computer screens—instantly. Conversations are held in real time, as though the person were in the room. Instead of talking, people type one sentence at a time back and forth to each other. There are chat rooms on all the commercial online services. America On-Line has chat rooms for individuals with disabilities, as well as several Down syndrome chat sessions, including "Inclusion Chat" and a "Sibling Chat." Check also for forums on CompuServe and Prodigy.

World Wide Web

More and more companies and organizations are setting up home pages on the World Wide Web (WWW) of the Internet. A home page is an online source for learning about the mission, services, and other resources available. The Internet and WWW can now be accessed through most of the commercial online services or directly through a local service provider. The home page of Down Syndrome Listserv includes links to other Internet resources including local Down syndrome associations, parental support resources, disability resources, and medical resources. The Uniform Resource Locator (URL) (i.e., the Internet address) for this Web site is http://www.nas.com/downsyn/.

Web sites related to specific topics can be searched using browsers such as Yahoo (http://www.yahoo.com/) or the WebCrawler (http://www.webcrawler.com/). Other WWW sites specific to Down syndrome are

- http://www.carol.net/~ndsc/ (National Down Syndrome Congress)
- http://www.macroserve.com/ACDS/ACDShome.htm (Association for Children with Down Syndrome)
- http://www.Webwiz.com/downsyndrome/ (Down Syndrome Organization of South Nevada)

CONCLUSIONS

The computer has the potential to provide continued learning and recreational experiences to adolescents with Down syndrome. In addition, it can provide them with opportunities for independent play, peer interaction, and creative expression. It is important that the hardware and software be carefully chosen so that the cognitive and motor demands are within the user's abilities and so that they provide activities of interest that are motivating and at the same time challenging. In addition, the Internet provides access to other resources and information regarding technology and how it can be used now and in the future.

REFERENCES

Meyers, L.F. (1988). Using computers to teach children with Down syndrome spoken and written language skills. In L. Nadel (Ed.), *Psychobiology of Down syndrome* (pp. 247–265). Cambridge, MA: MIT Press.
Pueschel, S.M. (1987). Visual and auditory processing in children with Down syndrome. In L. Nadel (Ed.), *Psychobiology of Down syndrome* (pp. 199–216). Cambridge, MA: MIT Press.

SUGGESTED READINGS

Alliance for Technology Access. (1994). *Computer resources for people with disabilities.* Alameda, CA: Hunter House.
Flippo, K.F., Inge, K.J., & Barcus, J.M. (Eds.). (1995). *Assistive technology: A resource for school, work, and community.* Baltimore: Paul H. Brookes Publishing Co.
Sussman, M., & Loewenstein, E. (1993). *Total health at the computer.* Tarrytown, NY: Station Hill Press.

Tanenhaus, J. (1991). *Home based computer program for children with Down syndrome: Computer software guide.* New York: National Down Syndrome Society.

Tanenhaus, J. (1995a). Computer learning in early elementary and postsecondary education. In L. Nadel & D. Rosenthal (Eds.), *Down Syndrome: Living and learning in the community* (pp. 197–203). New York: Wiley-Liss.

Tanenhaus, J. (1995b). DISKoveries. *Closing The Gap,* October/November, pp. 10–12.

Tanenhaus, J. (1995, December). Monitor. *Long Island Parenting News,* pp. 26–28.

Tanenhaus, J. (in press). *Computers: Tools for lifelong learning.* East Rockaway, NY: Technology for Language and Learning.

Appendix

Resource List

Organizations

Apple Computer	800-776-2333
Closing The Gap	507-248-3294
Council for Exceptional Children	800-CEC-READ
IBM	800-426-4832
National Lekotek Center	800-366-PLAY
RESNA	703-524-6686
Technology for Language and Learning	516-625-4550
The Arc	817-261-6003
Trace Research & Development	608-262-6966

Adaptive Equipment

AbleNet	800-322-0956
Academic Software	606-233-2332
Don Johnston Inc.	800-999-4660
Edmark Corporation	800-426-0856
IntelliTools	800-899-6687
R.J. Cooper & Associates	800-RJCooper
Sima Products Corp.	800-345-7462
TASH	905-686-4129

Software Companies

Attain	617-776-1110
Berkeley Software	510-540-5535
Broderbund Software, Inc.	800-521-6263
Casady & Greene	408-484-9228
Compton's New Media	619-929-2500
Compu-Teach	800-448-3224
Creative Multimedia	800-262-7668
Creative Wonders Electronic Arts	800-245-4525
Davidson and Associates	800-556-6141
Digital Impact, Inc.	800-775-4232
Discovery Channel	301-986-0444
Disney Software	800-688-1520
Dr. T's Music Software	617-455-1454
Graphix Zone	800-828-3838
Great Wave Software	408-438-1990
Grolier Interactive	800-285-4534
Grypon Software Corp.	800-795-0981
GTE Interactive Media	619-431-8801
HarperCollins Interactive	212-207-7462
Hartley Courseware	800-247-1380

Houghton Mifflin	800-733-7075
Humongous Entertainment	206-486-9258
Image Smith	310-325-1429
IMSI	415-257-3000
Individual Software	800-822-3522
Inroads Interactive	303-444-0632
Interplay	714-553-6655
IVI Publishing	800-952-4773
Laureate Learning Systems	800-562-6801
Lawrence Productions	800-421-4157
The Learning Company	800-852-2255
MacPlay / Interplay	714-553-6655
Maxis	510-927-3709
Mayer-Johnson Co.	619-550-0084
MECC	800-685-6322
Merriam-Webster, Inc.	800-201-5029
Microfax	800-676-3110
MindPlay, Methods & Solutions, Inc.	800-221-7911
Mindscape, Inc.	415-883-3000
National Geographic Society	202-828-5664
Nordic Software, Inc.	402-488-5086
Optimum Resource, Inc.	800-327-1473
Orange Cherry Software	800-672-6002
Parrot Software	800-727-7681
Random House, Inc.	212-751-2600
Sanctuary Woods	415-286-6000
Scholastic	800-541-5513
Sierra On-Line, Inc.	800-757-7707
Simon & Schuster Interactive	212-698-7000
Sound Source Interactive	805-494-9996
StarPress, Inc.	800-782-7944
Sunburst Communications, Inc.	800-321-7511
Theatrix Interactive	510-658-2800
Voyager Company	212-431-5199

16

Beyond High School

Postsecondary Education as a Transition Outcome

Elizabeth Evans Getzel
Karen F. Flippo
Katherine Mullaney Wittig
Douglas L. Russell

For many students with disabilities, postsecondary education provides an opportunity for further training and career preparation. Yet, for students with mental retardation, postsecondary education is not often tried or considered as a potential postschool outcome (Page & Chadsey-Rusch, 1995). Wagner (1989) reported that 14% of all students with disabilities attended postsecondary programs. Students with mental retardation were included in this group, yet had the second-lowest participation rate, at approximately 6%.

Postsecondary education programs are offered in a variety of settings including trade or business schools, vocational-technical schools, community colleges, and specialized training in business and industry (HEATH Resource Center, 1989; Wille-Gregory, Graham, & Hughes, 1995). Identifying potential training and education programs in the community is an important step in learning about the types of opportunities available to students with Down syndrome.

Careful consideration must be given to whether postsecondary education is an appropriate postschool goal for the adolescent involved. Long-range planning for the student with Down syndrome should include a discussion of all potential postschool goals, including participation in postsecondary programs. Because of the overall lack of participation in postsecondary programs by students with mental retardation, further research is needed to determine the outcomes or benefits of their participation (Page & Chadsey-Rusch, 1995). Students with Down syndrome who could benefit from the training or education that programs offer and from the social interaction with their peers should have the option of attending these programs beyond high school.

This chapter provides an overview of postsecondary education program options for adolescents with Down syndrome within the individualized education program (IEP) transition-planning process. Information is provided about who should be involved on the transition team, methods for exploring postsecondary programs, and the role of assistive technology in postsecondary education. A case study is also included to illustrate the planning process for investigating postsecondary programs with students with Down syndrome.

TEAM MEMBERS FOR POSTSECONDARY TRANSITION

The Individuals with Disabilities Education Act (IDEA) of 1990 (PL 101-476) identifies certain individuals who must attend IEP meetings (IDEA § 300.344). These participants are the student's teacher, a representative from the local education agency, parents, students, representatives from any other agency that is likely to be responsible for providing or paying for transition services, and other individuals who are identified by the parents or local school division. Each team member provides an important contribution to the planning process in determining appropriate postsecondary education programs for youth with Down syndrome. Examples of some of their contributions are described next.

Secondary School Staff Participation

Secondary school staff must identify the necessary skills and services that students will need to successfully enter postsecondary education programs. A primary barrier inhibiting students with disabilities from making successful transitions into advanced programs is the failure to develop or employ IEPs to clarify objectives and needed skills (Sarkees & Scott, 1985). It is particularly important that school staff become knowledgeable about postsecondary opportunities and support services because this transition option is not often considered for individuals with mental retardation (Page & Chadsey-Rusch, 1995). Secondary school personnel play a key role in developing curricula to strengthen the skills students need to make successful transitions into postsecondary settings (Boyer-Stephens, 1990). Some planning activities can begin in middle school with teachers, parents, and students developing IEP goals that reflect the requirements needed for postsecondary training (Brown-Glover, 1992).

Student Participation

It is important that students take an active role in their own educational planning. The IEP transition-planning process offers youth with Down syndrome an opportunity to develop an awareness of their strengths and needs and an opportunity to practice articulating their interests, aspirations, and choices. Self-awareness, self-advocacy, and independence contribute to feelings of self-determination (West, Barcus, Brooke, & Rayfield, 1995). Assisting students in developing self-advocacy skills as they prepare for their postsecondary education provides them insights about themselves and an understanding of how their training or education relates to future employment.

Family Participation
In selecting postsecondary education settings, families play a critical role. Families are influential in helping their children determine their career and lifestyle options (Morningstar, Turnbull, & Turnbull, 1995). Finances, achievement expectations, and perceptions of the degree of independence that their child exhibits are all factors in educational choices for students. For families of youth with disabilities, promoting skills of self-determination and perseverance for their son or daughter is an important part of the transition-planning process (deFur, Getzel, & Trossi, 1996). These skills need to be reinforced at home and at school. For example, choice making and decision making could be included in all aspects of a student's life, including decisions about after-school activities, clothes, meals, and the student's school schedule (West, Gibson, & Unger, 1996).

School Counselor Participation
Another important member of the transition team is the school guidance counselor. With postsecondary education as the primary transition goal, secondary transition planning may overlook the need for career guidance (deFur et al., 1996). However, career guidance services can help students with Down syndrome and their families understand what postsecondary options can best meet their needs.

School guidance counselors can assist the transition team in working with students to develop career goals and in helping to develop a framework for postsecondary education plans. Without an overall context provided by a career objective, the transition team may be restricted in its ability to identify specific supports and services in order for students to achieve their goals (deFur, Getzel, & Kregel, 1994). A study conducted to explore the experiences of students with mental retardation attending postsecondary education found that participants' IEPs contained no specific objectives under the goal of attending the local community college (Page & Chadsey-Rusch, 1995). Page and Chadsey-Rusch (1995) found that the absence of specific IEP objectives resulted in a lack of coursework at the community college related to future employment. Guidance counselors can help the team assist students to explore career goals and the type of experiences needed during high school to prepare them for postsecondary programs.

Vocational Instructor Participation

If students have participated in vocational education classes, the instructors can provide specific information about the training and skills the students have received. They can also provide information about the types of programs available in the community and about what students will need to prepare for further training in a postsecondary setting.

Vocational Rehabilitation Counselor Participation

Vocational rehabilitation counselors are another essential team member in transition planning, helping to obtain necessary future services and supports while students are in high school (Getzel & Kregel, 1996). Some of the services or supports that could be provided include 1) assistance for attending some postsecondary schools, 2) special equipment or assistive technology devices to assist in postsecondary education, 3) assistance with transportation or independent living needs, or 4) information for financial planning (Wehman & Revell, in press).

Community Representative Participation

Other team members necessary for effective transition planning are community representatives from community college and vocational schools. Although these representatives do not typically attend transition-planning meetings (deFur et al., 1994), they can provide an important link to postsecondary education settings by informing transition team members about the services and supports offered and about how best to meet the students' needs while attending their programs.

DETERMINING APPROPRIATE POSTSECONDARY PROGRAMS

Careful study must be made of the availability of postsecondary education programs for students with Down syndrome and of the programs' ability to meet the academic, social, and emotional needs of these students. As stated previously, postsecondary education and training can occur in a number of settings, including private schools, business and industry, or community colleges (Schloss, 1984).

When considering postsecondary programs, information and resources should be identified to assist in the decision-making process. Often learning about best practices in the area of transition for students with Down syndrome can help determine which programs are most appropriate. Ideas about trends in postsecondary programming can be obtained by contacting universities and asking questions about their practices and projects. Other ideas for collecting information or developing ties with community programs include 1) contacting area private industry councils to learn about training opportunities through the Job Training Partnership Act (JTPA;

1982) (PL 97-300), 2) learning about nationally funded projects to develop resources for best practices in vocational preparation and in the transition from school to postsecondary education settings, and 3) identifying resources to assist in locating postsecondary programs with established education and training opportunities for students with disabilities. One resource is the HEATH Resource Center, National Clearinghouse on Postsecondary Education for Individuals with Disabilities (Getzel, 1990).

LEARNING ABOUT POSTSECONDARY PROGRAMS

It is important to learn as much as possible about the postsecondary campus or training site in order to gain information about the school community and the supports available to students with Down syndrome. Students and their families should plan to visit the training program or campus; at that time, they should plan to talk with other students with disabilities who are enrolled in the school or program to learn about their experiences. Table 16.1 provides some suggested activities for exploring various postsecondary education options.

Program Structure

There are several areas to consider when gathering information about a particular program to determine whether it will meet the needs of students with Down syndrome. One of the first areas to explore is the way in which the program is structured. Does the community college or technical school have a program that is specifically designed to serve special populations? Is the program part of the regular curriculum with supplemental supports built into the coursework? Or is the program designed to serve students with disabilities through the supports and services available to all students attending the postsecondary school? For example, in the study conducted by Page and Chadsey-Rusch (1995), the students attended a postsecondary program without a specifically designed curriculum for them. The students enrolled in computer classes and a fitness course offered through the college. They were able to benefit from the support services offered through

Table 16.1.   Suggested activities for identifying postsecondary education programs

- Explore a variety of postsecondary options. Postsecondary education can include trade or business schools, voctional-technical schools, community colleges, and specialized training in business and industry.
- Review information about schools, looking at training or coursework offered, diversity, and size of student body, and the school's community (both academic and social environments).
- Visit potential schools and find out about available services and supports.
- Talk to students with disabilities attending postsecondary programs about their experiences.

Adapted from HEATH Resource Center (1989); Wille-Gregory et al. (1995).

the community college, including counseling, orientation class, and peer tutoring. Even though the students were attending the college as a result of a grant, the authors concluded,

> Although the procurement of a state model-demonstration grant enabled them to attend a community college, it was clear from the interviews with others that teachers, and even some community college personnel, were realizing that the community college experience could be an option for students with mental retardation. (Page & Chadsey-Rusch, 1995, p. 93)

If the program is designed to serve students with disabilities, several models have been developed to serve these students in a community college setting (Gugerty, Tindall, Gavin, & Gribbon-Fago, 1993). One model is a pull-out program designed for students whose chances of success would be limited even with intensive support services in mainstreamed programs. This type of program is more individualized and incorporates all aspects of a student's life, including housing, leisure, financial, medical, occupational, and transportation. One community college, for example, designed a pull-out program consisting of four components: occupational skill development, occupational support and personal management courses, student development services, and personal life management. Occupational skill development is achieved through technical college courses with support, specifically designed technical college courses, and supervised occupational training. Community-based training sites are used as part of the program's individualized occupational education. As part of their occupational support and personal management coursework, students enroll in classes that include career assessment and planning, daily living skills, self-advocacy, job-seeking skills, and community and leisure resources (Gugerty et al., 1993).

Another model program offers supplemental supports for students with disabilities enrolled in a technical program (Gugerty et al., 1993). Students participate in the regular training or educational program but receive additional supports to ensure their success. Services such as tutoring, coursework or environmental modifications, and career counseling and assessment are provided. One community college program that uses this model develops an individual technical plan to identify the services and supports that students need. Another program has been able to mainstream students with disabilities through a range of support options, including individual and small-group tutorials, taping of textbooks and other materials, counseling, reading of tests, assistance with housing, and coordinating services. The program offers an orientation day for students prior to entering the community college to ensure that all the necessary forms are completed and to enable students to meet the staff and tour the school.

A third type of model is designed to have students participate in the regular training program, with support provided directly in the classroom. Gugerty and colleagues (1993) described a program located at Contra Costa College in San Pablo, California. Students with cognitive disabilities requiring instructional modifications or supports are mainstreamed into a community college chef training program. Students with disabilities work with students enrolled in the Culinary Arts Program in the same kitchens and restaurants. Job coaches are an integral part of the program, offering support to assist students in understanding lecture material and incorporating learning techniques during hands-on demonstrations. The program targets the "better restaurants" as future employment options for students, rather than fast-food establishments, so that graduates' earnings will be higher.

Program Participants

The second area to explore when gathering information about a potential postsecondary program is, Who enrolls in the program? Some programs may state that they serve students with disabilities, but they may not have had students with Down syndrome enroll. Understanding who enrolls in the program will assist in exploring how students with Down syndrome are currently served or how students could be served in the future.

The IEP transition-planning team will need to examine what program accommodations are used and how student performance is evaluated. Asking questions about the instructional accommodations used by instructors when working with students with disabilities and how these students' performance is assessed yields insights on the appropriateness of the program for the individual student.

Program Outcomes

A final area that the team should consider is program outcomes. The team should review both the number of students who completed the program and, if they did complete, whether they were able to obtain employment in their field of training.

These types of questions were used by the Center on Education and Work at the University of Wisconsin–Madison when identifying postsecondary education programs that were effectively serving students with learning or cognitive disabilities (Gugerty et al., 1993). Table 16.2 summarizes some of the questions IEP transition team members could use when exploring programs in their community.

It is important to note that the programs previously described here had a process in place to assist students with disabilities to make the transition from secondary school to the postsecondary setting. If such a process

Table 16.2.   Suggested questions for obtaining information about postsecondary education programs

- How is the program structured?
- Are there academic requirements for the program?
- Does the program serve students with disabilities? Have students with Down syndrome been served?
- Are financial assistance options available for students with disabilities?
- How do students enroll in the program?
- What instructional accommodations are used by instructors?
- How is student performance evaluated?
- How many students with disabilities complete the program?
- How many students are working in their field of training?

Adapted from Gugerty et al. (1993).

is not in place, it will be critical for the IEP team to identify a postsecondary representative to participate on the team to help facilitate the transition of students. As stated earlier, these representatives are not typically present at transition meetings (deFur et al., 1994), but are important members as postsecondary options are being considered.

Tindall and Gugerty (1985) have provided suggestions that can help increase communication and understanding among service providers, educators, students, and families about postsecondary education as a transition option for students with disabilities. Their suggestions include

1. Form advocacy groups including parents, students, rehabilitation counselors, representatives from various postsecondary education and training programs, employers, and other interested community agencies to determine methods for improving or enhancing the transition of students with disabilities to postsecondary education.
2. Plan and conduct workshops to help participants identify their roles and responsibilities in the transition process. Participants could include parents, students with disabilities, vocational rehabilitation staff, JTPA staff, community college or technical school personnel, employers providing advanced training opportunities, and community agency representatives.
3. Collect and disseminate information about the variety of postsecondary education and training opportunities available to youth with disabilities.

ASSISTIVE TECHNOLOGY IN POSTSECONDARY EDUCATION

An assistive technology device is any device, piece of equipment, or product system, whether acquired commercially or off the shelf, modified or customized, that is used to increase, maintain, or improve functional capabilities of individuals with disabilities (Technology-Related Assistance for Individuals with Disabilities Act of 1988, PL 100-407). An *assistive technology service* can be defined as any service that directly aids an individual with a disability in the selection, acquisition, or use of an assistive technology device.

Students with Down syndrome and their families need to acquire information about assistive technology and services appropriate to their needs. By utilizing these supports, students can maximize their opportunities to participate in advanced courses or training (Birely, Landers, Vernooy, & Schlaerth, 1986). It is important when exploring postsecondary education programs to identify the instructional approaches that are used and to determine whether assistive devices and services can assist students with Down syndrome to gain access to information and increase skills.

A wide range of assistive technology equipment is available that varies substantially in cost and complexity. Unfortunately, a common perception is that assistive technology is highly technical, expensive, and difficult to obtain. This is wrong because there are two classifications of assistive technology. A low-technology device is passive or simple, with few moving parts (Mann & Lane, 1991); examples include picture books, Velcro materials, book holders, and magnifying glasses. High-technology devices are those that have a greater complexity and may have an electronic component (Inge & Shepherd, 1995). Environmental control systems, adaptive driving controls, and power wheelchairs are classified as high-technology devices.

Assistive Technology and Transition

Students who will need assistive technology in their postsecondary education program should have the technology requirements written into their IEPs. The skills and supports identified through school and work experiences will be helpful in prioritizing assistive technology requirements for young adults. Purchase of assistive technology to enable students to enter advanced training or education programs must be based on individual assessment and should be evaluated across environments. Teachers, employers, and other professionals cannot determine what an individual needs even if they have had prior experience with individuals with disabilities. Poor assessment practices have frequently led to abandonment of technology. A bad experience using a device or service may prevent the individual from wanting to use assistive technology in the future. Assistive technology devices are continually being updated and perfected. As individuals' knowledge increases and environments change, it is important to frequently assess needs and compare the effectiveness of new technology devices to those currently in use.

Assessing Assistive Technology Needs

Assessing students' needs for assistive technology should provide information to help guarantee students' success in the college or vocational training setting. In school environments, assistive technology should assist students in participating in class activities and in facilitating interaction with other students and instructors. Assistive devices should also help students learn new skills and achieve program outcomes.

For individuals with Down syndrome, as for those with other disabilities, a comprehensive approach to learning about the individual yields the best results. The assessment team should include individuals who know the individual well. For example, a team may include the individual and family members (who are the locus of control in the process), teacher, speech-language pathologist, psychologist, rehabilitation engineer, vocational rehabilitation counselor, social worker, and computer programmer. Ideally, professionals should have current training and experience with assistive technology, should work well on a team, and should be willing to conduct assessments in the individual's own environments rather than in a clinical setting. Examples of team functions are assessment of needs, identification of a variety of assistive devices and services, suggesting funding sources, and offering assistance both with training on the devices and follow-up that can include help with maintenance and repair and ongoing evaluation.

Once the student's needs and abilities are known and the environments analyzed, it is time to select the proper device. Guidelines for technology selection are 1) look for simple solutions—think of low-technology devices before high-technology devices; 2) consider the learning and work style of the learner; 3) consider the long-range implications of the disability; 4) examine each device carefully; 5) investigate all options; and 6) compare similar equipment from different manufacturers. Then answer the following questions (Rothstein & Everson, 1995; West, Mast, Cosel, & Cosel, 1996):

- Does the device achieve outcomes (e.g., task completion, improved social functioning)?
- Is the device age appropriate?
- After initial training, do the individual, family member, teacher, and employer understand how to use the device?
- Will the individual have the same needs over time?
- Does the technology fit the postsecondary education or training environment without being intrusive?
- If portability is a factor, how portable is the device?
- Is the device adaptable to a wide variety of situations and uses?

Prior to purchasing any device, an individual should have the opportunity to test out its effectiveness. Many rehabilitation engineering and regional assistive technology centers loan devices for this purpose. This testing period leads to wiser purchases and less abandonment of the technology.

HIGH TECHNOLOGY FOR LEARNING

Computer hardware and software undergo constant improvement. As emphasized in Chapter 15, computer access for students with cognitive disabilities can greatly enhance their learning and skill development. Computers can increase students' ability to profit from the curriculum, in addition to providing opportunities for social interaction, improving students' communication skills, and helping students to develop their personal productivity skills (Golinker, 1995). Educational computer programs can promote mastery of material using drills and practice. They can also provide tutorials, provide supplementary instruction, and increase personal productivity for youth with cognitive disabilities. Students are able to repeat a program until mastery. With computers, users can proceed at their own pace, make mistakes, receive immediate feedback, and not suffer embarrassment if they are unable to grasp the material.

Continuing advances in technology, including computer technology, are enabling students with disabilities to take advantage of an ever-widening variety of educational experiences. Students with Down syndrome can participate in inclusive programs that are customized to allow students to progress at their own speed. When exploring postsecondary education options, it is important to identify what technology is available to assist students in their learning.

Case Study: Matthew

Matthew is a 19-year-old student with Down syndrome. He has severe articulation disorder, with an apraxic component, and severe receptive and expressive language disorders. His speech disorder makes it extremely difficult for Matthew to be understood. Matthew is able to increase his comprehension when he maintains good eye-to-eye contact and eye-to-mouth contact with the speaker. He is able to perform tasks in a very routine manner, which allows him to function fairly independently. He has been enrolled in programs ranging from self-contained classes for students with disabilities to mainstreamed classes.

Matthew has been involved in many community activities and enjoys participating in sports. He plays basketball, has taken dance and gymnastic classes, and has recently been taking ice skating lessons. He has occasionally expressed an interest in participating in some of the clubs at school but has never attended any of the meetings.

At Matthew's IEP meeting, the team began reviewing the goals and objectives in his individualized transition plan (ITP). Matthew stated at the last meeting that he wanted a job to earn money to buy the things he wanted. His parents had agreed to incorporate more community-based experiences into Matthew's schedule. Most of his community experiences had involved local restaurants and bakeries. Matthew was interested in cooking and was completing a vocational education program in occupational home economics.

The vocational education teacher attending the IEP meeting stated that Matthew had done well but needed ongoing support to learn new material presented in class, as well as close supervision during initial hands-on demonstrations. After Matthew had learned a skill, he was able to work more independently. The special education teacher providing support to the vocational staff had designed cards that showed pictures of the recipes the class was working on. Matthew was able to follow directions with these special cards and needed only minimal prompting after learning the recipe.

Even though Matthew's speech is difficult to understand, he is very social and interacts with the other students in the class. The vocational teacher said that the high level of activity going on in the kitchen did not distract Matthew; however, his desire to talk with the other students did at times create problems. The instructor and the special education teacher were working on helping Matthew to stay on task more and to reduce the amount of socializing he was doing while working. The vocational instructor recommended that Matthew continue to receive training until he completed the program at the end of the next school year.

Matthew's parents were concerned that his employment options would not allow him to do the cooking and baking that he enjoyed. Through his community-based program, he was able to be involved in a number of different jobs related to food service. Matthew told his parents he did not like the dirty pans. Matthew's parents wanted him to have a job that allowed him to earn a good income and had career possibilities. The team talked about what possibilities were available for Matthew and what the next steps should be.

The vocational education teacher asked the team if they were aware of a program at the local community college that was designed for students with disabilities. Most of the members had heard of the program through information distributed by the college but were not sure if it would meet Matthew's needs. The vocational rehabilitation counselor explained that he had visited the program and thought it might be good for Matthew and his parents to see it. One of the programs offered was a culinary arts program that integrated the students into the regular classroom with supplemental supports. The team determined that Matthew and his parents should visit the program and that the team would reconvene in 3 months to discuss the program's potential for Matthew. The vocational rehabilitation counselor told the family that he would call the special needs coordinator at the college to find out when they could visit the program and meet the staff. Matthew's special education teacher wondered if a representative from the college could attend their next meeting to talk about the program and work with the team to make recommendations for Matthew's potential transition into it. Matthew's rehabilitation counselor said that he would find out if someone could attend.

Matthew's ITP contained objectives about exploring the community college program. The team members brainstormed for potential questions that Matthew and his parents could ask the staff while they were visiting. The team was interested in learning about the program's academic requirements, how students manage the transition into the program, the range of accommodations used, and how many students with Down syndrome had been served.

As part of his IEP objectives, Matthew will continue his vocational education class and will work in his consumer mathematics class on using his special measuring equipment that he obtained to assist him when preparing food.

CONCLUSIONS

This chapter has presented ideas for exploring postsecondary education for adolescents with Down syndrome within the IEP transition-planning process. Careful planning and preparation is needed to ensure that these students are able to succeed in meeting their educational, social, and emotional needs through participation in postsecondary programs. Further information is needed to learn the impact of students' participation in such programs in terms of meeting their personal goals; however, from a few studies that have been conducted, results indicate that individuals with mental retardation can benefit from participating in postsecondary schools in such areas as lifelong learning, self-esteem, and friendships (Page & Chadsey-Rusch, 1995; Uditsky, Frank, Hart, & Jeffrey, 1987). Through effective planning, development of appropriate supports, and a shared commitment, postsecondary education programs can provide adolescents with Down syndrome opportunities to pursue their dreams and goals.

REFERENCES

Birely, M.K., Landers, M.F., Vernooy, J.A., & Schlaerth, P. (1986). The Wright State University program: Implications of the first decade. *Journal of Reading, Writing, and Learning Disabilities, 2,* 349–357.

Boyer-Stephens, A. (1990). Transition to postsecondary education. *Missouri Lincletter, 13*(2), 1–3.

Brown-Glover, P. (1992). Applications for youth with mild mental retardation. In P. Wehman (Ed.), *Life beyond the classroom: Transition strategies for young people with disabilities* (pp. 237–260). Baltimore: Paul H. Brookes Publishing Co.

deFur, S., Getzel, E.E., & Kregel, J. (1994). Individual transition plans: A work in progress. *Journal of Vocational Rehabilitation, 4*(2), 139–145.

deFur, S.H., Getzel, E.E., & Trossi, K. (1996). Making the postsecondary education match: A role for transition planning. *Journal of Vocational Rehabilitation, 6,* 231–241.

Getzel, E.E. (1990). Entering postsecondary programs: Early individualized planning. *Teaching Exceptional Children, 23*(1), 51–53.

Getzel, E.E., & Kregel, J. (1996). Transitioning from the academic to the employment setting: The employment connection program. *Journal of Vocational Rehabilitation, 6,* 273–287.

Golinker, L. (1995). *The Assistive Technology Funding and Systems Change Project.* Washington, DC: United Cerebral Palsy Associations.

Gugerty, J.J., Tindall, L.W., Gavin, M.K., & Gribbon-Fago, B. (1993). *Serving students with learning or cognitive disabilities effectively in two-year colleges: Seven exemplary approaches.* Madison: Center on Education and Work, University of Wisconsin–Madison.

HEATH Resource Center. (1989). *Make the most of your opportunities: A guide to postsecondary education for adults with handicaps.* Washington, DC: Author.

Individuals with Disabilities Education Act (IDEA) of 1990, PL 101-476, 20 U.S.C. §§ 1400 *et seq.*

Inge, K.J., & Shepherd, J. (1995). Assistive technology applications and strategies for school system personnel. In K.F. Flippo, K.J. Inge, & J.M. Barcus (Eds.), *Assistive technology: A resource for school, work, and community* (pp. 133–166). Baltimore: Paul H. Brookes Publishing Co.

Job Training Partnership Act, PL 97-300, 29 U.S.C. §§ 1501 *et seq.*

Mann, W.C., & Lane, J.P. (1991). *Assistive technology for persons with disabilities: The role of occupational therapy.* Rockville, MD: American Occupational Therapy Association.

Morningstar, M.E., Turnbull, A.P., & Turnbull, H.R. (1995). What do students with disabilities tell us about the importance of family involvement in the transition from school to adult life? *Exceptional Children, 62*(3), 249–260.

Page, B., & Chadsey-Rusch, J. (1995). The community college experience for students with and without disabilities: A viable transition outcome? *Career Development for Exceptional Individuals, 18*(2), 85–96.

Rothstein, R., & Everson, J.M. (1995). Assistive technology for individuals with sensory impairments. In K.F. Flippo, K.J. Inge, & J.M. Barcus (Eds.), *Assistive technology: A resource for school, work, and community* (pp. 105–132). Baltimore: Paul H. Brookes Publishing Co.

Sarkees, M.D., & Scott, J.L. (1985). *Vocational special needs* (2nd ed.). Homewood, IL: American Technical Publishers.

Schloss, P.J. (1984). Postsecondary opportunities: The role of secondary educators in advocating handicapped young adults. *Journal of Vocational Special Needs Education, 7*(2), 15–19.

Technology-Related Assistance for Individuals with Disabilities Act of 1988, PL 100-407, 29 U.S.C. §§ 2201 *et seq.*

Tindall, L.W., & Gugerty, J.J. (1985). Improving interagency linkages for handicapped youth. *Journal of Vocational Special Needs Education, 7*(2), 9–14.

Uditsky, B., Frank, S., Hart, L., & Jeffrey, S. (1987). On campus: Integrating the university environment. In D. Baine (Ed.), *Alternative futures for the education of students with severe disabilities: Proceedings of the Conference on Severe and Multiple Handicaps: Alternative Futures* (pp. 96–103). Edmonton, Alberta, Canada: Publication Services, Faculty of Education, University of Alberta.

Wagner, M. (1989). *Youth with disabilities during transition: An overview of descriptive findings from the National Longitudinal Transition Study.* Stanford, CA: SRI International.

West, M.D., Barcus, J.M., Brooke, V., & Rayfield, R.G. (1995). An exploratory analysis of self-determination of persons with disabilities. *Journal of Vocational Rehabilitation, 5,* 357–364.

West, M.D., Gibson, K., & Unger, D. (1996). The role of the family in school-to-work transition. In G.H.S. Singer, A. Glang, & J.M. Williams (Eds.), *Children with acquired brain injury: Educating and supporting families* (pp. 197–220). Baltimore: Paul H. Brookes Publishing Co.

West, M.D., Mast, M., Cosel, R., & Cosel, M. (1996). Applications for youth with orthopedic and other health impairments. In P. Wehman (Ed.), *Life beyond the classroom: Transition strategies for young people with disabilities* (2nd ed., pp. 419–444). Baltimore: Paul H. Brookes Publishing Co.

Wille-Gregory, M., Graham, J.W., & Hughes, C. (1995, Spring). Preparing students with learning disabilities for success in postsecondary education. *Transitionlinc,* 1–6.

17

Legal Protections for Students with Disabilities

Salome M. Heyward

The majority of the legal mandates affecting adolescents with disabilities are those applicable to educational agencies. States and local school districts must provide services to children through 18 years of age and, if state law further provides, educational services may be extended through age 21 (Implementing Regulations [IDEA]: Assistance to States for the Education of Children with Disabilities, 34 C.F.R. § 300.300). Parents of adolescents will have their greatest involvement with the following laws that concern the state's and local school district's responsibility to provide educational services: the Individuals with Disabilities Education Act (IDEA) of 1990 (PL 101-476); Section 504 of the Rehabilitation Act of 1973 (PL 93-112; henceforth, Section 504); and the Americans with Disabilities Act (ADA) of 1990 (PL 101-336). These laws encompass the full spectrum of services, from early intervention programs for preschool children to transitional plans to prepare older students for adulthood. Therefore, it is important for parents, educators, practitioners, and all others who work with individuals with disabilities to have a general knowledge and understanding of the full panoply of rights and responsibilities within the educational arena. This chapter surveys those rights and responsibilities, including pertinent aspects of the legislation itself as well as court cases that have affirmed and clarified specific features of the law. Please note that the term *regular education* is used in this chapter because that is the term that was used at the time the cases and legislation discussed herein were decided or enacted, respectively.

LOCATION AND NOTIFICATION OF STUDENTS
School districts are responsible for locating, evaluating, and offering a free appropriate public education to all students with disabilities within its ju-

risdiction. This responsibility is not passive but, rather, is an extremely wide-sweeping one. It is not enough for school districts simply to wait for students to enroll and then present parents or guardians with information regarding school programs and responsibilities with respect to students with disabilities. Rather, as is discussed here, the school district must take a proactive stance toward outreach. It is important to note, also, that the district's responsibility is not limited to public school students who would avail themselves of a public education but also extends to students enrolled in private schools. The district must not only offer services to students placed in private schools but even if their parents decline to enroll them in public school the district must continue to make these services "available" to them.

> (a) If a child with a disability has FAPE [free appropriate public education] available and the parents choose to place the child in a private school or facility, the public agency is not required by this part to pay for the child's education at the private school or facility. However, the public agency shall make services available to the child . . . . (Implementing Regulations [IDEA], see 34 C.F.R. § 300.403)

Thus, the fact that a student is enrolled in a private facility does not deprive him or her of the right to be served in the public arena or to take advantage of services offered by a public agency. Furthermore, this obligation may require the provision of special education and related services to students while they are, in fact, enrolled in private facilities. In a 1995 case, *Cefalu v. East Baton Rouge Parish School Board,* a public school district was ordered to provide a student enrolled in a private facility with a sign interpreter.

How extensive do a district's outreach activities have to be? The goal is to ensure that parents of children with disabilities are provided full information regarding the district's responsibility to provide a free appropriate education and its availability. It is "information-giving so that parents and the handicapped may choose whether they desire to participate in the public program" (*David H. v. Spring Branch Independent School District,* 1983). Procedures that merely provide notice to those already served by the district, such as sending letters to parents of students enrolled the previous year, are insufficient. The procedures utilized must permit the district to reach those not currently served, including, for example, providing information to private schools, mailing brochures to the known parents of children with disabilities, public service announcements on television and radio, newspaper ads, placing brochures in offices of pediatricians, and surveying child care centers and kindergartens.

However, the district is not at fault if it fails to offer services to every child with a disability within its jurisdiction. As noted by the court in *David H.* (1983, at 1339), the legal mandate does not require that every unserved child be identified; rather, it requires that the district's actions be assessed in terms of the thoroughness and extensiveness of its efforts. The key is whether the procedures utilized reflect a good-faith effort to identify, locate, and notify unserved students and their parents.

WHO MUST BE SERVED AND WHAT SHOULD SERVICES LOOK LIKE?

The pertinent federal mandate provides that children who are of an age that the state is required to provide them educational services (i.e., ages 3–21) must be provided a free and appropriate public education regardless of the severity of their disabilities. Thus, school districts must ensure that "all children with disabilities, regardless of the severity of their disability, and who are in need of special education and related services are identified, located, and evaluated . . ." (Implementing Regulations [IDEA], 34 C.F.R. § 300.128). A number of questions come to mind regarding this mandate:

1. As the phrase "regardless of the nature and severity" implies, is this in fact an absolute standard?
2. What is an appropriate education?
3. Are the educational services in fact free without concern for overall cost?

The first two concerns are discussed next. The third concern, regarding cost, is discussed in a later section titled "Free Education."

Regardless of the Severity

The meaning of the phrase "regardless of the severity of their disability" was resolved judicially in *Timothy W. v. Rochester, New Hampshire, School District* (1989). In this case, the court of appeals rejected the district court's startling conclusion that if a child does not possess an ability to learn or benefit from educational services, a school district need not provide educational services to the child. The court had specifically held that "a handicapped student who does not have a learning capacity was not intended to receive special education." The court of appeals specifically rejected this interpretation of the "regardless of the severity" standard by ruling that the "district court erred in requiring a benefit/eligibility test as a prerequisite." The court outlined the responsibility of educational agencies under the mandate as follows:

> The language of the Act in its entirety makes clear that a "zero reject" policy is at the core of the Act, and that no child, regardless of the severity of his or her handicap, is to ever again be subjected to the deplorable state of affairs which existed at the time of the Act's passage, in which millions of handicapped children received inadequate education or none at all. In summary, the Act mandates an appropriate public education for all handicapped children, regardless of the level of achievement that such children might obtain. (*Timothy W. v. Rochester, New Hampshire, School District*, 1989, at 960–962)

Thus, the phrase "regardless of the severity" is to be given its plain meaning and does, in fact, impose an absolute responsibility to provide educational services to students with disabilities. Therefore, when school districts are faced with the task of providing services to students with disabilities with serious impairments, the question should never be whether the services must be provided, but, rather, how programs or services will be provided that address their individual educational needs. The severity of the impairment is simply one factor to be considered in deciding on the type of program that must be developed.

Appropriate Education

Educational services for students with disabilities cover a wide range of program offerings in addition to or in place of instruction in a regular education setting. Specifically, this refers to

(a)(1) . . . specially designed instruction, . . . , to meet the unique needs of the child with a disability, including—
  (i)   Instruction conducted in the classroom, in the home, in hospitals and institutions . . . and
  (ii) Instruction in physical education.
(2)   The term includes speech pathology, or any other related service. . . .
(3)   The term also includes vocational education. (Implementing Regulations [IDEA], 34 C.F.R. § 300.17)

However, the real question is what should these appropriate educational services look like? The services provided must confer educational benefit to the student, must meet the student's individual needs (including the need for related aids and services and assistive technology devices and services), and must provide for the needs of the student with a disability as adequately as the needs of people without disabilities are met. It is vitally important for parents to understand these three concepts—discussed, in turn, next—because they form the cornerstone of all services to students with disabilities.

Educational Benefit

Do school districts have to design and implement educational programs that will allow students with disabilities to reach their maximum potential? Frequently, disputes between parents and school districts regarding the appropriateness of educational services center around this very question. Understandably, parents want their sons and daughters to be offered the best possible educational program; thus, they have difficulty accepting school districts' offers that they believe fall short of that goal. What standard should be used to judge the quality of such programs? The U.S. Supreme Court, in *Hendrick Hudson District Board of Education v. Rowley* (1982), outlined the proper standard. In that case, a conflict developed between the parents of a student with a hearing impairment and school officials because the parents believed their daughter's educational program should emphasize cued speech, whereas school officials favored a total communication approach relying on sign language. The parents insisted that their program was the only one that would allow the student to benefit from the services offered to the maximum extent possible. School officials conceded that many experts believed that the program recommended by the parents allowed individuals with hearing impairments to reach their maximum potential but maintained that their approach would permit the student to benefit from the services offered and to function successfully in school. The Court rejected the assertion that the mandate to provide an appropriate education requires educational agencies to "maximize the potential of each handicapped child" (*Hendrick Hudson District Board of Education v. Rowley*, 1982, at 200). The Court defined an appropriate education as follows: "the 'basic floor of opportunity' . . . consists of access to specialized instruction and related services which are individually designed to provide educational benefit to the handicapped child." The Court specifically stated that access to educational services means "to confer some educational benefit," not to "maximize the potential of each handicapped child" (*Hendrick Hudson District Board of Education v. Rowley*, 1982, at 200). Therefore, while it may be true that the program proposed by parents could maximize the student's educational experience, the educational agency is not required to provide that program. The yardstick for parents is not whether the best educational program has been developed but whether the proposed program will "confer some educational benefit."

The next difficult question for parents to answer is How does one determine whether a child is receiving educational benefit? The success or failure of students in a "regular" education setting is measured in terms of grade levels culminating in graduation, whereas the educational programs of students with disabilities, in most instances, do not conform to such an orderly progression. Often those students perform under individualized education programs (IEPs) that reflect similar goals year after year, with the termination of their educational careers being marked by their reaching the legal age limit for the provision of public educational services. Therefore, on the continuum between the provision of minimum or no services and services that maximize potential, it is very difficult to determine where those services that "confer some educational benefit" fall. The Court acknowledged the difficulty of answering this question by noting:

> The [Education for All Handicapped Children Act of 1975, PL 94-142] requires participating states to educate wide spectrums of handicapped children, from the marginally hearing-impaired to the profoundly retarded and palsied. It is clear that the benefits obtainable by children at one end of the spectrum will differ dramatically from those obtainable by children at the other end, with infinite variations in between. . . . We do not attempt today to establish any one test for

determining the adequacy of educational benefits conferred upon all children covered by the Act. (*Hendrick Hudson District Board of Education v. Rowley,* 1982, at 202)

With the above statement, the Court established that a determination of whether benefit has been conferred should be made on a case-by-case basis. As a general rule, the Court noted that for students with disabilities in "regular" education settings the program provided "should be reasonably calculated to enable the child to achieve passing marks and advance from grade to grade." For all other students with disabilities, the program must be "personalized instruction with sufficient support services to permit the child to benefit educationally from that instruction" (*Hendrick Hudson District Board of Education v. Rowley,* 1982, at 203–204). It is important for parents to understand that in making the assessment of whether educational benefit has been conferred, both the courts and federal enforcement agencies pay deference to the purely pedagogic decisions of educators. Educational decisions are presumed to be correct in the absence of powerful evidence to the contrary. Courts generally respect the purely academic decisions of educators unless they are arbitrary or capricious, represent a clear statutory/regulatory violation, or reflect evidence of actual discrimination. Thus, parents who choose to contest a recommended placement or proffered services must do more than argue that their suggestions are more appropriate or better. However, school districts will not be permitted to provide educational programs or services that confer only *"de minimis"* or trivial advancement, nor will they be permitted to ignore overwhelming evidence that indicates that the program or services are not successful (see *Board of Education v. Diamond,* 1986; *Daniel R.R. v. State Board of Education,* 1989; *Polk v. Central Susquehanna Intermediate Unit 16,* 1988).

Individual Needs

Educational programs must be designed to meet the individual needs of students. The "touchstone" of an appropriate education is "individualization." The state's responsibility is to provide *"personalized instruction* with sufficient support services to permit the child to benefit" (*Hendrick Hudson District Board of Education v. Rowley,* 1982, at 203). School districts have been found in violation for adhering to policies and procedures that result in a categorical refusal to consider the unique needs of a particular student—for example, for refusing to consider or provide special education services for longer than 180 days and for providing identical services to all students with a particular disability without consideration of their individual skills, abilities, and needs. The standard is that any policy or practice that "inhibits consideration of the individual needs of [students]" violates federal statutes and regulations (see *Brazosport (Texas) Independent School District,* 1987; *Georgia Association of Retarded Citizens v.*

McDaniel, 1984). Furthermore, external factors including economic or administrative expediencies such as limited staff time or budgetary constraints cannot be used to dictate the nature or degree of services a student receives.

"As Adequately as the Needs of Nonhandicapped Persons Are Met"

The educational programs offered to students with disabilities must compare favorably to those provided to students in "regular" educational settings. The key is that the services provided each group of students must be comparable unless the individual needs of students with disabilities demand otherwise. As noted by the administrative law judge in *Missouri State Department of Education v. United States Department of Education* (1987), a case in which the state was charged with discriminating against students with disabilities as a class by providing them with only a 5-hour school day while providing all other students with a 6-hour day:

> To establish a violation of Section 504, it is necessary only to establish that there exists a class of handicapped children who are limited to a school day of five hours by a policy that is not based on an individualized educational program for each child as required by the Act. The quality of services provided must also be equal. Therefore, teachers must be trained and/or certified; adequate materials and classroom space must be provided; necessary teachers, therapists, and aides must be hired; sufficient educational choices must be offered; and so on.

Related Aids and Services

The educational services that must be provided include related aids and services (i.e., those that are "necessary for the student to benefit from educational instruction"). "Related aids and services" is one of those phrases used in the regulations for which no clear definition is provided. Examples of related services found in federal regulations include "developmental, corrective and other supportive services (including psychological, counseling and medical diagnostic)" and "transportation, . . . developmental, corrective, and other supportive services (including speech pathology and audiology, psychological services, physical and occupational therapy, recreation and medical and counseling services)" (Section 504 of the Rehabilitation Act of 1973—App. A, p. 493, and 20 U.S.C. § 1401 [17]). The Supreme Court in *Irving Independent School District v. Tatro* (1984) held that intermittent catheterization was a related aid or service and stated that the following two questions must be answered to determine whether the requested services are "supportive services necessary for the student to benefit from educational instruction": first, "whether the service is required to assist a handicapped child to benefit from special education," and, second, whether the service is "excluded from this definition as a medical service serving purposes other than diagnosis or evaluation" (*Irving Independent School District v. Tatro,* 1984, at 664, 672). The standard is that educational agencies must provide services that permit students to benefit from the educational services offered and not those that convert the district's or agency's primary function from providing educational services to one of medical practitioner.

Merely determining that the student cannot attend school without a service does not adequately answer the question. School districts are not required to provide services that are essentially medical in nature, even though they may provide meaningful access to education. There is a "medical services exclusion." For example, services of a physician beyond those for diagnostic or evaluative purposes are excluded, and school districts are not obligated "to provide a service that might well prove unduly expensive and beyond the range of their competence." Furthermore, whereas schools are required to hire experts such as "occupational therapists, speech therapists, psychologists, social workers," they are not required to provide "the services of a physician or hospital" (*Irving Independent School District v. Tatro,* 1984, at 673–674).

But how do school districts distinguish between services that are primarily educational in scope and those that are medical? The courts have used the extensiveness of the services required as a guide. Services that are "beyond the competence of school personnel" and require "constant, in-school nursing care" and would subject a school "to excessive costs and the burden of health care" need not be provided (*Detsel v. Board of Education,* 1986). For example, in *Detsel,* the need for a full-time attendant to provide life-sustaining tasks such as suctioning lungs and cardiopulmonary resuscitation was ruled to be the type of service that a school district was not required to provide. The standard is one of reasonableness. The interests involved should be balanced, considering the cost, the time involved, and the capacity of school health professionals to provide the service. Furthermore, the services must meet the educational needs of the student. Districts will not be permitted to avoid responsibility by improperly using the medical exclusion (i.e., incorrectly characterizing requested services/aids as medical, emotional, or noneducational). Courts and federal enforcement agencies look beyond the labels and assess the nature and scope of the requested services. Agency rulings have held that services such as physical therapy, speech-language therapy, occupational therapy, individual counseling, family counseling, and psychotherapy are related aids and services.

Free Education

In General Educational agencies are responsible for all costs associated with meeting the appropriate educational needs of students with disabilities. Agencies have been consistently found in violation of federal statutes and regulations for attempting to shift the burden of providing a free appropriate public education to parents. For example, they may not 1) impose a limit on the amount that will be paid for necessary services that serves as a blanket restriction that precludes consideration of a student's individual needs; 2) condition their payments on a student's parents assuming financial responsibility for certain services; 3) refuse to pay for necessary evaluations; 4) arbitrarily limit the amount of instructional services provided to students with disabilities; or 5) restrict service providers to teachers and aides rather than necessary professional experts. Furthermore, while it is permissible to require parents of students with disabilities to pay fees that are imposed on all parents, such as athletic fees, parents of students with disabilities cannot be required to pay more for similar services solely because their children have disabilities (*Riley v. Jefferson County Board of Education*, 1989).

There are circumstances under which it is permissible to consider cost in selecting an educational program or service. However, unless the school district is asserting that providing the program or service would impose an undue administrative or financial burden, "cost considerations are only relevant when choosing between several options, all of which offer an 'appropriate' education" (*Clevenger v. Oak Ridge School Board*, 1984).

Residential Placement   Under certain circumstances, districts are financially responsible for providing public and/or private residential placements. If a district does not itself provide students with disabilities with necessary requisite services, it must assume the cost of *any alternate placement* (Section 504, App. A, par. 23, p. 493). The principle issue of controversy between parents and districts is that of determining whether a residential placement is necessary. According to the court in *Vander Malle v. Ambach* (1987), the key question to be answered is "whether full-time placement may be considered necessary for educational purposes are [sic] whether the residential placement is a response solely to medical, social or emotional problems that are segregable from the learning process" (667 F. Supp. 1015, 1040). How does one distinguish among medical, social or emotional problems, and educational needs, and what happens when they are intertwined?

The court in *Parks v. Pavkovic* (1985) outlined a series of hypothetical cases in an effort to answer the above question. The court stated, in part,

In the first [case], a deaf and blind child, perfectly capable of living at home, is institutionalized on the basis of a judgment that he can get a better education in a more controlled environment . . . .

In our second hypothetical case, the child is in a coma and is institutionalized because he cannot be cared for at home . . . .

In the third case, an intermediate case . . . , the child cannot be cared for at home because of some purely physical problem, but because of that problem neither can he be educated unless he were institutionalized. (733 F. Supp. at 1404–1405)

The court stated that cases one and two were simple (i.e., living expenses should be provided for the student placed for purely educational reasons, whereas no such reimbursement would be required for the child in the coma who was "completely uneducable in his condition"). With respect to the third case, the court rejected the argument that districts should be excused from responsibility merely because "the child would have to be institutionalized quite apart from educational needs that also required institutionalization" (id. at 1404–1405). Thus, the prevailing principle is that if the student is only properly educable in a residential setting, the district is responsible for the cost of such a placement despite the fact that noneducational problems may also be involved. If a residential placement is required, room, board, and related services must be provided at no cost to the parents. While districts are not precluded from requiring that parents pay for services or products not related to the child's educational needs, they must use procedures that clearly isolate those noneducational items so that parents do not inadvertently pay for educational services. Furthermore, the district is also responsible for providing transportation services for students who it placed in or referred to a program not operated by it for purposes of providing them a free appropriate education. The important elements are 1) the student must be placed in or referred to the program by the district, 2) the services must be adequate, and 3) parents must incur no greater cost than if the student were placed in the district's program.

It is important to understand that if the district has offered an appropriate education and the parents, nevertheless, unilaterally place the child in a private facility, the district is not responsible for paying for the services. However, there are circumstances under which a district may be required to pay for a placement unilaterally made by parents. "Schools may be ordered to reimburse parents when the parents' unilateral placement of the student is the result of the district's failure to adhere to federal mandates" (*Florence County School District 4 v. Carter,* 1993). The district has a duty to pay if the following conditions are met (*Holland v. District of Columbia,* 1995):

1. The district violated a procedural requirement of the law.
2. The unilateral placement is an appropriate placement.
3. The cost of the placement is reasonable.

Educational Setting

Students with disabilities are served in a variety of educational settings: "regular," "regular" with supplemental aids and services; resource classes; self-contained, separate facilities; and homebound services. The essential question is How does one determine which of the available settings are appropriate? Federal regulations require that students with disabilities be educated in the "regular" education setting to the "maximum extent" appropriate to their needs. This raises two important priorities for districts: 1) providing an education that is appropriate to the needs of the student, and 2) educating the student with nondisabled students to the maximum extent appropriate (i.e., mainstreaming). The best way to conceptualize the connection between these two priorities is to view them as being indispensable to each other (i.e., the educational program is not appropriate if it is not offered in the proper setting).

A student with a disability may not be removed from the "regular" education setting unless the district can demonstrate that the needs of the student would be best served by placement in another setting (Section 504 of the Rehabilitation Act, 1973, App. A, ¶ 24, p. 494). If the student cannot perform in a "regular" setting, the district must select the setting closest to the "regular" educational setting that will provide the student an appropriate education. For placements that result in students with disabilities being segregated from their peers, districts must provide 1) clear evidence that placement in a "regular" education setting with supplemental aids and/or less restrictive placements was considered and found to be inappropriate and 2) specific reasons why the student must be educated in a more segregated environment.

A lot of tension between parents and school districts revolves around the question of the extent to which students with disabilities are educated in a "regular" education setting. Parents accuse districts of being too quick to segregate students with disabilities and thus deny them the opportunity to interact with their peers without disabilities. Districts are required to give serious consideration to including students with disabilities in the "regular" classroom; this consideration must be more than a token gesture. However, the mainstreaming mandate does not require districts to place all students in a "regular" setting, as argued by some. Districts are permitted to evaluate the "likelihood of success of mainstreaming" by reviewing the student's history of placements as well as relevant and legitimate documentary data (see *Poolaw v. Bishop,* 1995). They do not have to give students an opportunity to fail in the regular setting if it is clear that such a placement would not result in educational benefit. The following factors are considered in determining whether a student should be mainstreamed:

1. The educational benefit of full-time placement in the regular classroom
2. The nonacademic benefits of such a placement
3. The effect the student with a disability will have on the teacher and the other students in the "regular" class
4. The costs of mainstreaming the student (*Poolaw,* 1995, at 836)

EVALUATION AND PLACEMENT

Evaluation

The responsibility imposed on districts regarding the evaluation of students who are believed to need services is proactive. Before any action is taken regarding the initial placement of such students, a full evaluation of the students must be conducted. Furthermore, evaluations must also be conducted before each significant change in a student's educational program—this includes changing the nature of the services provided, as well as removing, reassigning, dismissing, or denying placements (Implementing Regulations [IDEA], 34 C.F.R. § 300.531). The change must be an alteration in the general education program, not mere variations in the program. The obligation to evaluate does not apply to minor alterations such as replacing one qualified teacher with another equally qualified teacher or adding 10–15 minutes to a student's transportation time. "A fundamental change in or elimination of a basic element of the educational program" must be identified for an evaluation to be required (*Lunceford v. District of Columbia Board of Education,* 1984). Examples of such changes include failure to implement a student's IEP, graduation, and suspension of a student from a school bus.

Parents are not permitted to interfere with the district in the performance of its evaluation responsibilities. They must permit the district to evaluate their children if they wish the district to provide necessary educational services. Furthermore, they cannot withhold permission to evaluate in an effort to force the district to rely solely on the independent evaluative data supplied by them. "The school system may insist on evaluation by qualified professionals who are satisfactory to school officials" (*Dubois v. Connecticut State Board of Education,* 1984; see also *Andress v. Cleveland Independent School District,* 1995). The student cannot be provided appropriate educational services if his or her parents deny the school system the right to evaluate or reevaluate. However, "a parent who disagrees with the school evaluation has the right to have the child evaluated by an independent evaluator, possibly at public expense, and the evaluation must be considered by the school district" (*Andress v. Cleveland,* 1995, at 178).

The evaluation procedures used must

a.   include tests and evaluative materials that are validated, administered by trained personnel, administered in a manner that the result accurately reflects the students' aptitude, achievement levels, skills and abilities rather than the limitations imposed by the disability and designed to assess areas of educational need,

b.   employ more than a single criterion for determining the appropriate placement of students,

c.   involve a multidisciplinary team or group of individuals in the process,

d.   ensure that students are assessed in all areas related to the disability including, where appropriate, "health, vision, hearing, social, emotional status, general intelligence, academic performance, communicative status and motor abilities." (Implementing Regulations [IDEA], 34 C.F.R. § 300.532)

The following are examples of evaluation procedures that violate the law: placement of students using IQ test scores as the sole criterion; using a district-developed checklist as an assessment tool that has not been validated; employing untrained individuals to test students and/or to interpret evaluative data; and refusing to offer necessary test accommodations, such as extended time or readers. Districts have also been found in violation of federal mandates for failure to conduct evaluations in a timely manner. Unreasonable delays deny students with disabilities meaningful access to educational services (*Foster v. District of Columbia Board of Education*, 1982). In addition, students must be reevaluated "at least every three years to determine their continuing eligibility for special education services" (Implementing Regulations [IDEA], 34 C.F.R. § 300.534). Students may be reevaluated more frequently if circumstances warrant or teachers or parents request it.

Placement Procedures
In making placement decisions, public agencies are required, by law, to

(1) Draw upon information from a variety of sources, including aptitude and achievement tests, teacher recommendations, physical condition, social or cultural background, and adaptive behavior;

(2) Ensure that information obtained from all of these sources is documented and carefully considered;

(3) Ensure that the placement decision is made by a group of persons, including persons knowledgeable about the child, the meaning of the evaluation data, and the placement options; and

(4) Ensure that the placement decision is made in conformity with the [least restrictive environment] rules. . .

(5) If a determination is made that a child has a disability and needs special education and related services, an IEP must be developed for the child. (Implementing Regulations [IDEA], 34 C.F.R. § 300.533)

The placement meeting is intended to determine the student's present level of educational performance, assess how best to meet the student's educational needs, identify the nature of educational services needed, establish educational goals, and identify the criteria that will be used to assess whether the student is achieving his or her educational goals. Based on this meeting, an IEP is developed for the student.

All significant factors that have an impact on the student's learning capacity must be considered during the placement process. One of the basic tenets of the federal mandates is that placement decisions should not result in "misclassification or misplacement" of students. Therefore, district procedures that restrict or interfere with the consideration of information that is necessary or relevant are unacceptable. For example, districts may not refuse to consider relevant evaluative data or reports offered by parents, fail to conduct necessary evaluations, or prohibit teachers from recommending certain services such as extended school-year services. However, the duty to consider all relevant information is not a license for parents to seek to dictate the nature of the placement proceedings and to substitute their judgment for that of the educators. Thus, once a district has properly evaluated a student and has considered all the relevant information and data, it will not be required to pay for additional evaluations simply because the parents disagree with the placement decision. Furthermore, the decision of whether to follow or implement particular recommendations of evaluators and experts is solely within the purview of the placement committee.

As noted, the placement committee should include a group of people knowledgeable about the student and his or evaluation data and placement options. The knowledge of the people must be specific and meaningful. The court's decision in *Hollenbeck v. Board of Education of Rochelle Township* (1988), a case involving the accommodation of a wheelchair athlete, is a good illustration of this point. The court noted that the committee participants in total were either inexperienced regarding athletics in general or "handicapped" athletics in particular, or had no knowledge regarding wheelchair athletes or the student's physical abilities and disabilities. The court also noted that some of the participants themselves doubted their ability to resolve the matter. In concluding that the requirement that placement decisions be made by a group of knowledgeable people had been violated, the court stated that "none of the participants fully understand the dynamics of track and field events let alone wheelchair track" (*Hollenbeck v. Board of Education of Rochelle Township*, 1988, at 667). Thus, it is clear that it is not sufficient to simply have individuals on the committee who are familiar with the child and have general expertise. Their knowledge must relate to the abilities and disabilities of the student with respect to the specific placement options being considered.

It is also important to remember that placement decisions must be the result of something more than a cursory review of the data and evidence. There exists a responsibility to "thoroughly investigate, analyze, and discuss pertinent issues" (*Hollenbeck v. Board of Education of Rochelle Township*, 1988, at 668). Districts must also document information and data considered during the placement process, including all placement options considered.

Due Process Procedures

Federal regulations require that districts permit parents to be active participants in the delivery of educational services. One of the basic cornerstone protections contained in the regulations to ensure the individual's right to full participation is the mandate that procedural safeguards be provided. As noted by the Supreme Court in *Honing v. Doe* (1988), such safeguards "guarantee parents both an opportunity for meaningful input into all decisions affecting their child's education and the right to seek review of all decisions they think inappropriate." The procedural safeguards that districts are required to provide are the right to inspect all relevant records with respect to the student's identification, evaluation, or placement; the right to prior written notice when an agency seeks to change or refuses to seek to change the student's identification, evaluation, or placement; the opportunity to present complaints regarding identification, evaluation, or placement; an impartial due process hearing; and a right to appeal the hearing decision (see Individuals with Disabilities Education Act [IDEA] of 1990, 20 U.S.C. §§ 1415[b][1][A], 1415[b][1][C], 1415[b][1][E], 1415[b][2], 1415[e]). The key to determining when these safeguards should be provided is whether the decision or action in question has a significant impact on the delivery of educational services to the student. Thus, actions that involve changes in the manner in which services are provided (direct versus indirect), substantial modification of the educational program offered (number of hours of services offered or changing a self-contained program to a resource program), modification of the performance objectives in the IEP, or initiation or discontinuance of services require that procedural safeguards be provided. Districts are not permitted to place conditions on, or otherwise interfere with, the provision of procedural safeguards. For example, a district may not refuse to permit parents to proceed to a due process hearing until the parents have participated in a mediation process.

Notice   "Parents are entitled to adequate written notice a reasonable time before the agency either (1) Proposes to initiate or change the identification, evaluation, or educational placement of the child . . . ; or (2) Refuses to initiate or change the identification, evaluation, or educational placement" (*Holland v. District of Columbia,* 1995, at 422). The notice mandate ensures that parents are given sufficient information within a reasonable amount of time to fully exercise their right to consent or disagree regarding placement decisions affecting their children. Therefore, the notice that is provided must be explicit and understandable. If the district fails to provide proper notice, it is not a defense that the parents obtained the information elsewhere and fully understood their rights. Conversely, if the district has taken all the necessary steps to provide effective notice, the district will not be held accountable if parents fail to understand and seek clarification.

Access to Records

(a) Each participating agency shall permit parents to inspect and review any education records relating to their children that are collected, maintained, or used by the agency . . . . The agency shall comply with a request without unnecessary delay and before any meeting regarding an IEP or any hearing . . . , and in no case more than 45 days after the request has been made. (Implementing Regulations [IDEA], 34 C.F.R. § 300.562)

Although parents must be provided the opportunity to examine relevant records, this requirement does not preclude the district from requesting that parents comply with nondiscriminatory administrative procedures regarding the records. For example, parents may be required to request permission to review the records in advance or to review them during prescribed time periods. The key is that the restrictions or limitations imposed on the parents of a student with disabilities must be the same as those applied to all parents. The district's policy must clearly reflect that the parents of a student with disabilities are not being treated differently solely on the basis of their child's having disabilities. The district may not, however, restrict actual access to relevant records. In addition, parents may not be required to provide justification for their need to review records, nor may the district make it so difficult for the parents to obtain the records that they are effectively denied access.

Hearing Procedures   Parents have the right to request a due process hearing and a subsequent administrative review (appeal) to resolve any disagreement regarding the delivery of services. This is an absolute right, and, as noted previously, the district may not seek to restrict it by failing to provide notice, refusing to participate, or delaying the implementation unnecessarily (*Honing v. Doe,* 1988, at 311–312). The importance of the right to seek due process cannot be underestimated. Without this right, the other procedural safeguards would be empty promises at best, because districts would retain unilateral authority regarding the delivery of educational services. Once a due-process hearing is requested, the child whose placement is at issue must remain in his or her present placement until the controversy is resolved, unless the parties agree otherwise. This "stay-put" doctrine protects students with disabilities and their parents from unilateral actions on the part of districts that would deprive them of their right to participate in the educational process.

The standard used to determine the appropriateness of the due-process procedures used by the district/state is that there must be "fundamental fairness" to the procedures as implemented. While parents continually raise concerns regarding the impartiality of hearing officers and reviewers, their decisions will not be overturned without substantial evidence of misconduct. Courts have held that there must be a "substantial showing of personal bias" in order to disqualify a hearing officer or obtain a ruling that a hearing is unfair (*Kattan v. District of Columbia,* 1988). Furthermore, courts will not substitute their judgment for that of educators if the district has complied with the procedural standards of the implementing regulations and the educational program developed is reasonably calculated to confer educational benefits (*Board of Education of Murphysboro v. Illinois State Board of Education*).

Parents are not the only individuals who initiate due-process proceedings. Under circumstances in which a district believes that a proposed course of action or program is best for the student, but the parents disagree, then the district should initiate due-process procedures. Districts may not acquiesce to the wishes of parents when acquiescence results in the denial of a free appropriate public education to the student. If the data, record, or documentation shows the educational professionals that the student's present placement or the parental requests are not appropriate, then the district is obligated to take whatever steps are necessary, including initiating a due-process hearing, to provide appropriate educational services. It is also important to note that parents are not permitted to bypass these administrative remedies under the IDEA in order to sue the school district in federal court pursuant to the ADA and/or to Section 504. Individuals seeking redress are required to exhaust their administrative remedies under the IDEA before bringing claims under the ADA and Section 504, as well as other federal statutes. This restriction is intended to ensure that the proper parties (i.e., parents and school districts) are given the greatest opportunity to resolve placement disagreements among themselves.

CONCLUSIONS

Although there are numerous federal statutes and regulations that provide protections to adolescents with disabilities, the starting point for anyone seeking to protect the rights of these individuals will under most circumstances be the IDEA. The IDEA provides the most specific and complete legal protections for students with disabilities, beginning with preschool and extending to transition programs from secondary education services. An additional federal program for parents to consult is the Program for Individuals with Developmental Disabilities, one component of which provides for the funding of state Protection and Advocacy systems. These systems have been extremely helpful in assisting parents to advocate for their children.

REFERENCES

Americans with Disabilities Act (ADA) of 1990, PL 101-336, 42 U.S.C. §§ 12101 *et seq.*

Andress v. Cleveland Independent School District, 64 F.3d 176, 178 (5th Cir. 1995).

Board of Education v. Diamond, 808 F.2d 876 (3rd Cir. 1986).

Board of Education of Murphysboro v. Illinois State Board of Education, 41 F.3d 1162, 1166 (7th Cir.).

Brazosport (TX) Independent School District, EHLR 352: 531 (1987).

Cefalu v. East Baton Rouge Parish School Board, 907 F. Supp. 966 (M.D. La. 1995).

Clevenger v. Oak Ridge School Board, 744 F.2d 514, 517 (6th Cir. 1984).

Daniel R.R. v. State Board of Education, 874 F.2d 1036 (5th Cir. 1989).

David H. v. Spring Branch Independent School District, 569 F. Supp. 1324, 1339 (S.D. Tex. 1983).

Detsel v. Board of Education of Auburn, 637 F. Supp. 1022, 1026 (N.D.N.Y. 1986).

Dubois v. Connecticut State Board of Education, 727 F.2d 44, 48 (2d Cir. 1984).

Education for All Handicapped Children Act of 1975, PL 94-142, 20 U.S.C. §§ 1400 *et seq.*

Florence County School District 4 v. Carter, 114 S. Ct. 361 (1993).

Foster v. District of Columbia Board of Education, EHLR 533: 520 (1982).

Georgia Association of Retarded Citizens v. McDaniel, 716 F.2d 902 (11th Cir. 1984), cert. denied, 469 U.S. 1228 (1985).

Hendrick Hudson District Board of Education v. Rowley, 458 U.S. 176 (1982).

Holland v. District of Columbia, 71 F.3d 417 (D.C. Cir. 1995).

Hollenbeck v. Board of Education of Rochelle Township, 699 F. Supp. 658 (N.D. Ill. 1988).

Honing v. Doe, 484 U.S. 305 (1988).

Implementing Regulations [IDEA]: Assistance to States for the Education of Children with Disabilities, 34 C.F.R. §§ 300.300 et seq. (1990).

Individuals with Disabilities Education Act (IDEA) of 1990, PL 101-476, 20 U.S.C. §§ 1400 et seq.

Irving Independent School District v. Tatro, 468 U.S. 883 (1984).

Kattan v. District of Columbia, EHLR 441: 207 (August 1988).

Lunceford v. District of Columbia Board of Education, 745 F.2d 1577 (D.C. Cir. 1984).

Missouri State Department of Education v. United States Department of Education, No. 84-504-3 (1987).

Parks v. Pavkovic, 733 F.2d 1397 (7th Cir. 1985).

Polk v. Central Susquehanna Intermediate Unit 16, 853 F.2d 171 (3rd Cir. 1988), cert. denied, 102 L.Ed.2d 970 (1989).

Poolaw v. Bishop, 67 F.3d 830 (9th Cir. 1995).

Rehabilitation Act of 1973, PL 93-112, 29 U.S.C. §§ 701 et seq.

Riley v. Jefferson County Board of Education, Case No. CV-89-P-0169-S (N.D. Ala. 1989).

Timothy W. v. Rochester, New Hampshire, School District, 875 F.2d 954 (1st Cir. 1989), cert. denied, 107 L.Ed.2d 520 (1989).

Vander Malle v. Ambach, 667 F. Supp. 1015 (S.D.N.Y. 1987).

IV

LIFE IN THE WORKPLACE

18

Transition from School to Work

Richard G. Luecking
Ellen S. Fabian

It is not an overstatement to suggest that the most critical social and instrumental activity for young adults in American society is work. Work, after all, provides an opportunity for developing professional networks, acquiring skills, purchasing essential and nonessential goods and services, and even making friends. The benefits of work for young adults have long been recognized, although only since the early 1980s have parents, students, and educators acknowledged the critical importance of work for young adults with disabilities, leading to the initiative that resulted in the federal Education of the Handicapped Act Amendments of 1983 (PL 98-199) regarding transition and transition policy.

The significance of work to young adults with disabilities, including those with Down syndrome, is now widely acknowledged, and the ability of programs to improve work access and opportunity for these individuals has evolved tremendously. Employment outcomes for youth with disabilities who exit schools do remain lower than those of their peers without disabilities (Wagner, Blackorby, Cameto, Hebbeler, & Newman, 1993). However, there is little doubt that transition research and practice since the 1980s have resulted in the ability to identify programs and services that improve these youths' chances to succeed once they leave school.

In fact, it is now possible for young people, regardless of the nature or type of disability or any categorical label, to fully expect that the culmination of their public education experience will be a job. This chapter describes the values and practices underlying successful transition from school to work programs and illustrates successful strategies and practices.

VALUES OF TRANSITION FROM SCHOOL TO WORK PROGRAMS

As mentioned, the transition from school to work initiative took shape beginning with the 1983 Amendments to the Education of the Handicapped Act and continued with the federal transition initiative led by the U.S. Office of Special Education and Rehabilitative Services (Will, 1984). These efforts were spurred by the results of follow-up studies of youth with disabilities after exiting high school. A majority of these studies found that youth from all disability groups were employed at a rate lower than that of the general population, with the employment rate tending to be about 65% (i.e., Edgar, 1988; Hasazi, Gordon, & Roe, 1985; Wagner, 1989). The documentation of poor employment outcomes and of postschool difficulties of these students stimulated the national initiative and led many states to enact transition policies and to promote local level efforts.

As a consequence of these developments, a growing body of literature has emerged describing best practices and programs in the transition from school to work. The most impressive of these school-to-work programs are based on a firm commitment to and belief in the philosophy that all individuals who want to work can make a productive contribution to society. Successful transition programs share a common core of programs and practices, as well as some underlying beliefs. Some of these basic values or beliefs include the following:

1. Consumer input (i.e., student and family) is central to all stages of successful transition planning.
2. Program practices should be based on meeting individual student needs, rather than fitting student needs into existing services.
3. An ecologic framework, taking into account environmental as well as personal factors that contribute to the success of a transition, is fundamental.
4. A strong commitment to community integration throughout the transition planning is important for eventual employment success.
5. Creative job development strategies predicated on a commitment to diversified employment opportunities and establishment of positive relationships with local business communities promote success.
6. A perspective on a student's overall development that incorporates future career planning and career growth fosters the idea that transition is not a static, but a lifelong, process.

SUCCESSFUL TRANSITION PRACTICES—WHAT WORKS

With research and practice in the area of transition dating back to the early 1980s, professionals and practitioners have been able to identify transition practices that are associated with positive outcomes. The following descriptions of best practices are not exhaustive, but are designed to assist families and practitioners to understand basic programmatic elements to incorporate into their transition planning and development efforts.

Longitudinal Planning

The wisdom of beginning early to identify opportunities for career exploration, vocational assessment, and vocational training—all of which are part of developing a viable career path—has long been recognized. In fact, this awareness led to the requirement of an individualized transition plan (ITP) for students in special education as early as age 14. Long-term planning efforts focused on specific goal outcomes (e.g., employment, desirable living situations, access to social activities) to improve the quality of students' lives after they exit school.

Long-term planning is most effective when it is actively influenced by students and their families and/or significant others. Families in particular play many crucial roles in transition planning, including attending planning meetings; actively participating in the development of individualized education programs (IEPs); advocating for desired instructional processes—especially those that occur in natural environments such as worksites, stores, and public facilities; providing educators with pertinent information about the student's preferences and interests; reinforcing skills learned in school by helping the student practice them in other environments; and supporting and encouraging the student's participation in specific vocational experiences.

Emphasize Careers, Not Labels

When school-to-work programs are organized according to the interests and aptitudes of each student, rather than by disability or categorical label, students tend to achieve better employment outcomes. The emphasis on career choice for people with Down syndrome and those with other developmental disabilities is a relatively recent phenomenon. Early theories of career choice were based on a relatively simple "matching" approach—the belief that the individual had certain traits (cognitive, psychologic, and behavioral) that would then fit with certain occupational factors (Parsons, 1967). For individuals with disabilities, though, this "trait and factor" approach was expanded to suggest that one could match occupations to disability. So, for example, people who were deaf were thought to be "suited" for jobs in noisy work environments, whereas other workers without hearing impairment might be distracted or stressed. Similarly, people who were blind were trained to be piano tuners and craftpersons, and people who had mental retardation were placed in highly repetitive jobs, which were believed too tedious for other workers. This type of matching of disability label to job tasks is demeaning and, fortunately, is no longer widely accepted. However, its vestiges are sometimes seen when people with disabilities are only offered access to certain types of entry-level jobs, or when more emphasis is placed on what a person cannot do, than on what his or her skills are.

Work-Based Learning Opportunities

Work-based learning includes career exploration, vocational assessment, vocational training, and paid work experience at employer worksites. The more work opportunities a student experiences, the more successful he or she is likely to be in postsecondary employment. Paid work is an especially critical component of educational curricula. Regardless of disability type or degree, students are significantly more likely to be employed as adults if they engage in real, paid work while in school (Hasazi et al., 1985; Tilson, Luecking, & Donovan, 1994).

Connection to Community
Resources Through Interagency Collaboration

The non–work-related life needs of students can significantly influence eventual adult employment. Family support, living arrangements, income, peer interactions, and other circumstances can markedly affect postschool outcomes. Student success is often contingent on linking of the student to necessary ancillary community resources. Also, as the student nears the end of his or her publicly supported education, there is an additional need to develop communitywide, collaborative, and cooperative processes among school and adult services. These services might include, for example, employment agencies, community living programs, local and state social services departments, state and local developmental disabilities agencies, and the state vocational rehabilitation agency. Other programs and services might include mental health agencies, Social Security offices, and other services available specifically for people with developmental disabilities.

Sustained Involvement of Employers

Employers are willing to invest the time and resources in workplace learning activities so long as they perceive direct benefit. However, employers' motivation to participate in transition programs must go far beyond good corporate citizenship. Opportunities to influence curriculum, to directly train prospective employees in the intricacies of their industry, and to receive effective consultation in work-force preparation are just a few of the possible benefits. Effective transition programs create these opportunities and regard employers as indispensable partners and valued customers.

STRATEGIES ASSOCIATED WITH
JOB DEVELOPMENT IN TRANSITION

Several successful strategies for implementing transition programs have been widely described in the literature (see, e.g., Siegel, Robert, Waxman, & Gaylord-Ross, 1992; Stark & Karan, 1987; Wehman, Kregel, & Barcus, 1985). In the course of the authors' own experience in developing and managing school-to-work programs at TransCen, the authors have utilized a set of effective practices and beliefs that have assisted over 2,000 students with disabilities to gain competitive employment experiences (Fabian, Luecking, & Tilson, 1994). Working with local school districts, the authors have helped to establish work-based opportunities for students throughout their secondary school years. These work-based development strategies are illustrated in the following case study and are then delineated in the subsequent text.

Case Study: Ben

Ben is a young adult with Down syndrome. Beginning at age 14, his IEP included objectives that involved improving Ben's social skills to prepare him for the adult world. Ben, his teachers, and parents began to discuss educational objectives that would eventually contribute to his employment. By age 16, he began a series of work-based onsite vocational training experiences. One of these included working in a large government office, operating a paper shredder and performing simple filing functions. Another vocational experience involved assisting in a hospital supply room unpacking and sorting materials, as well as at an insurance company office performing custodial functions.

These experiences were selected based on careers Ben wanted to explore and were based on businesses that were available as training environments. In essence, Ben spent much of his time participating in learning experiences that occurred in the community. During and after these experiences, Ben and his parents identified some of the specific tasks he really enjoyed, such as people contact and the opportunity to participate in a variety of tasks, as well as his preference for work environments where people gave him regular feedback.

In his last year of school, Ben's transition teacher helped him find a job with a local insurance company. She noted on several visits that a number of clerks were working there answering and sorting mail and processing claims. After discussing the tasks with the clerks, the teacher presented a proposal to the employer, whereby Ben would open and stamp the mail and the rest of the clerks would focus only on processing claims. In addition, Ben delivered the mail

---

to individual desks. As a result of this job creation, the insurance clerks were able to speed up their responses to customers, and Ben's work made a valuable contribution to the company.

By the time Ben exited school, he had been at the insurance job for 6 months. The transition teacher arranged for a local employment agency to follow Ben on the job, but Ben's co-workers and supervisor at the office also provided ongoing supervision and support to ensure that Ben performed well.

Ben's case study illustrates a variety of strategies useful in promoting quality jobs in the community for students with disabilities in the transition from school to work programs. Six of these strategies are described in the paragraphs following:

1. *Maintain a focus on career education and job choice.* One of the most significant factors in vocational success is the individual's belief that he or she can succeed. For students with disabilities, positive expectations of vocational success may have been curtailed by lack of experience, by lowered expectations of others, and by previous failures (Fabian et al., 1994). The first step in assisting people to make good vocational choices is to assess and develop positive interventions for improving their vocational self-images. Activities that may contribute to improving an individual's vocational self-efficacy and expectations include providing opportunities to try out real jobs in the community, ensuring that vocational tasks are challenging but achievable, and providing opportunities for meeting a variety of different people and observing them on the job. For example, in the case of Ben, teachers and parents took the time to ensure that Ben had access to a variety of vocational experiences and assisted him in identifying aspects of these job trials that were not appealing to him. Perhaps the most important strategy for improving an individual's vocational self-confidence is to ensure that the person's co-workers share a positive belief in his or her potential to make a contribution.

2. *Ensure that students with disabilities have adequate and varied social experiences.* Workplaces are social environments, and one of the major reasons that people with disabilities lose their jobs is not their lack of work skills but their inability to socially "fit into" the work environments. It is critical that students with disabilities, particularly those who may not have had a variety of community experiences, participate in varied social experiences so that they can acquire the interpersonal skills essential for succeeding in the work world. Ben, for example, had participated in a number of vocational internships where he encountered different people, made new friends, and engaged in various social experiences. Such expe-

riences also enable students, their families, and their teachers to identify work environments most suited to the individual's social competencies. After all, the social skills required to work in a bank lobby are different from those required to work on a loading dock.

3. *Prepare students for the job search.* Students with disabilities may have limited understanding of legislation regarding their entry into the world of work and may be reluctant to disclose their disability to employers. However, with the passage of the Americans with Disabilities Act (ADA) of 1990 (PL 101-336), it is now illegal for employers to discriminate against applicants who, with or without reasonable accommodations, are qualified for available positions. The Americans with Disabilities Act has important implications for job preparation.

It is clearly important to prepare students and their families to under-. stand and benefit from the provisions of the Americans with Disabilities Act. Such preparation includes 1) self-knowledge, including understanding of the individual's functional limitations, functional strengths, accommodations for learning styles, and other manifestations of his or her disability; 2) knowledge of specific occupational areas and jobs; and 3) self-advocacy, especially as it relates to presenting skills and strengths to employers and identifying and requesting accommodations.

In the case of Ben, for example, knowledge concerning his functional limitations and strengths was important in assisting him to prepare for a variety of careers. His case example emphasized job creation rather than modification, but the need for reasonable accommodations may have arisen if, for example, Ben had been able to perform some of the essential mail-related functions of the existing clerk's job, but not all of them. In addition, assisting Ben's co-workers and supervisors to convey information to him in a clear and structured way was another type of accommodation strategy that was discussed with the employer during the job interview.

4. *Develop creative employer marketing strategies.* Marketing efforts to employers should be based on marketing individual or programmatic services in the area of transition, not disability. In the example of Ben, the transition teacher first approached the insurance company by stating that she was a high school teacher who worked with students interested in careers in business and requested an appointment so that she might better learn specific occupations and jobs in order to prepare her students. During her visit to the insurance company, the teacher spent time observing a variety of positions, noting which of these might be performed by her students, and which might require additional modifications to conduct. Disability was not mentioned during this visit, except in the context of the employment interview when potential accommodations or job creation strategies were discussed. Instead, the teacher focused on developing a relationship with the employer, emphasizing her (the teacher's) potential

as a resource for recruiting and hiring new staff, and not her role in special education. Based on this relationship, and after subsequent visits and observations, the teacher was able to suggest creating a new job for Ben that would have the overall benefit of contributing to the productivity of the other workers.

5. *Help students prepare for employment interviews.* Preparing the student for an employment interview is an essential aspect of the job development process. Preparing for job interviews includes such activities as practicing answering potential interview questions, filling out job applications, making telephone calls to employers, learning social etiquette, and watching tapes that illustrate such activities. It is also important to consider preparing employers for interviewing students with disabilities. For example, employers might feel uncomfortable about talking to people with disabilities, or they might be worried about how to word some questions. Fabian et al. (1994) pointed out that assisting employers to prepare for an interview with a student applicant is as valuable a service as preparing the applicant.

6. *Negotiate accommodations with employers.* In the example of Ben, the teacher was able to make suggestions that improved the overall productivity of the office and enabled Ben to perform essential functions of a new job that contributed to the entire business. In some cases, students are able to perform some aspects of existing jobs, but not all of them. It is not necessary to engage the employer in arguments regarding what are "reasonable accommodations" under the Americans with Disabilities Act, but instead to approach the employer to discuss how the applicant's skills and employer modifications could be mutually beneficial.

7. *Develop strategies that are customer-responsive.* It is critical to remember that employers are customers of the job developer. Employers should have every reason to expect quality, responsive, and value-added service. Effective employment programs carry this message throughout all their operations and see it as critical to the entire employment process. As illustrated in the case of Ben, good job development strategies involve employers in the decision-making process and are mutually beneficial to the applicant as well as to the business. Job developers who try to "sell" a disability or who rely on employer charity in seeking job opportunities will not be effective in meeting that goal. Customer-responsive job development ensures that transition programs and students with disabilities are regarded as partners with employers, with tangible and valuable services to offer.

CONCLUSIONS

The transition from school to work for youth with disabilities, including those with Down syndrome, is a nationally supported initiative, with policies and programs carried out at state and local levels. After more than a decade of research, policy makers and practitioners can see the benefits to youth of engaging in transition planning in terms of improved employment outcomes for them and increases in their overall quality of life. Although transition programs and services may vary widely, fundamental belief in the ability of all people to make a contribution to businesses, together with creative planning and customer-responsive job development, will eventually ensure more uniform access to employment by youth with Down syndrome.

REFERENCES

Americans with Disabilities Act (ADA) of 1990, PL 101-336, 42 U.S.C. §§ 12101 *et seq.*

Edgar, E. (1988). Transition from school to community. *Teaching Exceptional Children, 20,* 73–75.

Education of the Handicapped Act Amendments of 1983, PL 98-199, 20 U.S.C. §§ 1400 *et seq.*

Fabian, E., Luecking, R., & Tilson, G. (1994). *A working relationship: The job development specialist's guide to successful partnerships with business.* Baltimore: Paul H. Brookes Publishing Co.

Hasazi, S.B., Gordon, L.R., & Roe, C.A. (1985). Factors associated with the employment status of handicapped youth exiting high school from 1979 to 1983. *Exceptional Children, 51,* 455–469.

Parsons, F. (1967). *Choosing a vocation.* New York: Agathon Press.

Siegel, S., Robert, M., Waxman, M., & Gaylord-Ross, R. (1992). A follow-along study of participants in a longitudinal transition program for youths with mild disabilities. *Exceptional Children, 58,* 346–356.

Stark, J., & Karan, O. (1987). Transition services for early adult age individuals with severe mental retardation. In R.N. Ianacone & R.A. Stodden (Eds.), *Transition issues and directions* (pp. 91–110). Reston, VA: Council for Exceptional Children.

Tilson, G., Luecking, R.G., & Donovan, M. (1994). Involving employers in transition: The Bridges model. *Career Development for Exceptional Individuals, 17*(1), 77–90.

Wagner, M. (1989). *Youth with disabilities during transition: An overview of descriptive findings from the National Longitudinal Transition Study.* Menlo Park, CA: SRI International.

Wagner, M., Blackorby, J., Cameto, R., Hebbeler, K., & Newman, L. (1993). *The transition experiences of young people wth disabilities: A summary of findings from the National Longitudinal Transition Study of Special Education Students.* Menlo Park, CA: SRI International.

Wehman, P., Kregel, J., & Barcus, J.M. (1985). School to work: A vocational transition model for handicapped youth. *Exceptional Children, 52,* 25–37.

Will, M. (1984). *OSERS programming for the transition of youth with disabilities: Bridges from school to working life.* Washington, DC: U.S. Department of Education, Office of Special Education and Rehabilitative Services.

19

Supported Employment

Providing Work in the Community

Paul Wehman
Wendy S. Parent
Darlene D. Unger
Karen E. Gibson

In the 1990s, the ability of education and rehabilitation programs for people with disabilities such as Down syndrome to achieve their intended purpose and improve the independence and productivity of U.S. citizens has been increasingly questioned (Dole, 1994). As the United States grapples with budget deficits and reexamines the role of the federal government in providing services to individuals with disabilities, the major federal programs that have been the cornerstone of educational and rehabilitation services are being heavily scrutinized. Within this environment, some policy experts (e.g., Weaver, 1994) are calling for privatization of rehabilitation services. Some congressional leaders (Dole, 1994) are calling for the overhaul or abolition of major legislation such as the Americans with Disabilities Act (ADA) of 1990 (PL 101-336) and the Individuals with Disabilities Education Act (IDEA) of 1990 (PL 101-476), along with a massive restructuring of the way federal funds are used by states for different disability programs.

The national debate on the role of the federal government in providing services to people with Down syndrome has dramatic implications for consumers and advocates. First, the concerns voiced by critics clearly reflect a growing belief that many of these programs have failed, that they are unable to improve the lives of the individuals they were intended to serve (Bowe, 1993). Second, the proposed changes in federal disability programs all focus on reducing federal expenditures in order to help reduce the nation's fiscal deficit. Third, and most important, it is reasonable to assume that people with disabilities, especially those with extensive disabilities, are at great risk of losing access to the limited level of educational and employment services currently available. In other words, it is increasingly likely that employment programs for people with mental retardation and other disabilities will decline, rather than grow, in the near future.

To help offset these social changes and philosophical trends that may ultimately damage the lives and opportunities of people with disabilities, it is important for successful programs that have generated meaningful outcome data over extended periods of time to document and disseminate their results. One such program is supported employment, an approach that focuses on helping chronically unemployed people with disabilities gain competitive employment with the necessary long-term supports. Supported employment is an effective service delivery strategy that has proven its ability to offer people with disabilities, especially those with Down syndrome, the extra help they need to adjust to a competitive jobsite. This chapter describes how the supported employment approach works, the role of natural supports with a job coach, and examples of businesses and support resources, in addition to including two specialized case studies demonstrating these principles.

OVERVIEW OF SUPPORTED EMPLOYMENT

The definition of *supported employment* in the Rehabilitation Act Amendments of 1992 (PL 102-569) has multiple features. Defined as paid employment for people with extensive disabilities for whom competitive employment at or above the minimum wage is unlikely and who, because of their disabilities, need ongoing support to perform their work, supported employment includes the following features: employment; ongoing support; jobs, not services; full participation; social integration; and variety and flexibility. Supported employment is a strategy for changing the mismatch between employment expectations for people with disabilities such as Down syndrome, as well as the typically limited options for their employment. Support is provided through activities such as training, supervision, and transportation. Supported employment is conducted in a variety of settings, particularly in worksites employing people without disabilities.

Supported employment combines employment and ongoing services. It is a type of employment, not a method of employment preparation or a type of service activity. It is a powerful and flexible way to ensure normal employment benefits; provide ongoing and appropriate support; create opportunities; and achieve full participation, integration, and flexibility.

Numerous positive benefits have been shown to accrue from supported employment programs. For example, the most obvious point in favor of competitive employment placement is the increased opportunity for greater wages and benefits (Thompson et al., 1992). With the tremendous cost of maintaining people with disabilities in centers that are nonvocationally oriented or that rarely lead to competitive employment, it is apparent that those consumers who can earn competitive level wages will be viewed with the most favor. These individuals will require less Supplemental Security Income (SSI) assistance from the federal government and, perhaps equally important, will clear the way for other consumers with more extensive disabilities.

Competitive wages will help to increase the independence of people with disabilities such as Down syndrome. The benefits may include insurance policies, medical insurance, dental insurance, and retirement. Of course, this range of benefits will not be available in all cases. Compared with the offerings of developmental centers and most sheltered workshops, however, there is a much greater likelihood of this type of fringe support.

The most obvious advantage of competitive employment wages and benefits may also be the most profound in the long run. Working all day for a total of $4–$5 is not a dignified remuneration for one's daily efforts. It is only natural that the individual eventually comes to view him- or herself as inferior to those without disabilities. Furthermore, people without disabilities who visit sheltered centers may leave with the perception that the economic value of a worker with disabilities is indeed only $4–$5 a day. This is an invidious and unfair conclusion.

Closely linked in importance to wages and benefits is the opportunity within supported employment to work among people without disabilities and not to be segregated with individuals with disabilities. This issue also includes the opportunity for people without disabilities to work daily with those with disabilities. In addition, the likelihood of friendships developing between those with and without disabilities is enhanced. Working with peers without disabilities provides opportunities for workers to learn to accept the criticism and ridicule to which all individuals must adjust. Continual insulation and protection from real work obstacles is a false panacea in the habilitation of individuals with extensive disabilities.

A hallmark of the 1980s in human services was educational inclusion—that is, inclusion of children and youth with disabilities into schools and classrooms along with their peers without disabilities. The underlying philosophy behind this move away from segregation has been the recognition that *all* students have the right to participate in normal activities in environments in which no stigma is attached. Whereas there has been steady progress in U.S. schools toward educational indecision, an extension of this philosophy into the workplace has been witnessed since the mid-1980s.

ROLE OF EMPLOYMENT SPECIALIST AND NATURAL SUPPORTS

The success of supported employment can be directly attributed to two important and unique features that distinguish it from other vocational options. The first of these features is the provision of individualized supports to assist people with Down syndrome, and other disabilities, to become equal participants in the competitive labor force. These supports generally focus on 1) identifying individuals' skills and interests (consumer assessment), 2) finding them jobs (job development), 3) teaching them how to do the job (jobsite training), and 4) providing needed assistance for as long as the worker is employed (ongoing follow-along services).

The second major feature is the role of the employment specialist or job coach who functions as a trainer, advocate, and facilitator in providing and coordinating the preceding supports (Sale, Wood, Barcus, & Moon, 1988; Wehman & Melia, 1985). The responsibilities of the job coach are varied, with primary emphasis on ensuring delivery of whatever work and work-related assistance individuals with disabilities need to become employed and maintain their jobs. A job coach, for instance, might oversee or provide for the following: training to get to and from work on the bus, an alarm watch to signal lunch and breaks, a picture book to assist with completing job duties, or advocacy and social skills training to facilitate relationships and promote development of friendships.

The individualized nature of the supported employment model in delivering needed supports in conjunction with the services of a professional job coach have been the major reasons that supported employment has been so widely accepted and promoted by consumers (Brooke, Barcus, & Inge, 1992; Parent, 1996), parents (Ferguson, Ferguson, & Jones, 1988; Hanley-Maxwell, Whitney-Thomas, & Pogoloff, 1995), employers (Kregel & Unger, 1993; Shafer, Hill, Seyfarth, & Wehman, 1987), rehabilitation professionals (Cook & Pickett, 1994–1995; Molinaro & Walls, 1987), and job coaches (Association for Persons in Supported Employment [5001 West Broad Street, Richmond, VA 23230]; Everson, 1991).

As a result of supported employment's success and popularity, the demand for it often exceeds the availability of services in many communities. Numerous individuals with Down syndrome and other disabilities who would like to work and could benefit from supported employment simply do not have access to the services and supports that would make their career goals a reality. It is not uncommon for a locality to report excessively long waiting lists for services—potentially up to 2 years or more—as individuals sit home or leave school waiting to receive the essential supports to allow them to work competitively.

One strategy that has proven extremely successful in assisting greater numbers of people with extensive disabilities to obtain their desired supports and to become competitively employed is to maximize the use of existing workplace and community supports in association with job coach support (Parent, Unger, Gibson, & Clements, 1994). The job coach continues to assume an instrumental role; however, rather than "doing it all," he or she arranges, coordinates, and monitors assistance from a variety of sources. For example, a parent may assist with filling out and submitting job applications, a co-worker may help a worker learn how to do his or her job, or a community member may drive an individual to and from work. Numerous advantages have been attributed to the provision of good supported employment services that rely on an array of support options, including naturally occurring community and workplace supports. These advantages include enhanced inclusion, greater business investment, reduced job-coach time, longer job retention, and better-quality services (DiLeo, Luecking, & Hathaway, 1995; Hagner & DiLeo, 1993; Murphy & Rogan, 1994; Nisbet, 1992; Parent et al., 1994).

The reliance on a variety of creative and innovative support resources expands the "cookbook" of options available to job coaches. Rather than responding to a need by automatically providing that assistance themselves, job coaches are responsible for assessing the situation with the individual with Down syndrome, sharing information about all possible support options, assisting the person to obtain the support of his or her choice, and providing ongoing assistance with whatever help is desired (Parent et al., 1994). Adhering to this approach during each component of the supported employment model is the best way to ensure that the individual's needs and choices are truly heard and responded to. Effective strategies for implementing this approach and for utilizing creative support options throughout supported employment service delivery are summarized next.

Consumer Assessment

The critical elements of the assessment process are for the job coach to really get to know the individual, build rapport, and determine what he or she truly wants. This is accomplished by meeting with the student and his or her family in a comfortable location; sharing information about supported employment, types of jobs, and potential support options; exploring supports and resources currently used by or available to the individual and his or her family; and encouraging their active participation in sharing ideas, in brainstorming options, and in making decisions. For example, in talking with the student and family it may be determined that flexible hours are an extremely important factor in job placement in order to accommodate the household's schedule. Similarly, the family may mention that they currently rely on members of their church and on neighbors to provide assistance on an as-needed basis.

In addition, community and situational assessments offer an opportunity for the job coach and potential employee to spend time in the community visiting local businesses (three or four 4-hour periods are recommended) to find out the individual's likes and dislikes in terms of job and support choices (Moon, Inge, Wehman, Brooke, & Barcus, 1990; Parent, Gibson, Unger, & Kane, 1995). Experience suggests that the best way to find out a person's strengths and interests is to have them participate in real experiences in actual environments, preferably in the individual's local community.

Job Development

Central to finding a job for an individual with Down syndrome is identifying the person's strengths, determining what people are available to assist with these efforts (e.g., parent, friend, teacher), and deciding the strategies to be utilized. For example, the individual may want to go with a friend to pick up job applications, have the parent assist with completing them, and have the job coach follow up with the employer contact. In addition, completing a functional résumé and attaching it to the application is an excellent way to present the individual's talents and abilities in a professional, competitive way.

The information presented to the employer and the manner in which it is presented are paramount to successfully obtaining the desired employment position. For example, if the individual is always punctual, point that out to the employer; if he or she is very happy and outgoing, emphasize what an asset these traits would be; if the person keeps working until a designated task is completed, focus on this commendable work habit. Determining the demands of the job and translating the potential employee's strengths in the context of what the job requires can help the employer look beyond the disability and realize the benefits associated with hiring a motivated employee who can make a valuable contribution to the company. It is important to investigate the types and degrees of support that are typically offered to employees in general or that could possibly be developed in an effort to begin matching the worker's needs to the natural business supports.

Jobsite Training

The key factors contributing to teaching an employee how to do his or her job include identifying all of the training options available; knowing the individual's learning style and preferences; assisting the worker to choose the best training and compensatory strategies; and arranging and monitoring the training. The job coach is ultimately responsible for ensuring that the individual performs the job to the employer's standards. However, standard company training procedure as is, expanded upon, or modified, is often adequate and effective at teaching the worker his or her job duties. A company, for example, may offer co-worker mentoring, videotape training, supervisor training, or other training options to new employees. Tapping into these resources in a manner that is meaningful to the individual is a critical role of the job coach. For instance, an employee paired to a co-worker mentor may need the job coach to instruct the co-worker on the best method of prompting the individual; a worker participating in a video-tape training who only learns well with hands-on experience would need additional instruction; or an individual provided with a company-sponsored checklist who could not read would need assistance with modifying the support to include pictures.

Once the desired training opportunities are selected and implemented, it is up to the job coach to assess their effectiveness by collecting jobsite training data (e.g., task analyses, production measures); supplementing the training needed using systematic instruction and other behavioral training techniques (Moon et al., 1990); and monitoring ongoing training needs and the adequacy of the available resources. In addition, the job coach must address numerous work-related issues either by providing his or her own assistance or coordinating existing community and workplace support resources. These issues include the many aspects of work that an individual with Down syndrome may need help with to be successfully employed, such as transportation, Social Security, getting along with co-workers, scheduling, punching in, responding to supervision, or handling certain infrequent job responsibilities.

Ongoing Follow-Along Services

The essential element in achieving thorough and stable long-term supports that truly meet an individual's ongoing, dynamic support needs is to be proactive and to consider everything. It is important that nothing be left to chance but, rather, that any potential support need, such as career advancement or seasonal changes, be anticipated and planned for. A variety of traditional and creative supports can be established to address a worker's needs; however, the detailed parameters of the support should be specified, including the person who will provide support, his or her responsibilities, method of contact, and any other pertinent information.

For example, an individual with Down syndrome employed for more than 10 years as a utility worker at a university performs his job duties using a picture book, an alarm watch, co-worker prompting, and supervisor monitoring. Figure 19.1 illustrates this individual's work schedule as a reference for other employees so that if they see him off task or in need of assistance they can communicate consistently and correctly with him regarding his job duties. In addition, specific support responsibilities that are assigned to other workers are outlined and posted on the wall (see Figure 19.2); this prevents a potential breakdown in support that is critically needed to ensure that the employer's standards are maintained.

8:00–8:30 A.M.	Check/empty trash and break boxes
8:30–9:00	Clean and polish stainless steel in dishroom
9:00–9:15	• Organize pans and fill sinks (simultaneously)
9:15–9:45	**Set timer for 30 minutes:** Spray pans and begin washing (while sinks are still filling)
9:45–10:00	**Timer sounds:** Check/empty trash and break boxes
10:00–10:15	**Watch beeps:** Breaktime (get drink only) **Watch beeps:** Return from break
10:15–10:30	Check/empty trash and break boxes
10:30–11:00	**Set timer for 30 minutes:** Spray and wash pans
11:00–11:15	**Timer sounds:** Check/empty trash and break boxes
11:15–11:45	**Set timer for 30 minutes:** Spray and wash pans
11:45–12:15 P.M.	**Watch beeps:** Lunchtime (get lunch and drink) **Watch beeps:** Return from lunch
12:15–12:30	Check/empty trash and break boxes
12:30–1:00	**Set timer for 30 minutes:** Spray and wash pans
1:00–1:15	**Timer sounds:** Check/empty trash and break boxes
1:15–1:45	**Set timer for 30 minutes:** Spray and wash pans
1:45–2:00	**Timer sounds:** Check/empty trash and break boxes
2:00–2:30	**Set timer for 30 minutes:** Spray and wash pans
2:30–2:45	**Timer sounds:** Check/empty trash and break boxes
2:45–3:00	Spray and wash pans
3:00	**Watch beeps:** Go home

Figure 19.1. David's work routine. (Developed by Karen Gibson, Rehabilitation Research and Training Center on Supported Employment, Virginia Commonwealth University, Natural Supports Transition Project [1995].)

TYPES OF JOBS AND SUPPORTS

In general, individuals with Down syndrome can work at many jobs in the community, provided they have the necessary support. The key to successful employment is that the potential employee's preferences and abilities match the required job duties for a specific position, in addition to the workplace culture and environment. For example, if an individual wishes to dress professionally for work by wearing a coat and tie, placing him in a job that requires him to wear jeans and sneakers would not lend itself to a successful job match. Also, if a position requires an individual to perform strenuous tasks of lifting heavy items at a fast pace, and the individual performs tasks at a slow, steady pace and has difficulty lifting heavy items, then that would not be a good job match. The idea that an individual with Down syndrome can only work at certain types of jobs, or that only certain types of businesses will hire the individual, needs to be dismissed. Based on the information the employment specialist has gathered from the assessment process, the employment specialist should present

J and H
- Monitor dish machine for appropriate temperature and working order.
- Monitor sink water, ask David to change if necessary.
- If excessive dirty dishes are observed and time allows, spray and stack them at the sink washing area.

M and C
- Ask David to do trash and boxes first thing in the morning before he reaches the dishroom. Observe to make sure he starts in your area.
- Check David's hat to make sure his watch is attached.
- Assist David in locating handiwipes if you observe him looking for them.

All Staff
- Pick up kitchen pans, utensils, and trays when walking through the dishroom and put them away.
- When walking through the dishroom, make sure David's timer is on (unless he is away from the area).
- When walking through the dishroom and David's timer sounds, monitor and prompt him to do trash and boxes.
- When David's watch on his hat beeps, monitor and prompt him to go on break or to lunch. If unsure of which activity, look at David's watch and it will tell you which it is.

Figure 19.2.   David's co-worker responsibilities. (Developed by Karen Gibson, Rehabilitation Research and Training Center on Supported Employment, Virginia Commonwealth University, Natural Supports Transition Project [1995].)

the individual with a variety of potential job options that match the individual's preferences and abilities.

Instrumental to the successful employment of an individual with a disability is the support provided by the community and workplace. As the job coach is exploring possible jobs, he or she should also be surveying the employment setting for potential support options or providers. For example, identifying an experienced employee whom other co-workers seem to rely on when they have difficulties or questions would be a potential support person for an individual with a disability. The employment specialist should clearly communicate the possible support needs of an individual to an employer during pre-placement activities. This allows the employer to identify the level and type of support the business might be able to provide. Most employers already have existing formal and informal support systems in place for individuals who are new to the business, such as company training videos and co-worker mentors. Businesses and employers provide training and support to all their employees in a variety of ways depending on the individual's needs and preferences and the feasibility of the support needed in relation to the business environment. The employment specialist, the individual with Down syndrome, key stakeholders in that individual's life, and the employer should work cooperatively to identify and develop supports that an individual with a disability could utilize. For example, most franchises or national retail chains typically provide an orientation session for all new hires, and the employment specialist should arrange for the individual to participate in whatever orientation and training is available to all new employees.

Often the employment specialist will sit through the orientation session with the new employee and assist him or her in completing any necessary paperwork. In other situations, the new employee may attend the orientation session unaccompanied by the employment specialist, and the employment specialist may prearrange to have the individual's paperwork completed by the parent or advocate prior to the orientation session. During the orientation session, the employer might also pair the individual with a disability with a senior co-worker to assist him or her during the orientation process and with training. In these instances, the employment specialist should facilitate the relationship between the co-worker mentor and the individual with a disability so that the employer takes the initiative in addressing potential support needs in the future, as would be the case for any of their employees. Knowing that the employer is vested in accommodating and supporting the person with a disability will contribute to successful employment outcomes for the individual.

In developing strategies to assist the individual to learn or to remember how to do the job, the employer and/or the employment specialist should utilize the information that the employer already has at his or her disposal. Most businesses already have standardized ways of training all new employees for a specified position, in addition to company-designed training manuals complete with job duties, checklists, and, possibly, picture cues. Either the employment specialist or the supervisor can modify existing company checklists or picture cues or adopt other compensatory strategies to meet the needs and preferences of the individual. The parents or teacher can also help by both suggesting compensatory strategies that have been successful in the past and developing these strategies. The amount of assistance provided by the employment specialist or other support provider will depend both on the needs and preferences of the individual with Down syndrome and the ability of the support to meet the worker's and employer's needs.

It is important for the employment specialist to consult with the employer and encourage his or her input in identifying and developing supports in the workplace. The employer knows the needs of the business best and is able to direct the job coach to existing supports. As stated, the supervisor or manager may be able to identify an experienced co-worker who could train the individual with Down syndrome or act as a mentor. The employment specialist should provide the employer whatever assistance is necessary to work with the new employee, but he or she should also model appropriate methods or techniques for training the individual in order for the co-worker to simulate those same techniques.

In some instances, the employment specialist may have to provide all of the initial training. Frequently, when an employment specialist spends significant time at the jobsite for initial training, other co-workers will offer to provide support to the individual. After arrangements have been made with the supervisor, this presents ample opportunity for the employment specialist to take a step back and monitor the training provided by the co-worker. It is crucial for the employment specialist to act as a liaison between the individual with a disability and the employer in helping to put in place supports that exist within the employment setting. Table 19.1 lists examples of types of businesses and positions that individuals with disabilities have been employed in, some of the individuals' support needs, the types of supports that were provided, and the role of the employment specialist.

Case Study: Eric

Eric was referred to a local supported employment program for a competitive job by his vocational rehabilitation counselor when he was 19 years old and attending self-contained special education classes at a public high school. Eric has Down syndrome, mental retardation requiring extensive supports, congenital heart disease, and a pacemaker. He has had numerous major surgeries including gall bladder removal, heart valve replacement, cardiac surgery, and multiple hospitalizations for pneumonia. Eric has substantial communication and verbal/comprehension weaknesses. His expressive language includes responses in one- and two-word phrases, and he has articulation difficulties. His receptive language skills are better, in that he demonstrates comprehension of simple directives typically through nonverbal means. He has difficulty with motor skills, especially finger dexterity. Eric becomes fatigued easily and must avoid strenuous work.

Today Eric is 21 years old, attends school, and is employed part time as a lobby attendant at his favorite restaurant earning $4.25 per hour. Because of his physical limitations, he works 3 days a week, 3 hours a day. The remainder of his week is spent in the classroom. In an effort to continue building his skills and work experiences, he participates in school-based work activities, which include horticulture, child care, and cafeteria work.

In determining Eric's job preferences, he participated in several assessment activities. The first was an assessment of his community, during which time he accompanied and directed two job coaches around his neighborhood. This not only gave the job coaches the

Table 19.1. Sample employment positions, support needs, types of support provided, and role of employment specialist

Type of business/position	Support needed	Support(s) offered by employer	Role of employment specialist
Hospital—Dietary aide	Assistance getting to and from the employee parking lot during evening hours	—Supervisor arranged for consumer to use hospital security to ensure that she got back and forth to her car safely during evening hours.	Employment specialist not involved
Hospital—Dietary aide	Initial job training	—Orientation meeting —Pairing with other co-workers —Supervisor-provided instruction	Providing additional support as needed
Hospital—Dietary aide	Remembering how to do the job	—Supervisor prompting of individual —Copy of all required job duties for the tasks that individual was assigned that night; these were provided for each position the individual might be responsible for at any given time.	Identifying support options; modifying checklist to meet needs and preferences of consumer; helping consumer use the support; ongoing monitoring of support
Restaurant—Parking lot and lobby attendant	Learning how to do the job	—Orientation meeting —Company videos —Pairing with other co-workers —Company checklists and job duty descriptions	Overseeing support arrangements; modifying company checklists by using picture cues; providing additional support as needed
Restaurant—Parking lot and lobby attendant	Clocking in and out for work	—Co-worker or supervisor clocks individual in and out based on information contained on card the employment specialist developed for individual.	Identifying support resources with employer and individual; training individual to use support; ongoing monitoring of support

Job	Support activity	Support strategy	Support options
Grocery Store—Bagger	Taking lunch and breaks	—Supervisor prompted individual to go on break and sets watch alarm for the time individual is to return to work.	Identifying support options with assistance from parent, individual, and employer; working together with individual and support provider
Grocery Store—Bagger	Performing infrequent duties associated with the position, such as price checks, restocking items, and gathering carts from the lot	—Employer assigned a co-worker mentor to employee so that individual could utilize the mentor for assistance when needed.	Helping individual to use support; working together with the individual and support provider; ongoing monitoring of support
Office Supply Store—Customer service associate	Transportation to and from work	—Employer assisted employment specialist with identifying co-workers who might be able to assist with transportation.	Identifying support options; sharing information and resources with individual and parents; working together with individual and co-worker to arrange schedules; making alternative transportation arrangements if support is not available
Office Supply Store—Customer service associate	Training individual to perform new tasks and providing follow-along services	—Employer identified co-worker mentor to assist individual and employer agreed to contact individual's parents if needs developed that employer could not address.	Advocacy; working with employer and parents to develop follow-along services; making alternative arrangements if support breaks down or individual chooses to no longer use support
Day Care—Teacher's aide	Reading the children's names above their individual storage units	—Photographs of each child were placed above each unit so individual could return items to appropriate unit.	Identifying support options; working with employer to develop supports and overseeing support arrangement
Day Care—Teacher's aide	Advocating for the employee and handling customer concerns	—Employer and co-workers advocated for individual when parents expressed concern over individual's ability.	Advocacy; ongoing monitoring of support

opportunity to conduct a job labor-market analysis, but they were able to observe Eric's familiarity with his neighborhood; identify locations Eric favored; and begin building a relationship with Eric by getting to know him and establishing rapport. Eric was given the opportunity to select a minimum of two situational work assessments, which would allow him new experiences and expose him to types of work with which he was not familiar. He and his family chose to try a light janitorial cleaning experience at a local fitness center because he enjoyed cleaning at home, and a lobby attendant position at a fast-paced restaurant. These experiences provided an excellent comparison of hands-on performance in two distinct environments. One demonstrated a busy, bright, noisy, customer-centered environment with general public interaction, whereas the other consisted of a steady, leisurely paced environment, with minimal interaction with the club members in a quiet location. Eric appeared to thrive with the customer contact because he was an extremely social young man. Even though his pace was somewhat slower than would be expected of this position, he was able to keep up with the demands of the job, and it was reasonable to believe that an accommodation and repetition through performance would improve his pace. The busyness of the job kept him on task, whereas he tended to slow excessively in the slower-paced job.

As a result of his performance during the assessments and after Eric had talked things over with his family and other key people in his life (including his case manager, teacher, and vocational counselor), he decided he wanted to be a lobby attendant. He was also able to identify where his first choice of employment should be which was his favorite restaurant near his home.

Eric required extensive accommodation regarding when and how long he should work given his physical limitations. In addition, he was involved in a number of social/recreational activities on the weekends that were important to him. Neither he nor his mother was willing to sacrifice these activities because of the improved self-worth and personal growth he experienced as a result of participating in these activities. This preference was expressed to Eric's potential employer when the employment specialist was developing a job for Eric. At first the employer reacted negatively, because he felt that all of his employees would rather be participating in social activities as opposed to working on the weekends. However, the employer was told that due to Eric's disability there were no alternative times for him to participate in these activities because they were only offered on the weekend. Eric's commitment to these activities was furthermore highlighted, as well as the benefits he received as a result of participating. The employer became impressed that given Eric's extensive limitations he sought to indulge in meaningful activities that added happiness and satisfaction to his life. He stated that he wished all of his employees were as committed to something, and he was happy to be able to help Eric achieve his goals. As a result, Eric was given the hours and days he wanted.

Once Eric was hired, many needs continued to surface that required support. In each case, numerous support resources were identified by brainstorming with Eric's family, co-worker, supervisor, case manager, friends, teacher, vocational rehabilitation counselor, and other people in Eric's life. Table 19.2 outlines many of Eric's needs, his first choice of support, and back-up supports that were developed to meet the identified needs.

Case Study: Mary

Mary is a 22-year-old woman who recently graduated from a special education center where she attended self-contained special education classes owing to her intellectual disabilities, inadequate expressive language, and emotional control problems. She has Down syndrome and a heart murmur, wears glasses, and is excessively overweight. She has mental retardation requiring extensive supports. Before graduating, Mary spent her last 4 years of school participating in community-based, integrated, paid work experiences. Mary resides with her mother, stepfather, and two stepsisters in a small home in a suburban area. Her mother does not work outside of the home.

Mary is employed as a part-time lobby attendant at a fast-food restaurant in her neighborhood. She works 4 hours a day, Monday through Friday, and earns $4.75 an hour. As part of her benefits, she receives a free uniform and reduced-price meals. When she is able to average 30 hours a week, she will be able to participate in the medical benefits program offered through the company and will receive paid leave. Mary is primarily responsible for keeping the tables and chairs clean during the lunch rush; supplying the tables with salt and pepper shakers and promotional displays; stocking the condiment stand; gathering trays from the lobby; preparing cleaning solution; wiping the food trays; washing the windows; keeping the floor clean; keeping the salad bar clean; cleaning in the bathrooms; and being courteous and responsive to the customers.

Prior to Mary's graduation and employment, she was referred to the supported employment program for placement into a supported competitive job. As part of the supported employment services that were provided, Mary participated in several assessments. On one of these she accompanied program staff during a community assessment of various job opportunities, including those at a local mall. While at the mall, Mary ate at her favorite fast-food restaurant, ordering her food independently and selecting condiments without assistance. Many of her skills were assessed at that time, such as her reaction to busy, large, and noisy spaces, as typified by the food

Table 19.2. Eric's support needs and support options

Identified need	First choice of support	Back-up support
Finding a job	Employment specialist	Parents/teacher/vocational rehabilitation counselor
Getting ready for work	Teacher assists	Friend/parent
Transportation	School	Specialized system/friend/parent
Getting into the store	Driver	Friend/parent
Punching in	Eric shows punched card to co-worker	Co-worker/supervisor
Negotiating duties	Supervisor determines	Employment specialist/parent
Arranging schedule	Supervisor determines	Parent/employment specialist
Learning the job	Co-worker	Employment specialist/teacher
Assistance with job	Co-workers prompt	Co-workers/supervisor
Infrequent job duties	Co-workers assist	Co-workers
Communication	Eric shows needs/wants	Co-workers' familiarity with Eric
Ordering lunch	Eric shows developed card to co-worker	Parent notifies of changes according to special diet
Handling Social Security	Parent	Independent consultant/case manager
Medical appointments	Parent	Sibling/case manager
Follow-along service	Employer monitors	Parent/service provider

court, as well as her social skills in small, confined, novelty stores. She was also observed as she browsed through numerous stores that she elected to visit in an effort to determine her likes, preferences, and method of making decisions.

Mary was furthermore given the opportunity to participate in situational work assessments to expose her to a variety of work experiences. She chose to bag groceries at a grocery store, which was prearranged by the supported employment program. Mary enjoyed the work, and her social skills with customers were excellent. Despite limited expressive language ability, she smiled appropriately at the customers and was outgoing. She was attentive to her work and performed tasks with accuracy. She got along well with her co-workers and was eager to continue working.

Mary's school work experience had also included 2 years in an elementary school cafeteria, as well as 2 other years working in a cafeteria at a county government complex. Because of her extensive work history, Mary did not opt to participate in other situational work assessments but chose, instead, to be observed in her job at the school cafeteria. After her assessments, Mary expressed the desire to work at her favorite fast-food restaurant. Mary, her mother, teacher, case manager, and vocational counselor asked the employment specialist to assist Mary with job development. The employment specialist contacted the restaurant Mary had selected and informed the manager about Mary and her overwhelming desire to work at that particular restaurant. After disclosing Mary's disability, the employment specialist learned that the manager had a successful experience working with a supported employee in the past at a different location. The manager was delighted that Mary had selected his store for employment and wanted to hire her immediately. An interview was scheduled for the following week. The employment specialist mentioned to the employer the potential need for accommodations during the interview, with the primary focus being communication and Mary's low intellectual functioning. Mary was accompanied to the interview by the employment specialist. She was given a tour of the store, and the essential duties of the job we explained or shown to her in a way she could understand. The manager offered Mary the job and she eagerly accepted.

Mary was delayed 2 months in starting her job because a uniform could not be located in her size, and she could not work without a uniform. When the uniform finally arrived, it had to be altered somewhat in appearance in order to fit her, requiring some flexibility on the part of the store manager. Throughout the 2 months, however, there was open communication between all parties. Even though at times it seemed Mary would not be able to work, the wait was well worth the time invested. Mary is now happily employed, and Mary and her family have developed strong relationships with her supervisor and co-workers. Everyone is very pleased with the outcome.

Table 19.3 outlines many of Mary's needs, her first choice of support, and back-up supports that were developed to meet the needs identified.

OBTAINING SUPPORTED EMPLOYMENT SERVICES

Often, people who want to work with help from supported employment services fail to obtain a job simply because they do not have the information to link them up with the primary agencies that can make it happen. These include the school systems, vocational rehabilitation agency, mental health/mental retardation agency, and supported employment programs. The following guidelines are offered to aid individuals with Down syndrome; their families; advocates; and rehabilitation, education, human service, and medical professionals who are interested in gaining access to supported employment services.

Explore Career Opportunities

The more information one gathers about different occupations, the better equipped one is to make career choices or to advise others regarding occupational decisions. For example, read the classifieds, visit businesses, talk to friends in other fields, explore career products, and invite guest speakers to describe their professions. It is important to not exclude job types, to avoid overlooking a potential career area or related interest that could be modified or molded to meet a person's particular skills.

Participate in a Variety of Experiences

For the professional, virtually every experience can be regarded as a new source of possible job types or support options that may be of use to someone with Down syndrome. The list of businesses, positions, and supports is endless, and every opportunity to find out about them should be exploited. As a consumer or parent, explore the community; participate in community work, training, volunteer, and social activities; talk with other parents and their sons or daughters about their experiences; and think about what people in your life can contribute as resources for career and support information.

Learn What Adult and Community Services Offer

Contact adult and community agencies and organizations, ask them about the services they offer, the eligibility criteria, and procedures for referral. As a professional, share all you know with the individuals and families with whom you come in contact. A lack of questions does not necessarily mean that the people who could benefit from services have all the information they need. Quite the contrary; often individuals do not even know what questions to ask to gain access to services they need. As consumers

Table 19.3. Mary's support needs and support options

Identified need	First choice of support	Back-up support
Determining job choices	Discuss assessments	Review past records/experiences
Finding a job	Employment specialist	Family/teacher/vocational rehabilitation
Getting ready for work	Mother assists	Sibling/friend/paid assistant
Transportation	Mother	Specialized public transportation
Work-related expenses	Mary	Family/SSA work incentives/vocational rehabilitation
Punching in	Mary with assistance	Co-worker/supervisor
Negotiating duties	Supervisor determines	Employment specialist
Arranging schedule	Supervisor determines	Parent/employment specialist
Learning the job	Videotape training	Co-worker/mentor/job coach
Performing the job	Compensatory strategies	Assistive equipment/co-workers
Infrequent job duties	Co-workers prompt	Supervisor/compensatory aid
Communication	Demonstration	Co-workers' familiarity with Mary
Social Security issues	Parents	Independent consultant

SSA, Social Security Administration.

or parents, do not be intimidated by professional jargon; instead, ask questions and persevere until you feel comfortable with the information obtained.

Find Out About Supported Employment

Contact the vocational rehabilitation agency and supported employment providers to find out about supported employment services in a locality, the referral procedures, and service delivery practices. By learning about supported employment, what to expect, the vast support resources that are available, and what outcomes can be achieved, a consumer, family member, professional, or advocate can participate more meaningfully in the decisions and choices that are made regarding employment for the person with Down syndrome. The best way to gain information about supported employment is to read written resources, talk with individuals and family members who have been involved with supported employment, visit supported employment providers and observe firsthand what can be offered, and attend local and national conferences with agendas that emphasize supported employment.

Arrange Services and Supports

Active involvement among all participants in planning and implementing supported employment is essential for the individual to achieve his or her career goals and to obtain the necessary supports. The critical first step in accomplishing this is to refer the individual to the vocational rehabilitation agency to request rehabilitation and supported employment services. Sharing of ideas, experiences, and skilled expertise through frequent written and oral correspondence by all parties is important to ensure that no competitive business or workplace, or community support or professional assistance, is overlooked. Only with interagency and intradisciplinary coordination, ongoing communication, creativity and open-mindedness, and advocacy by and for individuals with Down syndrome can their true and equal participation in the competitive labor force be assured.

CONCLUSIONS

Since its inception as a federal and state government–supported vocational rehabilitation program with the 1986 amendments to the Rehabilitation Act (PL 99-506), supported employment has afforded an increasing number of individuals with severe disabilities who were previously believed to be unemployable an opportunity to enter and compete in our nation's work force. Employment in community-based businesses and organizations is clearly an achievable goal for adolescents with Down syndrome. Supported employment and the use of resources that exist within community and workplace environments will assist people with Down syndrome in obtaining and maintaining competitive employment. It is through a collaborative effort of the individual, family members, rehabilitation and educational professionals, and other identified supports that individuals with Down syndrome can ultimately achieve their career goals.

REFERENCES

Americans with Disabilities Act (ADA) of 1990, PL 101-336, 20 U.S.C. §§ 1400 *et seq.*

Bowe, F. (1993). Statistics, politics, and employment of people with disabilities. *Journal of Disability Policy Studies, 4*(2), 83–91.

Brooke, V., Barcus, M., & Inge, K. (1992). *Consumer advocacy and supported employment: A vision for the future* [Monograph]. Richmond: Virginia Commonwealth University, Rehabilitation Research and Training Center on Supported Employment.

Cook, J.A., & Pickett, S.A. (1994–1995). Recent trends in vocational rehabilitation for people with psychiatric disability. *American Rehabilitation, 21*(4), 2–12.

DiLeo, D., Luecking, R., & Hathaway, S. (1995). *Natural supports in action: Strategies to facilitate supports of workers with disabilities.* St. Augustine, FL: Training Resource Network.

Dole, R. (1994, October 7). Employment for persons with disabilities. *Congressional Record.*

Everson, J. (1991). Supported employment personnel: An assessment of their self-reported training needs, educational backgrounds, and previous employment experiences. *Journal of The Association for Persons with Severe Handicaps, 16*(3), 140–145.

Ferguson, P.M., Ferguson, D.L., & Jones, D. (1988). Generations of hope: Parental perspectives on the transition of their children with severe retardation from school to adult life. *Journal of The Association for Persons with Severe Handicaps, 13,* 177–187.

Hagner, D., & DiLeo, D. (1993). *Working together: Workplace culture, supported employment, and persons with disabilities.* Cambridge, MA: Brookline Books.

Hanley-Maxwell, C., Whitney-Thomas, J., & Pogoloff, S.M. (1995). The second shock: A qualitative study of parents' perspectives and needs during their child's transition from school to adult life. *Journal of The Association for Persons with Severe Handicaps, 20*(1), 3–15.

Individuals with Disabilities Education Act (IDEA) of 1990, PL 101-476, 20 U.S.C. §§ 1400 *et seq.*

Kregel, J., & Unger, D. (1993). Employer perceptions of the work potential of individuals with disabilities: An illustration from supported employment. *Journal of Vocational Rehabilitation, 3*(4), 17–25.

Molinaro, D.A., & Walls, R.T. (1987). The paradigm shift in vocational rehabilitation. *Journal of Rehabilitation Administration, 11,* 44–48.

Moon, M.S., Inge, K.J., Wehman, P., Brooke, V., & Barcus, J.M. (1990). *Helping persons with severe mental retardation get and keep employment: Supported employment strategies and outcomes.* Baltimore: Paul H. Brookes Publishing Co.

Murphy, S., & Rogan, P. (1994). *Developing natural supports in the workplace: A practitioner's guide.* St. Augustine, FL: Training Resource Network.

Nisbet, J. (Ed.). (1992). *Natural supports in school, at work, and in the community for people with severe disabilities.* Baltimore: Paul H. Brookes Publishing Co.

Parent, W. (1996). Consumer choice and satisfaction in supported employment. *Journal of Vocational Rehabilitation, 6*(1), 23–30.

Parent, W., Gibson, K., Unger, D., & Kane, K. (1995). *Maximizing the use of community and workplace supports in supported employment: Case study illustrations.* Unpublished manuscript.

Parent, W., Unger, D., Gibson, K., & Clements, C. (1994). The role of the job coach: Orchestrating community and workplace supports. *American Rehabilitation, 20*(3), 2–11.

Rehabilitation Act Amendments of 1992, PL 102-569, 29 U.S.C. §§ 701 *et seq.*

Sale, P., Wood, W., Barcus, J.M., & Moon, M.S. (1989). The role of the employment specialist. In W.E. Kiernan & R.L. Schalock (Eds.), *Economics, industry, and disability: A look ahead* (pp. 187–205). Baltimore: Paul H. Brookes Publishing Co.

Shafer, M.S., Hill, J., Seyfarth, J., & Wehman, P. (1987). Competitive employment and workers with mental retardation: Analysis of employers' perceptions and experiences. *American Journal on Mental Retardation, 92*(3), 304–311.

Thompson, L., Powers, G., & Houchard, B. (1992). The wage effects of supported employment. *Journal of The Association for Persons with Severe Handicaps, 17,* 236–246.

Weaver, C. (1994). Privatizing vocational rehabilitation: Options for increasing individual choice and enhancing competition. *Journal of Disability Policy Studies, 5*(1), 53–76.

Wehman, P., & Melia, R. (1985). The job coach: Function in transitional and supported employment. *American Rehabilitation, 11*(2), 4–7.

20

Opportunities for Employment

Creative Approaches

David T. Helm
William E. Kiernan
Sara Miranda

A job provides both a means of economic self-sufficiency and an identity for an individual. Society assumes that adults will enter the world of work upon completing their education and become, in large measure, economically self-sufficient. Through work an individual can also expand his or her social network. Increasingly, social relationships and recreational activities are related either directly or indirectly to one's employment. One's job often serves to define one's role in society. Without work, many of the accepted adult roles for an individual are severely compromised. Unfortunately, for people who have a disability, employment options historically have been significantly limited. This chapter reviews changes in the role of employment for the adolescent with Down syndrome; it provides an overview of employment and training systems for people with disabilities; it identifies strategies that have proven effective for enhancing employment opportunities for people with disabilities; and, finally, it offers answers to frequently raised concerns from parents, family members, and people with disabilities relative to employment.

TRENDS IN EMPLOYMENT OF PEOPLE WITH DISABILITIES

Since the early 1980s there has been a growing recognition that employment for people with disabilities is a realistic option. Studies have documented that, through the effective matching of individual interests and strengths with employer needs, the provision of on-site training and supports, and, at times, the use of job coaches for ongoing supports, people who would formerly have been considered unable to work are entering and remaining in employment (Kiernan, McGaughey, Lynch, Morganstern, & Schalock, 1991; Mank, Oorthuys, Rhodes, Sandow, & Weyer, 1992; McGaughey, Kiernan, McNally, Gilmore, & Keith, 1994; Wehman, Kregel, & Shafer, 1989; West, Revell, & Wehman, 1992). During the 1990s, more than 105,000 people with severe disabilities have been reported working in supported employment, with about 30% of the more than 1.02 million individuals with disabilities served through the Community Rehabilitation Program system in either competitive or supported employment (McGaughey et al., 1994; West et al., 1992). Much of the interest in securing real jobs for people with severe disabilities accompanied the advent of supported employment (see Chapter 19). Supported employment originally focused on assisting individuals with more severe disabilities who were being served in day or sheltered workshops to move into real jobs with on-site supports (Kiernan & Stark, 1986; Rusch & Hughes, 1990; Wehman & Moon, 1988). This movement was fueled by a growing realization that placement and training on site was a more effective strategy than pretraining with subsequent job placement. Coupled with the changes in the economy from a manufacturing to a service base, there was a need to move the worker to the site rather than the work to the worker (Kiernan & Schalock, 1989).

A parallel emphasis was being developed around concerns expressed by parents about the need for better supports for their children with disabilities who were exiting schools and entering adult life (Turnbull & Turnbull, 1982). Research was demonstrating that students who had employment experiences while in high school were more likely to be employed, at the time *and* after leaving school (Hasazi, Gordon, & Roe, 1985). These results influenced the secondary school curriculum with many school districts adopting a vocationally oriented experience for these students (Hasazi et al., 1985; Wehman, Moon, Everson, Wood, & Barcus, 1988). However, the transition process was often complicated by an absence of real jobs after graduation for many of the students exiting school. Frequently the option was a waiting list or, for students with disabilities, placement in a sheltered workshop. Little in the curriculum connected the school experience with the actual options available through the adult service system (Wehman et al., 1988).

Although there has been an effort to increase the employment of individuals with disabilities in integrated settings through either supported employment or competitive employment, their unemployment rate remains at about 70% (McGaughey et al., 1994). Studies have reported that many people with disabilities who are not working, when asked, would enter employment if a suitable job were available (Harris, 1995). The technology to assist individuals to enter employment is available, yet many people with disabilities still do not have real jobs (Mank, 1994; McGaughey et al., 1994; Wehman & Kregel, 1995). Part of this dilemma reflects concerns expressed by individuals and family members in relation to employment, and part reflects the slow adoption of support strategies in real jobs by the professional education and rehabilitation communities. Both of these concerns are addressed in subsequent sections of this chapter. The following section provides a brief overview of the systems of employment and training that are available for adolescents with Down syndrome and other people with disabilities as they consider work as a realistic option for the future.

OVERVIEW OF EMPLOYMENT AND TRAINING SYSTEMS FOR PEOPLE WITH DISABILITIES

The early emphasis on employment of people with disabilities was directed at providing the individual who had experienced a traumatic injury with the necessary rehabilitative services in order to return to work. Federal and private rehabilitation efforts were directed at assisting the injured worker to return to work. The overriding focus of the rehabilitation effort was to save money by removing the worker who had been injured on the job from a dependency role and reinstating him or her into a production and employment role (Kiernan & Hagner, 1995).

It was not until the late 1960s and early 1970s that the rehabilitation field expanded its view to include services for those who had never been employed. Federal legislation specifically indicated that people with mental retardation and other disabling conditions from birth or those having a disability of early onset should be considered eligible for services so long as there was some reasonable expectation that employment would be the outcome of the rehabilitation effort. The Vocational Rehabilitation Act Amendments of 1965 (PL 89-333) opened the door for individuals with Down syndrome to be eligible for Vocational Rehabilitation services. Even with this change in legislation, many people with cognitive disabilities, particularly those with mental retardation requiring limited or extensive support, were not considered eligible for Vocational Rehabilitation services because there was no realistic expectation that they would be able to be employed. For many people with mental retardation and other developmental disabilities including Down syndrome who were accepted by Vocational Rehabilitation, the end outcome was closure into sheltered workshops (Whitehead & Marrone, 1986).

Many people with Down syndrome are served not by the public Vocational Rehabilitation system but by state agencies for Mental Retardation and Developmental Disability. This system has provided, and continues to provide, day and employment services for people with mental retardation, often utilizing sheltered and nonwork options, and it historically has placed much less emphasis on employment and more on community living and non–work-related activities. The criterion for eligibility is that the individual have a diagnosis of mental retardation. Some states have broadened their eligibility criteria to include the more comprehensive functional definition of developmental disabilities.

State agencies such as Mental Retardation and Developmental Disability, Mental Health, and Vocational Rehabilitation frequently contract for day and employment services with community not-for-profit agencies often referred to as Community Rehabilitation Programs. This system is varied, in that some agency programs are specific as to the range of services they offer—such as employment or community living services only—whereas others offer a broad array of services including early intervention, family supports, case management or service coordination, day and employment programs, recreation, and community living. Often the range of services offered reflects how prescriptive the actual contract might be. In the case of a supported employment contract, Community Rehabilitation Programs are only requested to provide this service for a designated number of individuals in real work settings. For other day services, the agency might provide work, community living, transportation, recreation, and other services.

Since the early 1990s, state agencies have made a greater effort to encourage the utilization of integrated employment (competitive and supported jobs) by requiring a certain percentage of those served through a contract to be placed in integrated jobs. This shift reflects the growing interest by both individuals with disabilities and sponsoring agencies to facilitate greater entry into the competitive labor market for all people with disabilities. More and more people entering the state Mental Retardation and Developmental Disabilities system are considered candidates for integrated employment. In 1993 the percentage of individuals with mental retardation served in integrated settings (30%) was nearly twice the percentage served in such settings just 2 years earlier (18%) (Kiernan, 1996).

With passage of the Individuals with Disabilities Education Act (IDEA) of 1990 (PL 101-476) an increased emphasis is furthermore being placed on development of vocational or adult life goals while the student is in his or her high school years. IDEA calls for development of a transition plan for all students with disabilities at age 16 and preferably at age 14 (see also Chapter 18). The transition plan should indicate what the student's long-term goals might be; some of the available resources; and the roles of school personnel, the public vocational rehabilitation agency, and other state agencies in the transition planning and implementation process. Transition planning is designed to coordinate resources to enable a smooth transition for the student from school to either postschool options or employment and other areas of adult life.

As the preceding description of employment and training systems has demonstrated, a substantial shift in program emphasis has occurred since the mid-1980s. This shift is characterized by an increased interest in developing programs and resources that meet the needs of the individual with disabilities, rather than fitting the individual into the existing service program. In addition, the growing interest in establishing a person-driven and ultimately a person-controlled system emphasizes the interests and preferences of the individual, rather than his or her impairments or the available slots that a state or community agency may have to fill. This shift furthermore has expanded the transition planning process to include the individual with a disability, family members, and friends as core members of the planning team.

Although the service resources noted previously continue to provide supports, the design of services is controlled much more by the individual and his or her family. The transition planning process has further acknowledged the need for employment planning to begin in middle school, or when the student is about 14 years old, with the student, family, and school personnel involving adult service representatives in planning and job development. The movement away from the purchase of workshop slots to on-site supports and creation of jobs to match individual skills and interests has led to a much greater interest in creating jobs or in creating jobs out of existing positions in areas best suited to the individual's skills.

The following section describes the change in the vocational or employment planning process from one emphasizing deficits and program settings to one focusing on individual preferences and the development of innovative supports for people on the job. Some of these support approaches have proven effective in facilitating the entry of adolescents with Down syndrome and other developmental disabilities into integrated jobs.

EFFECTIVE APPROACHES TO ENHANCING EMPLOYMENT OPTIONS

In addition to the expanded role of the individual and the recognition of competitive and supported employment as a viable option for people with disabilities, a shift has occurred in the emphasis of planning from a deficit design—or one that looks at what the individual is not able to do—to a design that considers the interests and preferences of that person and builds on his or her strengths. This shift has altered the service approach from one of "fixing the person" to one of adapting the setting, an approach referred to as *person-centered planning* (Butterworth et al., 1993; Smull & Harrison, 1992). Person-centered planning describes a group of closely aligned planning formats aimed at learning about and understanding how a person with a disability would like to live his or her life, what his or her hopes and dreams are, and what supports would be needed for that vision to become a reality. The individual's preferences, as well as choices and vision for the future, are the focus and the desired outcome for a person-centered planning approach.

A person-centered planning process contrasts with typical agency or educational planning, which tends to be formal, even legalistic, in nature. Too often the individual is not the primary actor in these meetings; in fact, some studies have reported that family, friends, and the individual whose life is being planned may not even be present at planning meetings (Irvin, Thorin, & Singer, 1993; Turnbull & Turnbull, 1982). Such formal meetings tend to be unidirectional, with the professional or paid staff providing all the information and recommendations to an inactive individual and his or her family. A person-centered planning process, however, is quite different and can yield a more satisfying and creative outcome. The expectations in a person-centered plan are that the individual is the core of the plan development, design, and coordination; that the participants are often personal friends, interested parties, and professionals; and that the individual is an active contributor in the discussion of the plan. The process does not focus on evaluation data or reports but, rather, on feelings and hopes, with the end product a consensus of what the individual and all those present would hope to see develop for the person.

Unlike many of the more formal and mandated planning processes, such as the individualized written rehabilitation plan, individualized transition plan, individualized service plan, and the like, the approach to developing a person-centered plan is varied. A number of processes have evolved under the broad title of person-centered planning. These processes have been termed "lifestyle planning" (O'Brien, 1987); "personal futures planning" (Mount & Zwernik, 1988); MAPs, or the McGill Action Planning System (Vandercook, York, & Forest, 1989); "outcome-based planning" (Steere, Wood, Panscofar, & Butterworth, 1990); "essential lifestyle planning" (Smull & Harrison, 1992); and "whole life planning" (Butterworth et al., 1993). Each of these approaches varies to some degree in focus or emphasis, but all share some generally defined principles, including the following:

1. The individual for whom the plans are being formed directs the process or guides the planning.
2. Family members and friends of the individual are included in all phases of the planning process, and there is a strong reliance on personal social relationships as the primary source of support to the individual.

3. The planning focuses on capacities and assets of the individual, rather than on limitations and deficiencies.
4. There is an emphasis on the settings, services, supports, and routines available in the community at large, rather than on those designed for people with disabilities.
5. There is recognition that such a planning process must tolerate uncertainty, setbacks, false starts, and disagreement (see Butterworth et al., 1993; Hagner, Helm, & Butterworth, 1996; O'Brien & Lovett, 1993).

The literature on person-centered planning provides a rationale for why this type of planning is important, how it can be effective, and how it varies from more formalized planning processes typically set up by providers creating legal or quasi-legal plans. The authors of the various approaches outline steps to implement the process, including model forms and exemplary practices such as checklists and interview formats (e.g., see Butterworth et al., 1993).

Although this chapter focuses on the concerns and outcomes of creative job options for adolescents with Down syndrome, person-centered planning can be applied to almost all aspects of one's life—as implied in the name of one such process, whole life planning. This type of planning process is not for all occasions, nor does it solve all problems. It has, however, proven to be an effective way to address many problems of focus and has provided positive direction in people's lives and careers (Marrone, Hoff, & Helm, in press). Person-centered planning can be particularly helpful when easy or straightforward job options may not be apparent to an adolescent with Down syndrome. As discussed later, such a planning process can lead to more individualized job development—at times job creation and in some instances job accommodation.

Since there is flexibility in such a planning process, it may be helpful to compare some of the key steps in two planning processes: whole life planning (Butterworth et al., 1993) and personal futures planning (Mount & Zwernick, 1988). Table 20.1 summarizes the key activities that occur within each of these steps.

Once a person-centered plan is developed, there is a need to identify jobs and to assist the individual in realizing his or her employment choice. In many instances the individual will identify areas of work interest that he or she wishes to explore. Those job interests often form job clusters on which job development will focus. The job development process thus becomes one of locating a company or employer with an opening in the desired area. Job placement would then be the final stage of this process.

A number of organized support structures mentioned previously, such as the public vocational rehabilitation system, the Department of Mental Retardation and Developmental Disabilities, or the local school system may

Table 20.1. Comparing two versions of person-centered planning

Whole life planning[a]	Personal futures planning[b]
1. *Organizing the planning process:* This step includes the who, when, and where of the meetings. Who should organize and facilitate the process should also be decided on in advance.	1. *Finding capacities:* Includes constructing a personal profile of the person: his or her history, relationships, places, choices, what works / doesn't work, ideas about the future.
2. *Developing a personal profile:* A comprehensive inventory of the places, people, and *activities* in a person's life is developed. The purpose is to gain a more complete picture of what the person likes to do, the people he or she likes to be with, where the person likes to spend his or her time, and clues as to the vision being developed.	2. *Discovering a vision and a plan:* A comprehensive review of the person's profile, the environmental trends, and images of a desirable future. Obstacles and opportunities are identified and strategies created, including systems change needs.
3. *Building a vision:* The central part of building a plan for the individual, this step synthesizes what the person likes to do, and what he or she hopes to be doing while attempting to draw on themes created in the profile.	3. *Building a circle through action:* This process develops a ``try-reflect-fix'' circle that builds increasingly more effective support for the person.
4. *Action planning:* This step ensures there is some accountability and that things will *actually* happen. People are assigned tasks to help achieve results.	4. *Working for systems change:* This phase specifies and works for changes in the service system to allow the most relevant assistance to be given to the individual.
5. *Supporting networks and plans:* In this step, the participants decide their next action: Will they continue to meet? When will they check in with each other? and How will they keep the process going?	5. *Continuation of process:* This allows participants to work together over time as equals across organizational boundaries.

[a]Adapted from Butterworth et al. (1993).
[b]Adapted from Mount and Zwernik (1988).

have job developers or placement specialists on their staffs. These individuals will typically seek out employers and monitor the job openings that are listed either on bulletin boards, through help-wanted sections of newspapers, or through individual networks.

Historically, most job development has been done through a placement person. More recently, however, there has been growing recognition of the benefit of using one's personal networks in job development. This is in fact the strategy that most people use when looking for employment. The network often includes asking family and friends to identify job openings, conducting informational interviews in companies that may have the types of work that are of interest to an individual, submitting open letters of interest in employment to a company, identifying friends or acquaintances who might be employed in selected companies, and other similar outreach efforts. Much of the literature has shown that this networking strategy is effective in many ways for people with disabilities. Upon identifying a job opportunity, a specific job interview is arranged so that the individual along with his or her representative, if desired, may meet with the company and file a formal application. This process sometimes is aided if the job developer or other representative contacts the employer beforehand to identify clearly the nature of the job as well as to advocate for the potential employee (Hagner & DiLeo, 1993).

In some instances, there will be a need to change or adapt some aspects of the workplace once the individual is hired. These accommodations are frequently small and may include, for example, reassigning certain jobs or tasks that may be difficult for the individual to do, consolidating tasks, or devising a sequence of performance for the worker. Some minor task redesign often allows the individual to better meet the employer's expectations and accomplish the tasks of the position. This activity is typically done for all employees when they first come on a job.

In other instances, there may be a need for a more dramatic job restructuring or job creation. In those instances, often there is considerable negotiation with the employer prior to a job offer being made. Through job creation, a position is created by identifying unmet or poorly met needs in the company and combining them to create a new position. Through job restructuring, existing jobs are modified by eliminating certain tasks or reassigning those tasks to others who have the relative skills and interest. Job restructuring can involve modifying working conditions such as work schedules, task sequences, or work area organization. Both job creation and job restructuring are strategies that require a more skillful and systematic approach to the job development process. Typically, in developing a job utilizing one of these strategies, the amount of time and effort required is greater than that of a direct placement or a direct job development effort. Clearly, in such instances, the ability and creativity of the job developer can play a vital role in securing employment.

In addition to modifying the job, adaptations or assistive devices may be necessary or advisable for a person with disabilities in the workplace. Assistive technology refers to objects or devices that assist an individual in completing tasks or activities more effectively or independently. Such approaches may include a wide range of possible solutions from generically available tools and devices such as an electronic stapler or high-intensity light to specialized adaptive equipment such as augmentative communication devices or computer adaptations. The majority of assistive devices are readily available and inexpensive and current data suggest that the cost to the employer of providing accommodation has been modest (Button & Wobschall, 1994). The Job Accommodation Network, a nationally supported network, provides employers with specific information on job modifications and assistive devices for employees with disabilities. This national center is a resource for employers as well as any person with a disability who may be seeking solutions to specific problems in the workplace.

An important development in employment services for adolescents with Down syndrome is the increased emphasis on involving natural sources of support in both identifying jobs and developing on-site assistance in the workplace. Natural sources of support include the individual's network of family and friends; co-workers and supervisors; and generic community resources such as churches, employment agencies, or service clubs (Nisbet, 1992). Such natural supports may occur spontaneously as in the example of a co-worker assisting an individual or may be facilitated through a human services consultation, as in the case of a job coach at the worksite (Hagner & DiLeo, 1993; Murphy et al., 1993).

The preceding discussion has outlined some of the strategies that are used for both identifying employment opportunities and assisting an individual to adjust to a job. The emphasis has been on establishing a person-centered plan utilizing the natural networks available to the individual. A job placement strategy often depends heavily on gaining access to those networks of support available to the individual and to family members, friends, or associates of that individual. The use of personal networks greatly enhances the ability to 1) identify interest, 2) identify employment opportunities, and 3) assist in matching the individual's interests to the employer's needs by providing natural supports within the work setting.

The following section reviews concerns expressed by adolescents with Down syndrome as well as family members regarding employment and its perceived risks. A brief overview of issues as well as possible responses and strategies to resolve these is provided.

EMPLOYMENT CONCERNS

Availability of Jobs

The concern is often raised that there are no jobs for adolescents, that unemployment of teens is high, let alone teens with disabilities. How can parents expect to assist their adolescents with Down syndrome in looking for jobs when people without disabilities cannot find jobs?

The unemployment rate, although an indicator of the number of people seeking employment, does not correlate highly with reduced access to jobs by people with disabilities. For all people, when there are many job seekers, the process of finding a job is more difficult. The use of personal networks is one on which many job seekers rely. This same network can work for individuals with disabilities as well.

As noted previously, in some instances new jobs are created, or existing jobs are reconfigured and a job-sharing arrangement is created. In other situations the adolescent decides to work as a volunteer at a place of employment, for a specific amount of time, in an effort to "get in the door." A job-search net is spread to include everyone the individual and his or her family and friends know in order to find elusive job opportunities. The networking strategies, job development, job creation activities, and targeted employment development based on individual needs and preferences often lead to real job opportunities for adolescents with Down syndrome.

Occupational Choice

Many young adults have not had opportunities for experiences that allow them to identify what their likes are or what types of jobs are available. How can parents or the individual know what kind of job to look for?

For the adolescent with Down syndrome, as with many adolescents, the concern may be a lack of knowledge about types of work in general. The educational experience and general community experiences in visiting worksites, talking with people in different occupations, and completing informational interviews may provide more specific information about real jobs in the community. By exploring what the person likes to do with his or her time, most person-centered planning processes have been able to generate ideas on jobs the adolescent might like to try. What is critical is to identify the individual's interests and preferences. What are his or her recreational interests? Are there any hobbies? What do family members do? Do they like to be around people? What types of settings do they like? These and many other questions help guide the creation of a work vision that allows people to begin to brainstorm solutions to this concern. The job exploration process is a lifelong activity. It includes the expectation that the individual with Down syndrome will be able to work; that the educational experience will provide him or her with firsthand experiences on which to build preferences; and that there are approaches for identifying, supporting, and maintaining work for that individual.

Transportation

Often there is concern that the adolescent is unaccustomed to using public transportation, and the parents cannot provide transportation to and from the jobsite. In some instances, there is a lack of knowledge about how to utilize public transportation, whereas, at other times, no public transportation is available. In many instances, the option of obtaining a driver's license is not possible. These situations can lead the individual and family to question whether a job is a possibility if there is no way to get there.

Transportation is one of the most frequently reported barriers to employment for people with disabilities. In fact, transportation problems need to be addressed for all of us. When no public transportation is available, some of the local options include advertising for car pools or ride sharing (newspapers, church or synagogue newsletters, shopping center bulletin boards, fellow employees), contracting with transportation services in the local community with either a local carrier or a private individual, or, in drastic instances, relocating one's residence to be near transportation. When public transportation is available, specific travel training may be necessary. Such training can use family members, friends, paid support resources, or other workers in the company.

Attitudes of Employers

Some people blame employers for the high rate of unemployment of individuals with disabilities claiming that no employer wants to hire a person with Down syndrome, or any disability, for that matter. National research does not support this concern, however (Harris, 1986, 1995).

A poll conducted of over 900 employers nationwide found that an overwhelming majority of managers give employees with disabilities a good or excellent rating on their overall job performance; the cost of employing people who are disabled is not a significant barrier; and most employers appear to be willing to consider the employment of more people with disabilities if they are qualified. Even better news is that employment opportunities for people with disabilities have improved since this poll, and with the advent of the Americans with Disabilities Act (ADA) of 1990 (PL 101-336), there is even less resistance to hiring people with disabilities. Parents may ask if *disabilities* (in the Act's title) really includes people with mental retardation. The answer is *yes*. Employers are interested in hiring good workers. When the skills of the individual are matched to an employer's needs and there is sufficient on-site support and training, many individuals with mental retardation can be good workers. The challenge is in marketing this concept to possible employers. Marketing can be done by anyone in the support network, including family, friends, and employment specialists. The process might involve heightening the employer's awareness about available on-site training and supports, providing examples of success stories, and highlighting a particular individual's strengths and accomplishments.

Job Security

In many instances, job changes occur. Some of these are voluntary (e.g., when an individual leaves one position and goes to another), and others are involuntary (e.g., a work force reduction or layoff). Either way, most employees will get involved in job-seeking and job-finding activities as well as receive some assistance either from the employer or from other resources in the job replacement process. Although layoffs are a major concern because of the potential instability or difficulty in returning to work, job change is a pattern of employment in this country, with the typical employee having an average of five to seven job changes in an employment history. The strategy for returning to work uses the same methods described earlier: personal networking, job creation, job development, and job supports. In a layoff situation, obviously, there are some potential resources including co-workers and former employers who may be able to play a role in identifying job opportunities. As workers are laid off, Community Rehabilitation Programs as well as the Vocational Rehabilitation system may also be able to assist.

Social Security Benefits

A number of provisions within the Social Security system allow people to maintain Social Security benefits (cash and medical) if they return to work, particularly those receiving Supplemental Security Income (SSI). The same provisions do not apply to those receiving Social Security Disability Insurance (SSDI); however, some efforts are afoot nationally to change this. Under the provisions of Section 1619(A) and 1619(B), an individual's Social Security cash payments are reduced $1 for every $2 earned until earnings rise above the Social Security allotment (Social Security Administration, 1987). In addition, medical benefits are available to individuals on Social Security until they reach a designated threshold, typically about $22,000 in earnings per year, although each state differs. When an individual is considering employment, it is important to contact the local Social Security office to inquire specifically about the nature of the work incentives and to obtain pertinent booklets and information.

Career Growth

Individuals with disabilities and their families often have the view that employers have limited expectations for people with disabilities, perceiving them as only able to function at entry-level positions within a narrow range of settings. Employer expectations, however, have changed over time, with an increased awareness that people with disabilities can produce in a wide variety of work situations. For individuals with mental retardation, the supported employment initiatives have greatly assisted in changing employer expectations (see also Chapter 19). However, there is a continual need to expand these expectations.

Job placement does not end with the first job, but must be continued throughout the individual's career. Most of us begin our work history with some entry-level work experience. Through additional training, accomplishments in the worksite, or specific supports, we may transfer into more rewarding and higher-paying jobs. Career growth is an important area to consider for people with disabilities. Unfortunately, this has been an area that has received much less attention than initial job placement. An emphasis on career growth emerges as a challenge because a number of programs begin to examine opportunities for expanding employment movement for people with disabilities in the work setting.

Personal Satisfaction

Some families contend that their son or daughter will be cared for financially and that therefore there is no reason for their child to seek employment. Money, however, is not the sole reward of employment. It is important to remember that employment provides a wide variety of other returns, including emotional, social, and developmental. Parents who claim that money is not an issue may actually be expressing lowered expectations for their child or apprehension that he or she would not be able to work. Parents want to provide security for all of their children, but when a child has a disability there is a tendency in some cases to seek greater security and to minimize risk. Nevertheless, it is important that the individual with Down syndrome have the opportunity to experience the multiple rewards of work.

Social Relationships

A major concern of many people who are working in segregated employment programs is that they will lose friends and relationships if they switch jobs. This fear can accompany any job change. It is important to reassure an individual that he or she can establish other friendships and that old friends can remain so in the future through telephone contact or planned get-togethers. Parents often raise concerns about their adolescent's vulnerability in a competitive work setting. These concerns may center around co-workers and include fears of teasing, scapegoating, and sexual exploitation. It should be recognized that risk taking accompanies participation in all community activities. Education for the adolescent with Down syndrome is the best way to alleviate these worries. Many individuals will already have experience and skill in responding to negative social interactions. All adolescents entering the workplace should already have received education in safe and responsible social-sexual behavior.

Job Complexity

Many jobs have multiple responsibilities that may vary during the week or be altered by the supervisor at a moment's notice. How can the new worker with Down syndrome adjust to such variability, let alone accomplish or succeed with all those responsibilities? All jobs change and evolve. If we think about our own jobs and how they have changed over the years, we can appreciate that job responsibilities rarely remain static. Yet if we know this might be a problem, it is not too difficult to structure the job clearly, with distinct and specific job responsibilities. Jobs can be engineered so that they are consistent and stable, so that both the worker and supervisor know what to expect on a daily basis.

CONCLUSIONS

This chapter has presented a case for parents and adolescents with Down syndrome to view employment in adult life as a realistic option. The changes in the approaches to transition and job placement have demonstrated that individuals with disabilities can be successful on the job when appropriate supports are provided. The involvement of the individual and family and friends, the use of personal networks, and the development of natural support resources have all contributed to people with disabilities gaining access to and maintaining employment. This chapter has also offered perspectives for parents to consider as they develop expectations for their son or daughter with Down syndrome. The active participation of the individual with Down syndrome in all aspects of job development and the use of expanded support networks in job identification as well as supports on the job are strategies that will play a significant role in realizing the personal dreams and aspirations of the adolescent with Down syndrome.

REFERENCES

Americans with Disabilities Act (ADA) of 1990, PL 101-336, 42 U.S.C. §§ 12101 *et seq.*

Butterworth, J., Hagner, D., Heikkinen, B., Faris, S., McDonough, K., & De Mello, S. (1993). *Whole life planning: A guide for organizers and facilitators.* Boston: Training and Research Institute for People with Disabilities.

Button, C., & Wobschall, R. (1994). The Americans with Disabilities Act and assistive technology. *Journal of Vocational Rehabilitation, 4*(3), 196–201.

Hagner, D., & DiLeo, D. (1993). *Working together: Workplace culture, supported employment, and persons with disabilities.* Brookline, MA: Brookline Books.

Hagner, D., Helm, D.T., & Butterworth, J. (1996). This is your meeting: A qualitative study of person-centered planning. *Mental Retardation, 34*(3), 159–171.

Harris, L. (1986). *The ICD Survey of Disabled Americans: Bringing disabled Americans into the mainstream.* Washington, DC: National Council on the Handicapped.

Harris, L. (1995). *The N.O.D./Harris Survey on Employment of People with Disabilities.* Washington, DC: National Organization on Disability.

Hasazi, S.B., Gordon, L.R., & Roe, C.A. (1985). Factors associated with the employment status of handicapped youth exiting high school from 1979 to 1983. *Exceptional Children, 51*, 455–469.

Individuals with Disabilities Education Act (IDEA) of 1990, PL 101-476, 20 U.S.C. §§ 1400 *et seq.*

Irvin, L., Thorin, E., & Singer, G.H.S. (1993). Family-related roles and considerations: Transition to adulthood by youth with developmental disabilities. *Journal of Vocational Rehabilitation, 3*(2), 38–46.

Kiernan, W.E. (1996). *Integrated employment: Status, approaches and challenges.* 1996 Collaborative Academy on Mental Retardation, President's Committee on Mental Retardation, Arlington, VA.

Kiernan, W.E., & Hagner, D. (1995). Rehabilitation counseling and the community paradigm. In O. Karan & S. Greenspan (Eds.), *Community rehabilitation services for people with disabilities* (pp. 255–276). Boston: Butterworth-Heinemann.

Kiernan, W.E., McGaughey, M.J., Lynch, S., Morganstern, D., & Schalock, R. (1991). *National survey of day and employment programs for persons with developmental disabilities.* Boston: Children's Hospital, Training and Research Institute for People with Disabilities.

Kiernan, W.E., & Schalock, R.L. (Eds.). (1989). *Economics, industry, and disability: A look ahead.* Baltimore: Paul H. Brookes Publishing Co.

Kiernan, W.E., & Stark, J.A. (Eds.). (1986). *Pathways to employment for adults with developmental disabilities.* Baltimore: Paul H. Brookes Publishing Co.

Mank, D. (1994). The underachievement of supported employment: A call for reinvestment. *Journal of Disability Policy Studies, 5*(2), 1–24.

Mank, D., Oorthuys, J., Rhodes, L., Sandow, D., & Weyer, T. (1992). Accommodating workers with mental disabilities. *Training and Development Journal, 46*(1), 49–52.

Marrone, J., Huff, D., & Helm, D.T. (in press). Person-centered planning for the millenium: We're old enough to remember when PCP was just a drug. *Journal of Vocational Rehabilitation.*

McGaughey, M.J., Kiernan, W.E., McNally, L.C., Gilmore, D.S., & Keith, G.R. (1994). *Beyond the workshop: National perspectives on integrated employment.* Boston: Children's Hospital, Institute for Community Inclusion.

Mount, B., & Zwernik, K. (1988). *It's never too early, it's never too late: An overview of personal futures planning.* St. Paul, MN: Governor's Planning Council on Developmental Disabilities.

Murphy, S., Rogan, P., Olney, M., Sures, M., Dague, B., & Kalina, N. (1993). *Developing natural supports in the workplace: A manual for practitioners.* Syracuse, NY: Center on Human Policy, Syracuse University.

Nisbet, J.A. (Ed.). (1992). *Natural supports in school, at work, and in the community for people with severe disabilities.* Baltimore: Paul H. Brookes Publishing Co.

O'Brien, J. (1987). A guide to life-style planning: Using *The Activities Catalog* to integrate services and natural support systems. In B. Wilcox & G.T. Bellamy (Eds.), *A comprehensive guide to* The Activities Catalog: *An alternative curriculum for youth and adults with severe disabilities* (pp. 175–189). Baltimore: Paul H. Brookes Publishing Co.

O'Brien, J., & Lovett, H. (1993). *Finding a way toward everyday lives: The contribution of person-centered planning.* Harrisburg: Pennsylvania Office of Mental Retardation.

Rusch, F.R., & Hughes, C. (1990). Historical overview of supported employment. In F.R. Rusch (Ed.), *Supported employment: Models, methods, and issues* (pp. 5–14). Sycamore, IL: Sycamore Publishing Co.

Smull, M., & Harrison, S.B. (1992). *Supporting people with severe reputations in the community.* Alexandria, VA: National Association of State Mental Retardation Program Directors.

Social Security Administration. (1987). *A summary guide to Social Security and Supplemental Security Income for the disabled and blind.* (SSA Pub. No. 64-030). Baltimore: Author.

Steere, D.E., Wood, R., Panscofar, E.L., & Butterworth, J. (1990). Outcome-based school-to-work transition planning for students with severe disabilities. *Career Development for Exceptional Individuals, 13*(1), 57–69.

Turnbull, A.P., & Turnbull, H.R. (1982). Parent involvement in the education of handicapped children: A critique. *Mental Retardation, 20*(3), 115–122.

Vandercook, T., York, J., & Forest, M. (1989). The McGill Action Planning System (MAPS): A strategy for building the future. *Journal of The Association for Persons with Severe Handicaps, 14*(3), 205–215.

Vocational Rehabilitation Act Amendments of 1965, PL 89-333, 1 U.S.C. §§ 101 *et seq.*

Wehman, P., & Kregel, J. (1995). At the crossroads: Supported employment a decade later. *Journal of The Association for Persons with Severe Handicaps, 20*(4), 286–299.

Wehman, P., Kregel, J., & Shafer, M.S. (Eds.). (1989). *Emerging trends in the national supported employment initiative: A preliminary analysis of twenty-seven states*. Richmond: Virginia Commonwealth University, Rehabilitation Research and Training Center.

Wehman, P., & Moon, M.S. (Eds.). (1988). *Vocational rehabilitation and supported employment*. Baltimore: Paul H. Brookes Publishing Co.

Wehman, P., Moon, M.S., Everson, J.M., Wood, W., & Barcus, J.M. (1988). *Transition from school to work: New challenges for youth with severe disabilities*. Baltimore: Paul H. Brookes Publishing Co.

West, M., Revell, W.G., & Wehman, P. (1992). Achievements and challenges: I. A five-year report on consumer and system outcomes from the supported employment initiative. *Journal of The Association for Persons with Severe Handicaps, 17*(4), 227–235.

Whitehead, C.W., & Marrone, J. (1986). Time-limited evaluation and training. In W.E. Kiernan & J.A. Stark (Eds.), *Pathways to employment for adults with developmental disabilities* (pp. 163–176). Baltimore: Paul H. Brookes Publishing Co.

V

LIFE IN THE COMMUNITY

21

The Role of the Family

Debra R. Langseth

In most families, parents and other family members typically find adolescence to be a trying time. Although the challenges of adolescence may differ significantly for families of adolescents with Down syndrome, many of the issues attendant to adolescence (e.g., the quest for independence, social activity within increasingly complex arenas and peer groups, dealing with puberty) will be encountered by all. Adolescents with Down syndrome may confront these issues at a later age or for a longer time, but the stage of adolescence can be neither avoided nor ignored. It is a crucial time of growth and trial in the passage to adulthood. Moreover, regardless of whether an adolescent is experiencing a trying stage, parents and family members must assume many roles simply because their adolescent's age forces issues to the forefront at home, at school, and in the community.

ADVOCATES, SERVICE COORDINATORS, AND EVALUATORS

Parents must remain strong advocates for their adolescent's education, determining, for example, whether to encourage further academic development or, instead, to request a functional curriculum that may better meet the future needs of their son or daughter. The family may instead request that their son or daughter enter job-training activities or programs for full- or part-day programming. All too often families are asked to make immediate decisions, in front of a team of professionals, so that they feel pressured into agreeing with a team's recommendations. Such on-the-spot decision making may or may not be appropriate and productive. Instead, families need to advocate for their adolescent from a position of strength, which may mean asking whatever team is requesting a decision to wait until family members have had time to review all the facts, as well as their feelings and emotions, about the specific request. Throughout the decision-making process, the adolescent's preferences and choices should be sought and, whenever possible, honored. It may also mean that after making a decision and watching the adolescent's performance, parents and other family members may want to change the decision.

When presented with changes in educational or work options, families must wrestle with their hopes, fears, and potential disappointments. It can sometimes be difficult for parents to remain strong advocates for their adolescent's job-training program when, for example, they are faced with the thought that their child may be riding a city bus to get to a work training site in the community. Concerns about exposure to failure, danger, exploitation, or ridicule may be the family's first thoughts when presented with these possibilities. Parents and other family members must consider new opportunities for the adolescent with Down syndrome, facing their apprehensions and evaluating the potential for gain as well as harm that is involved.

Families can find it even more difficult to look at their youngster's situation and determine that he or she is not continuing to make progress—for instance, in mathematics or reading skills, or in a certain therapy, or on a specific medication, or with a behavior or communication program. This may mean readjusting personal hopes and expectations for their child's progress. Although educators or medical personnel may continue to suggest specific courses of action, the parents must advocate for what they think is best for their adolescent. Parents should ensure that each family member understands all aspects of the professional's recommendations, consider their son's or daughter's preferences, as well as their personal opinions, and then feel confident that they are truly acting in the best interests of their adolescent with Down syndrome.

In the area of socialization, parents may also act as service coordinators and advocates for their adolescent with Down synrome. Parents frequently identify the need for social interaction with peers who do not have disabilities while controlling fears that their son or daughter may be taken advantage of, belittled, harassed, or physically hurt. In such a capacity, they may advocate and arrange for inclusion in community sports leagues, religious activities, theater projects, parties, or outings to restaurants.

In the process, parents may feel that they are playing the role of referee in what may appear to be ongoing struggles to ensure that the best interests of their adolescent are met while minimizing conflict between the various teams. For example, parents may need to weigh their adolescent's request to participate in a sports activity against possible medical limitations (the medical team), or they may need to evaluate the pros and cons of a job-training program (the vocational team), or they may need to assess participation in other community activities (the social or recreational team).

In such instances, the parent of an adolescent with Down syndrome may need to function in the role of an arbitrator and skilled negotiator.

SERVICE PROVIDERS AND ROLE MODELS

Parents and families of children with disabilities are role models to other family members, to friends, and to the community at large. As such, they can be highly instrumental in positively influencing society's actions and attitudes toward people with disabilities. For example, the family will be closely observed by the general public when teaching new skills; when dealing with and correcting inappropriate behaviors; when communicating with the adolescent in sign language; when listening and responding to his or her sometimes hard-to-understand speech; and when encouraging and assisting the adolescent with Down syndrome to achieve to the best of his or her abilities.

In *Count Us In*, a book dictated by two adolescents with Down syndrome to their mothers, Mitchell Levitz, one of the adolescents, states to his friend Jason and their mothers that one role of parents is to teach children about family values:

> One of the important values they give to the children is about love, commitment, responsibility, and how important you are to others. . . . It is really about how much love and compassion you have. That's what really counts about values. (Kingsley & Levitz, 1994, pp. 97–98)

Families determine and model the values they believe are important for their children. Parents' willingness to candidly address issues that their adolescent raises, as well as to introduce other topics that they feel it important to discuss, instills a sense of trust and provides an avenue for further communication between parents and adolescent. Families demonstrate their personal values on an ongoing, daily basis and can positively influence their son or daughter through conversations and actions that demonstrate honesty in emotions; communication styles; money management; work ethics; prejudice or bigotry; politics; and relationships with friends, family, and strangers. Although the family continually models desired values and behaviors, parents of an adolescent with Down syndrome typically find that they must actually teach the desired behaviors and skills that reflect their values.

Hygiene

Parents must often teach basic hygiene skills such as bathing, washing hair, brushing teeth, applying makeup, hair care, clothing selection, and so on. Many of these daily tasks are modeled from an early age; but when their child with Down syndrome reaches adolescence, parents may need to alter the teaching process to increasingly emphasize skills, behaviors, and attributes that will help their adolescent "fit in" with peers. Each parent needs to determine the most effective method for teaching these skills. For some adolescents, verbal reminders or a pictorial or written checklist may be needed; for others, hands-on assistance may be needed initially; and for some, parents may need to do the task for a long time.

Adolescence, of course, brings significant changes in terms of physical growth, appearance, sexual development, and moods. Parents need to inform their son and daughter about these changes before they occur in order to alleviate the concern, distress, or alarm that they may cause. The onset of menstruation in girls and the development of secondary sexual characteristics in both girls and boys are examples of the many bewildering changes *all* adolescents must confront. To understand the nature of these changes and how best to cope with them, the adolescent needs specific and detailed information and instruction.

Personal hygiene training provides an opportunity to discuss privacy and discreet communication. A daughter and son should be instructed about the appropriate time and place, as well as conversational partner, for discussing topics such as masturbation, menstruation, or wet dreams. Although the school likely provides some sexual education, the adolescent's parents should also plan a private time to talk with the adolescent about "good touch and bad touch" and to instill personal and family values about sexuality. Again, honest communication is needed to reassure a son or daughter about the facts versus what he or she might have heard from the peer group. Personal hygiene training also provides an opportunity for continuing dialogue about feelings and questions the son or daughter may have about his or her body changes.

As sons and daughters enter adolescence, their cute behaviors of childhood can become stigmatizing. Adolescents, for example, who hug and kiss adults at their first acquaintance, or who pat the bottoms of people as they pass by, may be setting themselves up for exploitation or censure. "While acceptable at one stage of life, [such mannerisms are] suspect and misinterpreted later" (Callanan, 1990, p. 382). Thus, the parent's role as teacher continues—this time, teaching socially appropriate behaviors.

Communication

Adolescents with Down syndrome do not always speak clearly and may have a difficult time getting their message understood by relatives, friends, teachers, job coaches, or store clerks.

> Because communication is the essence of relationships . . . there is a need to
> . . . focus both on teaching [people with disabilities] acceptable methods for
> expressing their needs and on teaching the significant others in their lives how
> better to assess the communicative intent of their behaviors. (Karan, Lambour,
> & Greenspan, 1990, p. 88)

The family will likely need to spend time teaching their adolescent how to convey his or her thoughts and needs in a nonstigmatizing manner. At times, the adolescent may resort to using negative behavior instead of words to convey his or her meaning. In such cases, a behavior program may be developed to help provide guidance to the family, school, and jobsite. The primary emphasis of such a program should be on assisting the adolescent to learn alternative means of communicating his or her desires, thereby negating the need for inappropriate behavior.

A family's reactions to communication styles (verbal and behavioral) and their attempts to understand the communicative intent will be modeled by the family's friends and peers and may well determine how an individual is accepted in his or her community. At times, the adolescent's communicative intent can be purely attention seeking, with an emphasis on trying to be cool and accepted by a group of adolescents without Down syndrome.

In *Count Us In* (Kingsley & Levitz, 1994), Jason Kingsley, an adolescent with Down syndrome, talks about pulling the fire alarm at school because some friends without disabilities told him to do so. He admitted that he knew his actions were wrong, but he wanted to get the attention of a group of kids. Instead, he was suspended from school for 5 days. The family's reactions to pranks such as Jason's will undoubtedly involve discussion about the pros and cons of his behaviors and while modeling and teaching values as well as desired alternate behaviors. What can be particularly frustrating for parents and family members is that "parents must not only encourage good choices, but also discourage bad ones. . . . We are required to discipline someone who is of a chronological age to be disciplining himself" (Trainer, 1991, p. 160).

Understanding the intent of a person's verbal or nonverbal communication is a challenge. At the same time, the individual with Down syndrome may also have difficulty understanding the communicative intent and nuances of language used by individuals without Down syndrome. For example, in *Differences in Common*, Trainer (1991) described difficulties with literal interpretations that individuals with Down syndrome tend to have. For instance, as a youngster, Trainer's son had been told that one car should not hit another car. When given the opportunity to drive bumper cars at a local carnival, he therefore became outraged that cars were hitting his bumper car (p. 89). In another example, Trainer's son was at work and was observed to be saying:

> Damn it! Damn it! . . . He looked sort of stricken, grab[bed] himself, and wet his pants. . . . The reason he wet himself wasn't hard to figure out. . . . A courtesy clerk, someone who loads groceries into customers' cars, is not to leave his duty post unless it is covered by another employee. Ben understands this, maybe too well. (Trainer, 1991, pp. 201–202)

The problems that can arise from such literal translations are obvious for supervisors at worksites; yet such literalness can also pose a problem with friendships and family members, as well as with participation in activities with the general public. Family members learn to accept and anticipate the literal understanding. In turn, they must provide education and modeling to others about their son's or daughter's specific language capacities.

Self-Esteem

The importance of helping the adolescent with Down syndrome to develop a high self-esteem cannot be stressed enough. Specific strategies for promoting self-esteem were discussed in Chapter 8. This subsection emphasizes the family's unique role in enhancing self-esteem.

During adolescence, the teenager may begin asking family members "Why can't I . . ." questions. These questions may include, "Why can't I drive, get a car, get married, have children, live on my own?" and so forth. The teenager may also state, "I wish I didn't have Down syndrome." The parents' and family's responses to these questions help the adolescent explore his or her own self-acceptance.

Families may encourage the adolescent to develop job skills such as meal preparation, household cleaning and management, and safety in the home and community. These are all skills that increase self-esteem, help the adolescent develop goals regarding his or her career, and ultimately move the adolescent toward greater independence. Each adolescent's (and family's) concept and goal of greater independence varies with the individual; yet family assistance in reaching the attainable goals is essential to helping the adolescent with Down syndrome develop a high positive self-regard.

Another area in which parents and families can help their adolescent with Down syndrome is in assisting him or her to learn to give back to the community. It can be emotionally difficult to continue to receive services or help from someone else. Instead, self-esteem can be enhanced by volunteering in the neighborhood, at community and religious activities, at school, and so forth. Self-esteem is bolstered when a person has useful activities and functions to perform.

Thus, the parents' function as service providers and as role models is extremely important in the overall development of the adolescent. "If parents have a positive perception of their children, it will be sensed by them and they will feel loved and accepted" (Pueschel, 1990, p. 215). One hopes that the adolescent not only will feel loved and accepted but will also be capable of demonstrating love and acceptance toward others.

RISK TAKERS

At the birth of a child with Down syndrome, parents have often been told that their child may only be able to achieve the cognitive skills of a "normal" 3- or 5-year-old. This may not be a particularly accurate or useful prediction. Nevertheless, as the child with Down syndrome grows older and enters adolescence, it becomes clear that cognitive development lags behind the physiologic changes that are occurring. Moreover, as the adolescent starts asking questions about dating, getting married, or driving a car, it is easy to forget that even children of 3 or 5 years old are conscious of and affected by the values and desires of their peers. Parents once again find that they must reexamine personal beliefs, understandings, hopes, and fears about their child's growing up and must make decisions about the types of risks they will allow themselves and their adolescent to take. In other words, the role of *both* parents and adolescents intensifies. Parents may again also find that their negotiating skills are both useful and strenuously taxed.

Dating, Marriage, and Children

As stated previously, by the time the youngster with Down syndrome reaches adolescence, he or she should understand male and female anatomy, sexual development, and reproduction. In early adolescence, however, the real issue is "romance, complete with hugging, hand holding, whispering, blushing, giggling, a little kissing, birthday presents, phone calls, and caring" (Trainer, 1991, p. 151). This stage means that parents should prepare for interminable telephone calls between the adolescent and his or her peers.

As the adolescent grows older, along with the telephone calls and dating, there may be excited talk about getting married and having children. At some point, there will undoubtedly be talk about going beyond hand holding and kissing to sex. As the romance appears to be heating up, a frank discussion about birth control and safe sex should also occur, perhaps at home with parents or at a medical practitioner's office in conjunction with a routine physical examination. Again, personal and family values will play an important part in discussions about dating, sex, marriage, and children. It is often difficult for parents to contemplate that someone they have worked so long and hard to safeguard is taking determined steps toward independence, including demonstrating an interest in developing intimate relationships.

The "Why can't I . . ." questions, discussions, and strategies noted previously can present opportunities for planning greater independence. As mentioned earlier, each adolescent's quest for independence and each family's perspective on independence will vary. Some or all of the topics discussed in the subsections following may be encountered during this ongoing search.

Driving or Using the City Bus

Transportation becomes an issue of increasing importance as teenagers, with and without Down syndrome, become more involved in social or sports activities. Teenagers tend to feel that they need greater independence in transportation. Although taking a city bus, where available, provides a sense of freedom, it is not considered nearly as cool as being in control of one's own transportation. As a result, the desire to be like one's peers and to drive or own a car is great.

With regard to public transportation, families may talk about differences in abilities between their adolescent with Down syndrome and his or her peers. Families may also share their fears for the safety of their son or daughter, as well as for that of other drivers or pedestrians; they may also express concern that their adolescent might not be able to read bus routes and might get lost. Families may at this time also suggest realistic goals whereby the adolescent can achieve success in areas other than driving a car or having independent transportation.

Voting

As the adolescent with Down syndrome approaches age 18, families may begin talking about the right to vote. Each adolescent and his or her family will need to determine the adolescent's competence in making an informed decision about for whom to vote. Much of this discussion and the final decision may result from conversations and values modeled by the family. If the adolescent initiates discussions about voting, the family has an opportunity to assess his or her interest in and knowledge of the political realm. An adolescent who does not yet appear ready to make informed voting decisions but wants to vote may be encouraged to wait to vote until the next election, thereby, ensuring that the parents have an opportunity to further discuss with him or her the election process, the candidates, how to vote, and so forth.

Living at Home versus Alternate Living Options

As an adolescent approaches graduation from high school (usually at age 21, when his or her right to a free and appropriate education ends), he or she may begin talking about wanting to live independently, to move out, and to be away from parents. However, the adolescent may need to live at home simply because there may not be personal or state funds available to help support him or her in a group home, apartment, or supported living situation. In this regard, by the time their son or daughter reaches his or her teens, parents should have already contacted local and state organizations to determine future residential and vocational options for their son or daughter.

Parents may decide that moving out of the family home must be contingent on the adolescent's levels of proficiency in areas such as personal hygiene, household maintenance, social behavior, money management, work ethics, transportation, home and community safety, medical care, and sound judgment. If financial assistance from state or local agencies is an issue, parents who find that it is indeed time for their son or daughter to move out of the house will want to contact their local resource centers to determine necessary procedures to facilitate the process of gaining access to support and services. Parents should also inquire—for their own sake as well as to be able to inform their son or daughter—about the length of the waiting lists for housing and other services.

Safety

In preparing their son or daughter to move out of the family home, one of the concerns that looms largest for parents is that of personal safety. Have they taught their youngster to be safe in the community, given the perils of modern life?

In today's society, adolescents of any age, with a disability or without, must be alert to their vulnerability to sexual abuse. Often adolescents with Down syndrome are very agreeable, trusting, and willing to please. Parents and family members need to teach their adolescent about when to open the door while at home; what to do when approached by someone in a car while walking down the street; what to do when someone other than their doctor says "take off your clothes"; what to do when harassed on the bus; what to do when offered alcohol or other drugs; or what to do if someone tries to rob, mug, or assault him or her. Unfortunately, safety precautions and sound judgment need to be taught repeatedly to prepare the adolescent for a worst-case scenario.

In the course of this instruction, parents must also work through their own feelings and fears while ensuring that the adolescent's spirit is not stifled. Although no one is immune from bad accidents or incidents, through training (including discussions and role playing), the likelihood of such occurrences can be reduced. Reducing the odds of undesirable outcomes is certainly one of the roles of the risk taker. Learning to become comfortable with those odds may be a lifetime struggle; yet accepting the odds and continuing to stress independence may bring great joy and happiness to the parent, family, and young adult with Down syndrome.

FINANCIAL PLANNERS/FUND-RAISERS

When planning for the financial security of their own retirement, parents usually want to plan for the financial security of their children. When planning for the financial well-being of the adolescent with Down syndrome, parents must take into account dwindling federal, state, and local funding sources. Some of the legislative appropriations for reduced-rent certificates, utility assistance, food stamps, Supplemental Security Income (SSI), and medical care are threatened with reduction. When weighing financial planning alternatives, the family must determine if their son's or daughter's government benefits may be affected by whatever financial plan they establish, and thus, whether their child's quality of life may be better without assistance from some type of family inheritance or other income.

If the choice is to establish a financial inheritance for the adolescent, perhaps first and foremost, the parents should write a will. The will allows the parents to determine how their estate is to be established and can ensure that taxes paid on the inheritance are minimal for the child with Down syndrome and other siblings. In addition, the parents may choose to purchase life insurance or to leave a lump sum of money to the child. Another option is to establish a trust, in which case an attorney who is familiar with tax law in the state in which the adolescent with Down syndrome lives must be consulted to ensure that the desires of the parents and the needs of the child will be met for the life span.

Guardianship is another area to consider when planning for the future of the adolescent with Down syndrome. Typically, the parent remains the guardian until the child is 18 years of age. At age 18, parents are no longer guardians unless they petition the court to have a guardian appointed. There are options of having a guardian appointed to assist with finances, personal property, medical decisions, or all aspects relating to the life of a person after age 18. Therefore, "guardianship is a serious matter, since it involves a major loss of personal rights and freedoms and can result in reducing a handicapped individual's opportunities to grow and gain independence" (Callanan, 1990, p. 413). Again, the state laws where their adolescent lives or may live after age 18 should be checked when considering guardianship.

Family discussions about guardianship are likely to be as intense as the discussions about getting a driver's license, getting married, or having children. Each family must make the decision it feels is best for their own son or daughter with Down syndrome while wrestling with the rights possibly denied by appointing a guardian and the independence possibly gained by not appointing a guardian.

SUPPORTERS OF FAMILY QUALITY OF LIFE

In addition to meeting the needs of their adolescent with Down syndrome, parents face the challenge of meeting the needs of other children in the family as well as their own needs. Yet, balancing the needs of all family members is crucial.

> Balance is the key to success. The child with a disability should not be the focal point any more than any other one family member should. The focus must change over time as family needs change—and that is the ultimate quality of life: when the focal point of the family moves from person to person because everyone has an equal quality of life. (Crutcher, 1990, p. 19)

Some families experience stress regarding household maintenance, the physical care of all family members, behavior problems of the adolescent, and so forth. Yet, other families appear to have developed ways to deal with the associated stress of raising a family member with a disability. Research indicates that some families

> have been able to reframe their child's disability into a positive referent or a fairly routine component of their day-to-day activities. . . . To the extent that a negative behavior is predictable and recurring, even a serious behavior problem may become fairly routine and minimally stressful. (Orr, Cameron, & Day, 1991, p. 449)

Families who are successful at reframing their perception of stressors tend to rely on various resources and coping styles, including the personal well-being and health of the primary caregivers and the immediate family, spiritual strength, financial stability, extended family resources, formal and informal support groups, and other social contacts who can provide support when needed. Each individual's reactions to stressors, and his or her utilization of resources and coping styles for dealing with stress, determine that person's quality of life. Despite researchers' attempts to quantify "quality of life," each family member, including the adolescent with Down syndrome, determines his or her personal definition of it; thus, quality of life may vary widely within one family.

Another salient aspect of family life is the relationship between the adolescent with Down syndrome and his or her siblings. Siblings may have complex feelings about having a brother or sister with Down syndrome; yet, they may not always communicate these feelings. These feelings may include anger about giving up special activities; frustration about having to care for the sibling or assume extra household responsibilities; embarrassment (sometimes as a result of teasing) about having a sibling with Down syndrome; or a self-imposed "need" to overcompensate for their sibling's inabilities. At other times, the sibling may feel a need to assume a protective role or to try to ensure that the sibling gets a fair opportunity in various activities (e.g., as a result of school groups mocking the adolescent or saying he or she is too slow, too fat, or too hard to understand to be part of a group dance, sport, trip). Within the family dynamics, a time of increased stress may occur when a younger sibling surpasses the adolescent in skills (e.g., a 16-year-old gets a driver's license, but the 17-year-old adolescent with Down syndrome does not have one). A parent's response to the preceding situations can model and reiterate family values and expectations.

In comparison to siblings still living at home, siblings who have left the family home may not be as involved in the day-to-day status of their sibling with Down syndrome. But this does not mean they are not concerned about their family.

Although adult siblings may appear detached at times, make no mistake, they are still emotionally involved with their brother or sister. If nothing else, they are bound to worry about what the future will be like when their parents are no longer around to care for their sibling with mental retardation. Ann in particular has given the future a lot of thought. She's asked me whether I think that sometimes—maybe often—siblings mouth sweet platitudes (He's the best thing to happen in our family—there must be a reason—she's so loving—they're such joyful children, etc., etc.) because it is easier than admitting some of the true feelings which can take over now and again. Feelings like resentment, anger, sorrow, unwanted responsibility (it's your kid, you had him, I didn't). How do you come to terms in deciding what you owe to yourself in your own life and what you owe to your brother or sister?. . . . We have told Ann again and again that she cannot and must not put her life on hold in order to cater to Ben. (Trainer, 1991, pp. 111–112)

In addition to siblings being concerned about their lifelong role as a brother or sister of a person who has Down syndrome, there may also be concern that they may have a child with a disability.

It is, therefore, imperative that siblings and concerned relatives consult well-qualified genetic counselors who are aware of current findings in this rapidly developing field as well as the ethical, legal and social implications of advising about important personal decisions in this area. (Berman, 1995, p. 446)

Medical and ethical decisions regarding genetic testing are personal decisions in which the sibling's family doctor, genetic counselor, and perhaps religious leader will likely play important roles.

Given the changing and continual demands on all family members, extended family, friends, work, and other affiliations, the various parent and family roles described in this chapter can at times seem overwhelming. At those times, families may need to ask for additional support. Almost all states have some sort of formalized Family Support Program that provides services for people with developmental disabilities. Some states offer a menu of support services such as respite care, therapies, and parent training. Other states offer a cash subsidy (from $200 to $700 per month), which can be used to "purchase needed services that cannot be paid for through other programs" (Slater, Bates, Eicher, & Wikler, 1986, p. 246). A few states offer cash directly to the family to be used at the family's discretion. Research indicates time and again that families that have the most control over the types of support they can choose tend to be the most satisfied.

Local chapters of The Arc (formerly the Association for Retarded Citizens of the United States) or the National Down Syndrome Society may assist in locating support groups or formal Family Support services. The Sibling Information Network is another resource group for families and siblings. In addition, some families may have access to support services from other community agencies. Organizations and agencies that provide support are encouraged to use a family-centered support model that implements

comprehensive policies and programs that provide emotional and financial support to meet the needs of families. . . . [and that design] accessible service delivery systems that are flexible, culturally competent, and responsive to family-identified needs. (Edelman, Greenland, & Mills, 1992, Handout 1)

The benefits of person-centered support programs for all family members cannot be emphasized enough.

CONCLUSIONS

A family's role in helping their adolescent with Down syndrome mature as a young adult is many-faceted. Families advocate, juggle priorities, and continually evaluate their son's or daughter's progress and satisfaction with school, the job-training site, medical staff, recreational leaders, and so on. Parents' roles as service providers and role models are certainly not new; however, parents may find they need to increase the intensity of teaching skills to their son or daughter and to the community at large as their adolescent matures.

As one's son or daughter approaches adulthood, the parent's role of risk taker (as well as that of the adolescent) may initially seem fraught with danger (e.g., tackling issues such as sexuality, driving, voting, or moving out of the family home). In helping the adolescent assert his or her independence, the parents need to consider the financial stability of the entire family, their adolescent's rights to federal and state benefits, and guardianship.

Finally, while meeting the needs of the adolescent with Down syndrome, parents must also ensure that the needs of their other children, as well as their own, are met. A collaborative and family-centered effort with professionals and informal family support networks should not be overlooked as an option for meeting the needs of the family, to facilitate achieving and maintaining an appropriate quality of life for all family members.

In closing, the parents of Jason Kingsley and Mitchell Levitz also played many roles as their children grew. They offered the following summation of raising adolescents with Down syndrome:

We have learned over the years not to have limited expectations for our sons. We wish for them the same things we wish for our other children: good health; a sense of satisfaction in their work; caring family and friends; and, possibly, the security, companionship, and fulfillment of an enduring love relationship. (Kingsley & Levitz, 1994, p. 181)

REFERENCES

Berman, P.W. (1995). *Brothers and sisters: A special part of exceptional families* [Book review]. *American Journal on Mental Retardation, 99,* 445–446.

Callanan, C.R. (1990). *Since Owen*. Baltimore: Johns Hopkins University Press.

Crutcher, D.M. (1990). Quality of life versus quality of life judgements: A parent's perspective. In R.L. Schalock & M.H. Begab (Eds.), *Quality of life perspectives and issues* (pp. 17–22). Washington, DC: American Association on Mental Retardation.

Edelman, L., Greenland, B., & Mills, B.L. (1992). *Building parent/professional collaboration*. St. Paul, MN: Pathfinder Resources.

Karan, O.C., Lambour, G., & Greenspan, S. (1990). Persons in transition. In R.L. Schalock & M.H. Begab (Eds.), *Quality of life perspectives and issues*. Washington, DC: American Association on Mental Retardation.

Kingsley, J., & Levitz, M. (1994). *Count us in*. New York: Harcourt, Brace & Co.

Orr, R.R., Cameron, S.J., & Day, D.M. (1991). Coping with stress in families with children who have mental retardation: An evaluation of the double ABCX model. *American Journal on Mental Retardation, 95*, 444–450.

Pueschel, S.M. (1990). *A parent's guide to Down syndrome: Toward a brighter future*. Baltimore: Paul H. Brookes Publishing Co.

Slater, M.A., Bates, M., Eicher, L., & Wikler, L. (1986). Survey: Statewide family support programs. *Applied Research in Mental Retardation, 7*, 241–257.

Trainer, M. (1991). *Differences in common: Straight talk on mental retardation, Down syndrome, and life*. Rockville, MD: Woodbine House.

22

Community Support and Participation

Getting Over a Fear of Heights

Jan A. Nisbet
with Theresa Crowley and Nick Crowley

The term *community* has become synonymous with the effort to include individuals with disabilities such as Down syndrome in those places, events, and activities that most of us have the opportunity to enjoy. In the broadest sense, community includes neighborhoods, clubs, work, entertainment, schools, celebrations, get-togethers, and family. In the narrowest sense, it refers to those environments and activities that happen outside of and in relation to school, home, and work. McKnight (1995) listed three kinds of associations that express and create community: 1) formal associations with officers elected by members; 2) gatherings of citizens who solve problems, celebrate, and enjoy a social compact; and 3) gathering places that also include transactions such as stores, restaurants, and businesses. Regardless of the breadth of the definition, most of us desire some form of community, particularly when the opportunity exists to determine the nature of our participation. Because we are individuals, both the scope and nature of our participation, as well as the way we interpret those experiences, varies.

McKnight (1995) has attempted to describe the decline in community in the past several decades as positively correlated both with the growth in the service economy and with the increasing necessity for dual family incomes, thereby inhibiting volunteerism, which historically has been dominated by mothers or women (old-fashioned gender roles) who are not working. Putnam (1993, 1995) has contributed to many of McKnight's conclusions and has further argued that the degree of citizen participation or "civic virtue," an ingrained tendency to form small-scale associations that create a fertile ground for political and economic development (Lemann, 1996), is related to the nature of governmental structures:

> Classic liberal social policy is designed to enhance the opportunities of individuals, but if social capital is important, this emphasis is partly misplaced. Instead we must focus on community development, allowing space for religious organizations and choral societies and Little Leagues that may seem to have little to do with politics or economics. (p. 22)

By way of example, Putnam pointed out that from 1980 to 1993 league bowling decreased by 40% and the number of individual bowlers rose by 10%. He also presented evidence that voter turnout, church attendance, and membership in voluntary and other associations is down; for instance, as Lemann (1996) also pointed out, volunteering decreased by one sixth between 1974 and 1989.

There is no doubt that members of the disability community, researchers, and practitioners have focused on community as the "cornerstone of community services" (Kendrick, 1994, p. 365). However, Kendrick and others have argued that community is not off the hook on social devaluation and neglect, and that this reality must be confronted as inclusive communities are sought. This tension between the idea of community as a supportive web of associations and relations versus a place fraught with anonymity and hostility (Taylor, Bogdan, & Lutfiyya, 1995) forces professionals, communities, families, and consumers to balance voluntary supports with thoughtful services that support self-determination. "Funded services are crucial to helping people remain in their communities and have control over their lives, but without ordinary relationships, no amount of services will make a person safe" (Ducharme, Beeman, DeMarasse, & Ludlum, 1994, p. 355). The bigger question, however, is how to ensure that young people with disabilities, including those with Down syndrome, have the greatest chance to be members of associations and to have relationships that result in community participation. The answer seems obvious, in that community membership is developmental and requires time.

Those of us who grew up in small towns know that membership is not immediate. The establishment of trust, intention, and interest requires months and, more often, even years. Living in a neighborhood, attending school, participating in school and community functions, being a member of a team or club—all pave the way to the ultimate goal of community membership. Any exclusion from participation requires some form of remedy or the realization that some individuals are more likely than others to be community members and participants. It is this realization that makes full inclusion an *essential* ingredient of future membership. Without full inclusion, associations require additional planning and, in some situations, development. Circles of support (Mount, Beeman, & Ducharme, 1988), one form of community association, are for some a remedy for segregation and disrupted participation, as well as a form of proactive planning for others who are well established in their communities but require a formal acknowledgment of their voluntary responsibility. Circles of support have been adopted throughout the United States and Canada and have broad utility as a transition-planning tool that exists outside the service system.

To better understand the perspective of families and young people with disabilities, this author asked a colleague, Theresa Crowley, and her 16-year-old son Nick, who has Down syndrome, to write about their ideas and experiences regarding inclusion and community. Their expressions follow.

Getting Over a Fear of Heights
by Nick Crowley

As a teenager in high school, I am in my second year. I am a sophomore at Londonderry High School. There is a difference between me and the other kids in my school. A lot of the other kids tend to learn faster than I do. I learn slowly because of Down syndrome. This means that I was born with an extra chromosome, which makes it hard for me to learn as fast as the other kids.

I start school every morning at 7:30. When I get on the bus, the kids are usually talking among themselves, about what they are doing, but they don't talk about me. Most of the people at school don't know that I have Down syndrome, and that is one of the things I like about high school. When I was in first through seventh grades, I was in a special program called PAL and AIM. These are the letters that stand for special class. But since eighth grade I have been in the mainstream classes with regular students and teachers. I didn't like being segregated from the kids in the mainstream while I was in the other classes. The thing that I mostly like about being in the mainstream now is that I can be with my friends and work harder on the types of things that are interesting, like biology. I have earned the name Dr. Crowley from my biology teacher, Mr. Gosselin.

One of the teachers at the high school is the football coach. He once saw his opponent's head manager, who had Down syndrome. He started to have kids with Down syndrome as managers for his team, too. When the coach came to the junior high looking for people who were interested in signing up for football, I went up and signed up. He asked me if I would like to be one of the managers on his team. I said yes. That was then, this is now; I am the head manager of the Division II champions, 2 years in a row. Once at my (individualized education program) meeting I found out about a school that teaches core carpentry. I was very interested in wanting to learn how to build things, like sheds. I had to take a computer test to be able to get into this school. After I started going, at the beginning of my sophomore year, I thought it was wicked fun, because we set up the whole thing into a business that includes a president and two vice presidents. I am the vice president of advertising and marketing. And the rest of the class is the crew. We get to tell the instructors what to do. One of the instructors is a residential carpenter, the other is a teacher.

I feel like this is one of the steps I need to take to accomplish my goal to become a carpenter. Being a carpenter is what I want to do for a living when I finish high school. I have made a few things out of wood by helping my uncles, Jay and Cy. A couple of things we have built are my clubhouse, our deck on our house, and Jay's whole house. This is what first got me interested in being a carpenter. The second step I hope to accomplish is getting over a fear of heights. I am going to gradually go up many different ladders that get higher, and even go on roofs. I am sure that I will be able to do this with my mom, my dad, and my uncle Jay urging me to try hard and not be nervous.

As I get older I would like to live in my own apartment with my cousin Matthew. He is 5 years younger than me, so, when we are both old enough, we will have our own jobs and support the apartment until one of us gets married. I am sure that might be hard for me, finding the girl I would want to marry. I might be too shy or get embarrassed because of my stutter. Most of the girls I am interested in already have boyfriends, and the only girls that are free are the kind I am not really interested in.

When I live with my cousin, he and I will split the chores. I'll do all the cleaning, and he'll do the cooking and some other stuff. I do much better with cleaning because I am a good organizer, and I like cleaning. Matt already knows how to cook a lot of things, and I don't. But I do know how to eat tons of things. Matt may have to remind me when to stop eating, or I will look like two, maybe three, sumo wrestlers put together.

If I do get married and have a family, I might decide to go live in Texas. Not for any job that I would be interested in, but because I hear there is great hunting down there and I love to hunt whenever I have free time. Even though I am already 17, I don't have my own car yet. Some of the seniors at school have cars because they took driver's ed before. My mom has signed me up for driver's ed during the spring, so I do think I will get a car someday. I think it will be great to learn to drive, because I feel like I'm the only person left who doesn't have his own car.

Sometimes I have questions about my adult life. These have to deal with the fact that I'm the only person I know who has Down syndrome as an adult. I think that with a bit of guidance I can live on my own and have my own house. But without guidance I would have to live with someone else, like my sister Taylor. Then how could I deal with a wife and maybe kids? I hope that things will all turn out right on the first try and not get screwed up. Because I'm afraid that if they get screwed up too many times, I might give up and live my whole life with my parents. Some of the things I have tried to do, like learning math, I never seem to be able to get. And I can't seem to stop stuttering, no matter how many times I try to stop and think about it. So those kinds of things sometimes I just give up on. But who knows what might happen to a person when he grows up? I think that, with enough chances, things will get better and better for my life.

My Son Nick

by Theresa Crowley

Nick is 17 years old. He is an honor student, a sophomore at London-derry High School, and head manager of the football team there. He has big brown eyes, a charming smile, and a devilish sense of humor. He also has Down syndrome. What Nick wants for himself is simple. He wants to sleep late on Saturday mornings. He wants to learn to drive. He wants to find a girlfriend who enjoys movies, in-line skating, and eating pizza the way he does. He wants to graduate from high school and go to college. Since he was 4 years old, he has wanted to be a carpenter.

What Nick needs in order to achieve his goals in life is not quite so simple, though. He will need more time than the average guy his age to learn to drive. He will probably need to take driver's ed ... more than once. And to find a girl with the same skills and interests he has will be much more difficult than for most boys. Most of the girls at school are sociable and consider Nick a friend but not dating material. This is a bit frustrating for him. Like most teenage boys, Nick is attracted to the head cheerleader and the girl who dates the captain of the football team. It is a delicate and awkward subject to discuss. Yet, it is important that Nick understand the reality of the situation.

Nick functions on a somewhat different level from the other students at his high school. He is one of more than 1,300 students, but he is the only one with Down syndrome. To say he is unique would be an understatement. Nick has many friends and hundreds of peers, but he does not have any true contemporaries. This, I think, will be one of the most difficult issues for Nick in his transition from student to adult: meeting and making friends with people who, like himself, are slightly different from the mainstream. People who are, on the one hand, very capable individuals, yet, on the other hand, may have a below-age-level understanding of the constantly changing social situations and decisions they face each day.

We have been in this town for most of Nick's life. He went to kindergarten here, and he was a cub scout and a boy scout here. He has taken 4 years of karate lessons, classes in drama, and has been involved in the local 4-H camp as a junior counselor. Nick is a part of this community. Yet, he has never met another teenager just like himself. We have not seen or heard of any organized social group or activities for people with learning disabilities.

As for Nick's goal to graduate from high school and go to college, I'm sure he will do both. It will take a while, no doubt, but he will succeed. It is because of Nick's ambition and focus and the fact that he has always given us just slightly more than we have expected of him that we decided to put him into high school courses that would lead him to graduate with a diploma instead of a certificate of completion.

I was forewarned by one of Nick's biggest advocates, his junior high case coordinator, that I might have to fight to get Nick into some of the classes he would need, according to federal standards, to get a high school diploma. We had never heard of ''diploma versus non-diploma track'' course selection. It hadn't occurred to us that Nick might go through 4 or 5 years of high school and *not* get a diploma. For Nick, this would make no sense. He needs a diploma to get into college.

I went into his initial (individualized education program) meeting determined to convince them that Nick has the potential to accomplish what is needed to get a diploma. It took several conferences between the special education people, teachers and counselors from the junior high and high school, my husband, Nick, and myself, to convince them to allow a student with learning disabilities to attempt courses like U.S. history, biology, and English literature. After some manipulation, confrontation, and acceptance of stipulation, we all agreed that it was certainly worth letting him try. A student can begin high school on the diploma track, and, if it becomes too difficult, he or she can switch to the nondiploma track; but the opposite is not true. Because of time constraints, once on the nondiploma track, a student cannot decide to switch to diploma; so, it was imperative that Nick start out on the right track.

It was Nick's past grade reports and recommendations from former teachers that carried the most weight. That, and Nick's own voice about how important school is to him, about how decisive and determined he is to work hard and look ahead. This is the first time a coded, special education student has been on the diploma track here, and everyone involved wants to see Nick succeed. He is advised to enroll in carefully selected classes—those that offer the most open and flexible learning environment with the most willing teachers.

This opportunity to prove that he is not necessarily *disabled,* but, rather, *differently abled,* may turn out to be one of the most beneficial services provided by the school system to any student. It is not often that a special needs student gets to be a role model or a groundbreaker for others. Another important facet of Nick's education process has been vocational testing and training. Vocational testing is usually offered to students during the summer before their junior year of high school. For most, this is age 16 or 17. For Nick, this would have been at age 18. We felt that waiting this long would have meant missing 2 very valuable years of learning. Again, we had to convince the school department to change the usual game plan and allow Nick to be tested as a freshman, so that he would be ready for placement as a sophomore.

The vocational aptitude test was presented to Nick, on the computer, just before the end of his freshman year. Since he had decided so many years ago that he was going to be a carpenter, he sped through the test, simply zeroing all areas of interest or aptitude except those that had to do with woodworking or building. The results came back with CARPENTER stamped all over it.

So, for his sophomore year, his course selection included two classes at the vocational-technical school in basic carpentry skills. After five classes each morning at the high school, Nick takes a bus to the next town, where he participates in classes designed to mirror the operation of a small manufacturing company that designs, builds, markets, and sells outdoor sheds. He acts as vice president of the company and maintains an A average. The experience he gains now will be invaluable in the future.

Speaking of experience, work experience has been one area where, until very recently, there seemed to be little hope. At age 17½, Nick had been unable to get an after-school job. He had interviewed at several of the local fast-food restaurants and convenience stores without any luck. The director of the 4-H camp, where Nick volunteered for summer work, told me that he gave a great interview. She reported that he came across as very confident and capable. She was thrilled to hire him as a junior counselor, for three summers. Yet none of his other interviews produced the same results.

What Nick needed was someone to set up an interview, and explain to the employer beforehand that though Nick did have some learning difficulties, and would be slower to train, he would be a very hard-working and enthusiastic employee. This would not have the best impact coming from his mother or father, so a job counselor was our best resource. The high school offers job counseling to students by academic year—that is, starting with the seniors and working down to the freshmen. At that rate, Nick would probably get his first session with a counselor at about age 20. That would never do, so, once more, we made calls to try to get things adjusted to take advantage of services at the best time for Nick. After getting some very specific guidance, he got an appointment, an interview, and a job as a front-end clerk at a local supermarket.

And here, I think, begins Nick's real transition from child to young adult. He has had a lot of support from a lot of people. He has a clear picture of his goals and is ambitious to work toward them. He has always had many advocates in his corner pushing and pulling to see that he has a chance to take advantage of every opportunity that is available.

For all of his life, I have tried to be an active participant in both Nick's social and educational experiences. But as I look ahead, I see less, not more, in the way of opportunities and programs that will be there for him to take advantage of. In preparing to write this, I spoke to the special education coordinator in our town about just what is in the works for young adults as they finish up their high school years, reach the age of 21, and are no longer provided for by federal regulations.

His answers were a bit unsettling. He said he didn't know of anything in this area. There are ''special, closed programs,'' he said, but most of the people he has seen leave the school system just seem to drop out of sight. Most likely, he thought, they are just staying at home: Maybe they have a part-time job, in a segregated facility; but he wasn't sure. ''It's a shame, really,'' he said to me, ''but I just never see them or hear from them much after they go home to their families; they just stay there.''

Surely, this isn't all there is. It sure isn't enough for Nick. But if the local department of education isn't aware of programs or projects that are in place for people with disabilities, then who is? Where are these programs? How do I find out about them? Will I be forever looking, watching, or pushing for a suitable situation for my son?

I hope I will be there for him, to support and encourage him, for a very long time. But I wonder if I will always have to step in and ask for special consideration or additional support for Nick. I will if I have to, for as long as I am able; but it seems that society as a whole might do more to help special citizens fit in comfortably. This may sound a bit like ''pie in the sky,'' but I think it is a very attainable goal that will provide immeasurable benefits to our most valued resource—families.

Nick and his mother and family have worked hard to be where they are. Full inclusion of a student with disabilities in high school is hardly the rule. A strong, supportive family is more common. Nick has a better chance than his peers with Down syndrome who attend school in another community to live a full life in his community. But he and his parents have fears and concerns: jobs, love, marriage, children, living, driving, transportation, and isolation. Their concerns are no different from those of any parent. What is different is the fear and its intensity. It is this fear that both moves and supports human services and frequently displaces community and voluntary associations. McKnight (1995) presented three ways that the excluded can be included: 1) heroic efforts on the part of the individual to forge his or her own path, 2) family and friends who see a good life is not only a services life, and 3) community guides who bring a person into the web of associational life. The preceding approaches may also be appropriate for any of us who have experienced exclusion. In the end, however, this author believes that it must be the community that recognizes the fear and exclusion, embraces it, and acknowledges that it too can benefit by being responsible for and encouraging inclusion. Perhaps this is naïve and idealistic. Nevertheless, in the meantime, there are three ways that the disabilities field can encourage community involvement and participation: 1) support full inclusion in child care, education, employment, and housing; 2) practice effective strategies designed to strengthen community involvement; and 3) encourage policies and practices based on the principle of self-determination.

SUPPORT FULL INCLUSION

Much has been written in the literature about inclusive child care, education, employment, and housing—addressed in this volume as well. The purpose here, however, is simply to emphasize that full inclusion is the clearest way to prevent exclusion and to support community participation. Voluntary associations often emerge from experiences and intimate knowledge of people. Knowing this, we must recognize that our earliest forms of association are often in the form of play groups, scouts, sports, student councils, school newspapers, after-school and summer jobs, and neighborhood after-school and weekend activities. To be part of them, we must be part of our schools and neighborhoods. This means that children with disabilities should go to school with their brothers, sisters, and neighbors.

PRACTICE EFFECTIVE STRATEGIES

Amado (1993), after reviewing several community inclusion projects to assist people with disabilities to interact with others in the community, outlined several principles and steps to success, as follows.

Principles for Community Inclusion

1. Act as though almost anything can happen when people with disabilities, their families, friends, and community members work together toward a common purpose and vision.

2. Start small, one-to-one, in order to learn and to ensure that individuals are involved to the fullest extent possible.
3. Plan and implement based on a view of a person's capacities, rather than of his or her impairments.

Steps to Success
1. Identify interests, gifts, and contributions of the person.
2. Explore and identify possible community connections by a) identifying places where these interests can be expressed, and b) identifying opportunities for community relationships that allow chances to see the same people over time and opportunities for social exchange and interaction.
3. Look for potential welcoming places such as community choirs, social justice groups, small family-owned businesses, and so forth.
4. Explore the local community, its history, leaders, and associational life including personal business, leisure and recreation, hobbies, continuing education and personal development, clubs and organizational activities, and volunteerism.
5. Look for interested people who may want to be involved with the person with a disability.
6. Introduce the individual with a disability to other individuals and to groups.
7. Continue to support relationships between the individual with disabilities and others over time.

ENCOURAGE POLICIES AND
PRACTICES BASED ON SELF-DETERMINATION

Like Nick and Theresa Crowley, people with disabilities are not passive recipients of the service system and community members. They are, and have the potential to be, fully self-determining individuals. Self-determination assumes that people with disabilities, whether individually or in concert with family and friends, have control over decisions and resources. Practices and language attesting to the importance of person-centered planning have emerged since the mid-1980s. Only since the mid-1990s, however, has an individualized budgeting process been demonstrated (Nerney, Crowley, & Kappel, 1995) that encourages choice of services and supports. Unfortunately, the way our service system is organized and funded frequently impedes the decision making and preferred lifestyles of many people with disabilities. Interests driven by group rates, slots, Medicaid policies and regulations, and vendors have superseded, in some cases, the realization of a naturally supported job in a business, membership in a community chorus, home ownership, and intimacy. Today people with disabilities and their families face the looming force of managed care, based on acute models of care that can claim but little experience in developing community associations and relations. For Theresa Crowley and Nick Crowley, principles of self-determination must be embedded in any system of long-term care. Otherwise, conversations about community involvement and participation will be further impeded. To this end, Taylor, O'Brien, Nisbet, Shumway, and Klein (1996) developed the position statement on managed care and developmental disabilities presented in the Appendix to this chapter.

CONCLUSIONS

What do young people with disabilities have to look forward to? Today there is a much wider recognition of the contribution of individuals with disabilities in neighborhoods, the workplace, postsecondary education, and other aspects of community life. In the best of worlds, we would like transition from school to adult life to be a natural event devoid of extensive paperwork, goal setting, objectives, and subobjectives. Unfortunately, in most parts of the United States, we are not there yet. In the best scenario, an individualized transition plan continues to serve as a tool to focus the attention of school personnel, families, youth, communities, postsecondary education, human services and supports, and employers on the fact that adulthood is imminent. In the worst, an all too familiar scenario, it serves as a tool to focus on the facts that high school prepared students for very little and that the adult services world is unprepared to support the inclusion of young adults in typical communities. Waiting lists continue to grow, in part because of the reliance on the human services system for answers. There is no one solution. However, self-determination is a concept that may provide direction for youth, families, educators, and human services professionals. When families and people with disabilities have the ability to directly control their resources and use them to support their decisions, we will move closer to a time when waiting lists for a student's transition from school to adult life are passé. Nerney and Shumway (1996) described the principles embedded in self-determination as follows:

Freedom: The ability for individuals with freely chosen family and or friends to plan a life with necessary support rather than being forced to purchase a program.

Authority: The ability for a person with a disability (with a social support network if needed) to control a certain sum of dollars in order to purchase these supports.

Support: The arranging of resources and personnel, both formal and informal, that will assist an individual with a disability to live a life in the community rich in community association and contribution.

Responsibility: The acceptance of a valued role in a person's community through competitive employment, organizational affiliations, spiritual development, and general caring for others in the community, as well as accountability for spending public dollars in ways that are life-enhancing for persons with disabilities. (pp. 4–5)

Nick Crowley and his family have actively sought full and rich experiences that will likely lead to a productive adult life for Nick. In many ways, their experience reflects these principles. Today in New Hampshire and elsewhere, public policy makers are struggling with how to give people direct control over resources such as Medicaid dollars. In the absence of this fundamental policy change, self-determination and successful transition from school to adult life will be rhetoric rather than reality.

REFERENCES

Amado, A.N. (1993). Steps for supporting connections. In A.N. Amado (Ed.), *Friendships and community connections between people with and without developmental disabilities* (pp. 299–326). Baltimore: Paul H. Brookes Publishing Co.

Ducharme, G., Beeman, P., DeMarasse, R., & Ludlum, C. (1995). Building community one person at a time. In V.J. Bradley, J.W. Ashbaugh, & B.C. Blaney (Eds.), *Creating individual supports for people with developmental disabilities: A mandate for change at many levels* (pp. 347–360). Baltimore: Paul H. Brookes Publishing Co.

Kendrick, M. (1994). Public and personal leadership challenges. In V.J. Bradley, J.W. Ashbaugh, & B.C. Blaney (Eds.), *Creating individual supports for people with developmental disabilities: A mandate for change at many levels* (pp. 361–372). Baltimore: Paul H. Brookes Publishing Co.

Lemann, N. (1996, April). Kicking in groups. *Atlantic Monthly*, 22–26.

McKnight, J. (1995). *The careless society: Community and its counterfeits.* New York: Basic Books.

Mount, B., Beeman, P., & Ducharme, G. (1988). *What are we learning about circles of support: A collection of tools, ideas and reflections on building and facilitating circles of support.* Manchester, CT: Communitas.

Nerney, T., Crowley, R., & Kappel, B. (1995). *Affirmation of community.* Keene, NH: Monadnock Developmental Service.

Nerney, T., & Shumway, D. (1996). *Beyond managed care: Self-determination for people with disabilities.* Unpublished manuscript, The Robert Wood Johnson Foundation National Project on Self-Determination and People with Developmental Disabilities.

Putnam, R. (1993, Spring). The prosperous community. *American Prospect, 13*, 35–43.

Putnam, R. (1995, January). Bowling alone. *Journal of Democracy*, 65–79.

Taylor, S.J., Bogdan, R., & Lutfiyya, Z.M. (Eds.). (1995). *The variety of community experience: Qualitative studies of family and community life.* Baltimore: Paul H. Brookes Publishing Co.

Taylor, S.J., O'Brien, J., Nisbet, J.A., Shumway, D., & Klein, J. (1996). *The imperative of managed care.* Syracuse University, Center on Human Policy, Syracuse, NY; Responsive Systems, GA; University of New Hampshire–Durham, Institute on Disability.

Appendix

POSITION STATEMENT ON MANAGED CARE AND DEVELOPMENTAL DISABILITIES

New health care policies—most notably, the concept of "managed care"—will present new challenges and opportunities for children and adults with disabilities and their families. Managed care in the broadest sense refers to the organizational arrangements that alter decisions that would otherwise be made by individuals or providers. The underlying assumption of managed care is to limit unnecessary service utilization while not withholding necessary care. However, there is no evidence that managed care organizations can successfully provide flexible, community based, and inclusive supports to people with disabilities. Yet the country seems to be rapidly moving toward managed care approaches that are based on an acute care model rather than a community-oriented long-term care approach. The risk is that people with disabilities and their families will be the victims of untested approaches that will negate the positive experiences and supports that lead to inclusion, self-determination, and community membership.

Managed Care and Developmental Disabilities

WHEREAS: Individuals with developmental disabilities should be able to exercise the same degree of choice about where and with whom to live as nondisabled persons in American society.

Families of children with developmental disabilities should receive the services necessary to maintain their sons and daughters at home.

From Taylor, S.J., O'Brien, J., Nisbet, J.A., Shumway, D., & Klein, J. (1996). *The imperative of managed care.* Syracuse University, Center on Human Policy, Syracuse, NY; Responsive Systems, GA; University of New Hampshire–Durham, Institute on Disability; reprinted by permission.

Families of children with developmental disabilities should have maximum choice and control over the nature and types of services provided to them.

Adults with developmental disabilities—or, in exceptional circumstances, their guardians—should be able to select the agencies or individuals from whom they will receive support.

Adults with developmental disabilities should receive supports and services based on their individual preferences and choices.

People with developmental disabilities should have the same opportunities as other American citizens to own and/or lease their own homes.

AND WHEREAS: Administrative decisions regarding supports for adults and children with developmental disabilities, or their families, should be made as close as possible to the people being served and, specifically, in the communities in which they live.

Minimally adequate dialogue with individuals with disabilities and parents, or the public, has typically not occurred in the decision making or the implementation planning in relation to managed care contracting.

The predominant models and techniques of managed care are derived from the acute and short-term treatment field of medicine. Their applicability to nonmedical arenas has not been tested.

Basic evaluation data is lacking as to the feasibility, problems, or needed considerations in converting social supports oriented systems, such as the developmental disabilities systems, to managed care.

Implementation efforts in public managed care contracts have been so extraordinarily optimistic that there has been repeated and significant underestimation of the lead time necessary to assure operation transition, client safeguards, and budget management.

Significant access problems for high-risk populations have been experienced in managed care, leading to problems of underservice and inadequate service for persons with complex and long-term conditions, as well as for persons of ethnic and racial minorities.

Loss of personal contact and of relationships has occurred as managed care contracts have repeatedly removed local decision making about care, and have turned control over to remote managers.

People with developmental disabilities and their families are not commodities, and entities must not attempt to realize unreasonable benefits from addressing their needs.

THEREFORE, WE, as representatives of associations or as individuals, endorse the following principles when managed care is implemented:

Managed care provides supports and services that people need to live successfully in their local communities.

Managed care should discourage placement in congregate facilities and encourage services that support people with developmental disabilities to live in their own homes and to participate in the everyday life of their communities as citizens, workers, and students.

Managed care must allow decisions regarding appropriate services to be made in local communities and by people knowledgeable about and chosen by the specific individuals and their racial and ethnic heritage to be served.

Among the options available through managed care must be vouchers and subsidies that enable people with developmental disabilities or their families the choice to directly purchase services from either certified agencies or private individuals.

Funding for services under managed care must be sufficient to support people with the most intensive needs to live in the community.

Cost savings realized through the more efficient administration of services must be committed, first, to addressing unmet needs in the community.

Managed care organizations must demonstrate a commitment to the community it serves.

Managed care should not supplant community associations and relations. On the contrary, it should support the full participation of youth with disabilities in all aspects of community life. For it is inclusion, participation, and association that provide the basis for a healthy community.

23

Promoting Quality of Life Through Recreation Participation

Linda A. Heyne
Stuart J. Schleien
John E. Rynders

By developing our leisure repertoires, we learn new skills, strengthen our physical and mental well-being, and build our self-esteem (Heyne & Schleien, 1994; Schleien, Meyer, Heyne, & Brandt, 1995). Without an adequate leisure repertoire, individuals may experience feelings of isolation and social withdrawal (Schleien & Meyer, 1988). In many cases, the absence of meaningful leisure lifestyles results in the development and perpetuation of maladaptive or aggressive behaviors (Gaylord-Ross, 1980; Kissel & Whitman, 1977; Wehman & Schleien, 1981).

Leisure skill curricular content has not been accorded sufficient attention, time, resources, and energy in most education programs (Schleien et al., 1995). Moreover, special education and general education curricula have not adequately addressed the use of after-school and postschool recreation environments and the pursuit of leisure activities in which individuals with developmental disabilities participate or might participate in the future (Schleien, Ray, & Green, 1997).

This chapter was supported in part by the Research and Training Center on Residential Services and Community Living through Cooperative Agreement H133B30072, funded by the National Institute on Disability and Rehabilitation Research, U.S. Department of Education. The opinions expressed herein do not necessarily reflect the opinions of the U.S. Department of Education, and no official endorsement should be inferred.

What is recreation participation like for adolescents with Down syndrome? Research indicates that their involvement in recreation activities tends to take place at home, to lack variety, and to be sedentary in nature. For example, a study of the recreation pursuits of individuals with Down syndrome, as reported by their parents, revealed that their leisure activities consisted chiefly of watching television, listening to music, playing alone with hobbies or games, and spending time with family members (Rynders & Horrobin, 1995). According to Rynders and Horrobin, the total number of hours per week that these young adults spent in passive, sedentary leisure activities (i.e., watching television, listening to recordings and to the radio) averaged approximately 5 hours per day, 7 days per week, per person. Clearly, spending this amount of time in physically inactive pursuits must be a contributing factor in the obesity of many individuals with Down syndrome.

COMMUNITY RECREATION PARTICIPATION

Adolescents with Down syndrome may resist physical activity not only because of a tendency to be overweight but also because they often experience difficulty performing both complex fine and gross motor skills (Bruininks, 1974). When their physical and motor limitations are coupled with communication difficulties—abilities frequently important in group-oriented community recreation programs—it is easy to see why their recreation participation rate is often low (Putnam, Werder, & Schleien, 1985; Rynders & Schleien, 1988).

It might be tempting to suggest that the underparticipation of adolescents with Down syndrome in community recreation and sports is due primarily to characteristics of Down syndrome; it is more likely, however, that the low rate of community recreation participation, especially inclusive recreation participation, is largely due to a lack of opportunity. Since the advent of the Americans with Disabilities Act (ADA) of 1990 (PL 101-336), the right of adolescents with Down syndrome to participate in activities at their neighborhood recreation agencies has been protected, and all public agencies must provide reasonable programmatic and physical accommodation to support the individual's participation. However, in many areas of the United States, practice has not kept pace with legislation, and agencies find themselves in need of additional in-service training regarding inclusion strategies and techniques in order to comply with the ADA (Schleien et al., 1997).

In a related vein, inclusion of youth with Down syndrome in community recreation means more than merely providing opportunities for their *physical* inclusion. Recreation, especially inclusive community recreation, has been identified as the optimal environment for the development of social relationships and friendships for children, youth, and adults, with or without disabilities (Green & Schleien, 1991; Schleien et al., 1997). In order for community recreation programs to satisfy both the *physical and social* participation needs of adolescents with Down syndrome, agencies must adopt systematic inclusion strategies. A description of some of these techniques is presented in the upcoming section on "Strategies to Promote Recreation Participation."

SIGNIFICANCE OF LEISURE EDUCATION

Although youth with developmental disabilities, including those with Down syndrome, have often been trained in ball skills (Kazdin & Erickson, 1975; Whitman, Mercurio, & Caponigri, 1970), table games (Wehman, 1977; Wehman, Renzaglia, Berry, Schutz, & Karan, 1978), independent free play (Wehman, 1977), social play (Paloutzian, Hasazi, Streifel, & Edgar, 1971; Strain, 1975), and the functional use of a community recreation center (Schleien & Larson, 1986) and a bowling alley (Schleien, Certo, & Muccino, 1984), to name a few, there is a relative paucity of literature focusing on *leisure* education programs for this population. Even though recreation has been identified as a related service in the Education for All Handicapped Children Act of 1975 (PL 94-142) and its reauthorization, the Individuals with Disabilities Education Act (IDEA) of 1990 (PL 101-476), recreation has yet to be established as an educational service in public schools (Ashton-Schaeffer, Bullock, Shelton, & Stone, 1995).

Leisure education can play a vital role in the education and community life of adolescents with Down syndrome (Heyne & Schleien, 1994; Schleien et al., 1995). For example, successful mastery of recreation skills can build a teen's self-confidence and sense of self-esteem. Meeting and interacting with people can enlarge a youth's social network, promote friendships, and introduce teens to dating. Participation in physical activities (e.g., jogging, weightlifting, skiing, basketball) can increase eye–hand coordination, fine and gross motor skills, agility, dynamic and static balance, muscular strength, and cardiovascular endurance. Artistic activities such as drawing, dancing, or learning to play a musical instrument can encourage a teen to express his or her talents and creativity. Gaining a sense of autonomy, an important developmental task during adolescence, can be achieved as teens take increased risks and venture away from home to participate in new activities, develop their independent recreation schedules, and widen their social contacts.

In addition, important collateral skills (e.g., communication, transportation, self-help, money management) can be developed through recreation participation. For example, adolescents with Down syndrome can learn to use public transportation to travel to a local YWCA or YMCA, pay for refreshments at a concession stand, or ask for assistance from a stranger when they need it. These benefits, combined, can contribute greatly to a young person's overall quality of life, versatility, and confident sense of self. Table 23.1 summarizes the benefits of recreation participation for youth with Down syndrome.

The following sections discuss strategies for planning, implementing, monitoring, and evaluating recreation participation by adolescents with Down syndrome. These practical strategies are illustrated with case examples of youth with Down syndrome who have successfully participated in a variety of recreation and sports activities, including weightlifting, figure skating, dramatic arts, sports, Special Olympics, and hanging out with friends in inclusive settings.

STRATEGIES TO PROMOTE RECREATION PARTICIPATION

Recreation participation requires the performance of a series of specific skills, ranging from simple one-step tasks to complex combinations of skills. Correspondingly, and similar to learning other functional life skills (e.g., vocational, domestic, community), learning recreation skills necessitates targeted, systematic instruction and repeated practice (Schleien et al., 1995). The strategies to promote recreation participation that are discussed here—also known as promising professional practices in inclusive recreation (Schleien, Light, McAvoy, & Baldwin, 1989; Schleien et al., 1997)—include individualized needs and preference assessments, environmental and task analyses, individualized adaptations to maximize participation, the use of behavioral teaching techniques, and the monitoring and evaluation of participant progress. Combined, these practices have come to be viewed as a "package" of strategies to promote recreation participation—and, in particular, inclusive community recreation participation.

These strategies apply to the full range of recreation and sports activities that may be enjoyed by adolescents with or without Down syndrome. The activities have the flexibility to be experienced either independently, with a companion, or in a group. Furthermore, the strategies promote the

Table 23.1.   Benefits of recreation participation

- Builds self-esteem and self-confidence
- Encourages the development of social relationships and friendships
- Develops fine and gross motor skills
- Promotes physical fitness
- Nurtures creativity and self-expression
- Increases independent functioning
- Develops collateral skills (e.g., communication, transportation, money management, self-help skills)
- Promotes overall quality of life

enjoyment of recreation activities across multiple settings—home, school, and community environments—as reflected in the behavior of teens without disabilities.

Individualized Assessment of Needs and Preferences

The first step in involving an adolescent with Down syndrome in recreation activity is to assess his or her recreation needs and preferences. The needs and preferences of these youth vary greatly, of course; therefore, it is imperative that assessments be approached on an individualized basis. Assessments should accentuate and capitalize on a teen's abilities, potential, talents, and personal preferences, rather than focusing on skills an individual may not possess.

Needs Assessment   Assessment information is best gathered from a variety of sources—that is, people who know the participant well and can provide a well-rounded picture of his or her life. The adolescent with Down syndrome, his or her parents or caregivers, other family members, teachers, peers, clergy, and related services professionals can all contribute information. The adolescent, parents, and family members are usually the best initial sources of information; hence, as a first priority, it is important to establish trusting relationships with them. Information should be gathered with a respect for and understanding of the family's culture, beliefs, and routines. A family's right to privacy must also be honored, and one should avoid burdening family members with a barrage of intrusive, personal, or irrelevant questions (as has often happened in the past during intake interviews with parents of children and youth with disabilities) (Heyne & Schleien, 1994).

A comprehensive assessment of an adolescent's needs would include information in the following areas: 1) recreation goals; 2) recreation preferences and interests; 3) current recreation participation and performance, including natural talents and aptitudes; 4) social and communication competencies and needs, including modes of communication, the nature of peer relationships, potential companions for recreation participation, effective social reinforcers, behavioral concerns, and whether the individual tends to recreate alone or with others; 5) physical and medical considerations such as motor abilities, physical handling or touching by others, mobility, physical fitness, needs, seizure disorders, and sensory impairments; 6) preferred leisure activities of the individual and the individual's family; and 7) personal resources for recreation participation, such as equipment, materials, and facilities (e.g., games, tennis courts, hiking trails, community recreation centers, shopping malls) that are available to the individual on a regular basis at home or in the community.

Recommended instruments that have been developed for conducting recreation needs assessments include the Client Home Environment

Checklist (Wehman & Schleien, 1981); the Home Leisure Activities Survey (Schleien et al., 1995); and the Participant Interest Survey (Schleien et al., 1995).

Preference Assessment   When conducting assessments, it is crucial that the individual with Down syndrome participate as fully as possible in the assessment process. The freedom to choose one's own leisure-time activities is an essential ingredient of recreation and leisure. In fact, Dattilo and Barnett (1985) have argued that, without choice in the use of one's free time, true leisure cannot be experienced.

Historically, people with developmental disabilities have had few opportunities to freely choose their recreation pursuits. Traditional activities of bowling, swimming, and arts and crafts, often offered in segregated settings, have typically comprised the extent of their leisure repertoires (Schleien & Werder, 1985). Yet research shows that, when given opportunities to participate in diverse, age-appropriate, and popular activities, individuals with disabilities tend to prefer the same varied recreation activities as their peers without disabilities (Matthews, 1980; West, 1981).

Although providing opportunities to make recreation choices is essential, there may be several practical difficulties in assessing the recreation preferences of adolescents with Down syndrome. For instance, a youth may be unable to express his or her preferences verbally or in a way that can be understood by a leisure educator (e.g., parent, certified therapeutic recreation specialist, classroom teacher). Often individuals who have significant multiple disabilities demonstrate few functional preferences that produce positive outcomes, and building upon the preferences that are expressed might encourage nonfunctional, stereotypic behavior or participation in age-inappropriate pastimes (Dattilo & Mirenda, 1987). In addition, many adolescents with Down syndrome have been exposed to such a narrow repertoire of activities that they are unaware of the full measure of options available to them. Lack of exposure, then, translates into both lack of participation and lack of self-initiation in preferred activities (Heyne & Schleien, 1994).

To overcome these obstacles, behavioral observation techniques offer useful methods to accurately assess the recreation preferences of youth with Down syndrome. For example, an individual may be presented with an array of recreation opportunities, selected as a result of the needs assessment procedure (Wehman & Schleien, 1981). Activities may be selected from among games (e.g., bocce, darts, cards, video or computer games), hobbies (e.g., photography, pottery, playing guitar, crocheting, baseball card collecting), or sports and physical activities (e.g., aerobics, tae kwon do, softball, weight training, rock climbing, clogging). An observer can then note the youth's response to the activities, whether positive or negative.

It should be noted that many adolescents with Down syndrome will be able to verbalize their preferences sufficiently. For those teens who lack expressive language skills, however, observations should be attuned to any of the following indicators of an individual's preference for or rejection of an activity or play material: 1) affect of the participant, indicated by smiles, frowns, and increased (or decreased) concentration or interest; 2) attraction of the participant to particular materials over others, evidenced by approaching, reaching for, touching, and manipulating preferred objects and discarding rejected objects; 3) duration of eye contact (i.e., visual acuity) with the recreation materials; and 4) duration of active engagement in the activity or manipulation of the materials. When observing an individual, one must also stay attuned to the person's idiosyncratic expression of preferences and dislikes, which might be manifested, for example, by increased gestures, stereotypic behaviors, vocalizations, having a tantrum, or withdrawal. Once preferred activities have been identified, one can proceed to target particular activities for leisure instruction (Schleien et al., 1995).

Guidelines for Activity Selection

When selecting activities to teach adolescents with Down syndrome, three areas of concern should be kept in mind: lifestyle, individualization, and environmental. Criteria for each of these categories are outlined on the Leisure Activity Selection Checklist (see Figure 23.1). The *lifestyle* criteria encourage the selection of activities that reflect the lifestyles of youth without disabilities. Activities should be chronologically age-appropriate—that is, peers without disabilities would typically enjoy them (Wehman & Schleien, 1981). Chronological age-appropriateness and lifestyle relevance are particularly important when developing curricula for teens, who have their own set of preferred activities apart from children and mature adults. If activities that are referenced for teens without disabilities are selected for leisure instruction, peers without disabilities will likely be attracted to join a youth with Down syndrome in the activities. Lifestyle criteria also address an activity's potential to be enjoyed both independently and socially, on a regular basis, in multiple situations, and across the life span.

A lifestyle criterion that is not included in the Leisure Activity Selection Checklist (Figure 23.1), but is implied, is the functionality of activities. A skill is considered functional if it is used frequently throughout the individual's daily routine at home, school, work, or in the community (Brown et al., 1979). Functional skills are important for developing a teen's independence and sense of competence across life's many situations, challenges, and contexts. Examples of functional leisure skills would be grasping a mouse to play a computer game, calling a friend on the telephone, lifting weights, tossing a Frisbee, or speed walking to energetic music played on a portable compact disc player.

Leisure Activity Selection Checklist

Participant: _____ Date: _____ Completed by: _____

Instructions: For each activity circle "yes" or "no" for each criterion. Tally the number of "yes" responses for each of these subsections and record them on the appropriate line. Tally the overall score for each activity. Activities that receive a score of 11–14 points are generally considered appropriate for instruction.

	Activity		Activity		Activity	
Lifestyle: A concern for selecting activities that are socially valid and that will facilitate typical play and leisure behaviors, as well as provide opportunities for increasingly complex interactions.						
1. *Age Appropriateness.* Is this activity something a peer without a disability would enjoy during free time?	yes	no	yes	no	yes	no
2. *Attraction.* Is this activity likely to promote interest of others who frequently are found in the participant's leisure-time environments?	yes	no	yes	no	yes	no
3. *Environment Flexibility.* Can this activity be used in a variety of potential leisure-time situations on an individual and group basis?	yes	no	yes	no	yes	no
4. *Degree of Supervision.* Can the activity be used under varying degrees of caregiver supervision without major modifications?	yes	no	yes	no	yes	no
5. *Longitudinal Application.* Is use of the activity appropriate for both an adolescent and an adult?	yes	no	yes	no	yes	no
Individualization: Concerns that address the activity's flexibility to accommodate and meet the unique needs and abilities of individual participants.						
1. *Skill Level Flexibility.* Can the activity be adapted for low- to high-entry skill levels without major modifications?	yes	no	yes	no	yes	no
2. *Prosthetic Capabilities.* Can the activity be adapted to varying disabilities (sensory, motor, behavior)?	yes	no	yes	no	yes	no
3. *Reinforcement Power.* Is the activity sufficiently novel or stimulating to maintain interest?	yes	no	yes	no	yes	no
4. *Preference.* Is the participant likely to prefer and enjoy the activity?	yes	no	yes	no	yes	no
Environmental: Concerns related to logistical and physical demands of leisure activities on current and future environments and free-time situations.						
1. *Availability.* Is the activity available (or can it easily be made so) across the participant's leisure environments?	yes	no	yes	no	yes	no
2. *Durability.* Is the activity likely to last without need for major repair or replacement of parts for at least a year?	yes	no	yes	no	yes	no
3. *Safety.* Is the activity safe (i.e., would not pose a serious threat to or harm the participant, others, or the environment if abused or used inappropriately)?	yes	no	yes	no	yes	no
4. *Noxiousness.* Is the activity not likely to be overly noxious (noisy, space consuming, distracting) to others in the participant's leisure environments?	yes	no	yes	no	yes	no
5. *Expense.* Is the cost of the activity reasonable? That is, is it likely to be used for multiple purposes?	yes	no	yes	no	yes	no

Area of Concern Scores
1. Lifestyle _____ _____ _____
2. Individualization _____ _____ _____
3. Environmental _____ _____ _____

Total Activity Score _____ _____ _____

Figure 23.1. Leisure Activity Selection Checklist. (Adapted from Schleien, Meyer, Heyne, & Brandt (1995).)

The *individualization* criteria (see Figure 23.1) addresses the activity's capacity to accommodate and meet the unique needs and abilities of individual participants. The activity must allow participation by a person who has entry-level skills as well as accommodate an individual with high-level skills, without substantial modification. The activity must also clearly match the interests of the participant, as emphasized in the previous section on preference assessments.

Environmental guidelines for activity selection focus on the physical and logistical aspects of recreation activities and on the implications for their current and future use during free time. Activities and materials with high potential for instruction are, for example, durable, safe, reasonable in cost, easy to store, not overly noisy, adaptable for multiple purposes, and available to the participant across several leisure environments.

Environmental and Task Analyses

An environmental analysis inventory provides a systematic, comprehensive approach to teaching targeted leisure skills and facilitating recreation participation in home, school, and community settings (Certo, Schleien, & Hunter, 1983; Schleien et al., 1997). Essentially, the inventory enables a leisure educator to itemize all the skills necessary to perform a particular recreation activity, step-by-step from start to finish, paralleling as closely as possible the way a person without a disability would perform it. Figure 23.2 reproduces part of a recreation inventory for inclusive participation as a sample of the initial steps of an environmental analysis inventory for participating in an exercise class at a community recreation center.

There are several advantages to using the environmental analysis inventory. First, the inventory offers an individualized approach to leisure skill instruction. Second, the task-analytic nature of the instrument allows one to break activity sequences down into steps that adolescents with Down syndrome at any ability level can perform successfully and, thus, master more easily. Third, the inventory outlines all the skills required for performance within the entire context of the activity, in whatever environment the activity may occur. Fourth, directions for special teaching techniques and individualized adaptations can easily be incorporated into the inventory. Fifth, once an inventory for an activity is developed, instruction may be consistently implemented by a parent, caregiver, or any number of service providers. Finally, the inventory provides a convenient checklist for measuring participant progress from one instructional session to the next (see the subsection on "Evaluation" later in the chapter).

In Figure 23.2, the left-hand column outlines the steps required to participate in an exercise class at a neighborhood recreation center. Upon developing this task analysis, a *discrepancy analysis* is then conducted. That is, if a participant is able to perform a step independently, a + is

RECREATION INVENTORY FOR INCLUSIVE PARTICIPATION (RIIP)
PART II: ACTIVITY/DISCREPANCY ANALYSIS

Leisure Skill Inventory

Inventory for Participant with Disability

Activity/Skill: __Exercise Class__

Name: __Debbie Cox__

Leisure Setting: __Hiawatha Recreation Center__

Directions: Below, give a step-by-step breakdown of those *basic* and *vital* skills a person without disabilities would need in order to participate in the activity. Include all components (e.g., breaks, using restrooms, drinking fountain, telephone).

Directions: Read the step(s) in left column. If participant can perform the step, mark a plus (+) in the center column. If the participant cannot perform the step, make a minus (−) in the center column. If the participant's performance is marked (−), identify a teaching procedure or adaptation/modification for that step in the right column. Upon completion, go to Part III: SPECIFIC ACTIVITY REQUIREMENTS.

STEPS (Activity Analysis):	−	+	Teaching Procedure, Adaptation/Modification, Strategy for Partial Participation
1. Enter the recreation center.		+	1.
2. Acknowledge recreation staff and others, if appropriate.	−		2. Initially, group home staff will appropriately model interactions with rec. staff and others. (Staff may not be available.)
3. Locate and proceed to the multipurpose center.	−		3.
4. Locate coat rack along the wall and proceed in that direction.	−		4. Initially, group home staff will model and assist Debbie in this step.
5. Take coat off, hang on coat rack or place it with other belongings (e.g., sport bag, purse) along the wall.	−	+	5.
6. Find a space on the exercise mat and proceed in that direction.	−		6. Initially, group home staff will model and assist Debbie in this step.

Figure 23.2. Recreation Inventory for Inclusive Participation (RIIP): Activity/discrepancy analysis. (From Schleien, S.J., Ray, M.T., & Green. F.P. (1997). *Community recreation and people with disabilities: Strategies for inclusion* (2nd ed., pp. 94–96). Baltimore: Paul H. Brookes Publishing Co.; reprinted by permission.)

#	Step		Notes
7.	Wait for class to begin.	+	7.
8.	Optional: Appropriately speak with others and stretch out.	−	8. Appropriate role modeling needed.
9.	When class starts, listen to and follow instructor's directions.	+	9.
10.	Do warm-up exercises.	+	10.
11.	Do strength training exercises.	−	11. Debbie may have difficulty with some of these exercises. The instructor will provide modified exer. or assistance as needed.
12.	When instructor offers a break, use drinking fountain if necessary.	+	12.
13.	Do aerobic exercises.	−	13. Assistance/modification, as needed.
14.	Check heart rate (3 x).	−	14. Assistance/modification, as needed.
15.	Do cool-down exercises.	+	15.
16.	Upon completion of class, help put mats away.	−	16. Appropriate role modeling/teaching may be needed.

327

Figure 23.2. *(continued)*

STEPS (Activity Analysis):	+	–	Teaching Procedure, Adaptation/Modification, Strategy for Partial Participation
17. Optional: Talk to other participants			17. Group home staff will appropriately model interactions with others.
18. Optional: use drinking fountain/ restroom, if necessary.			18.
19. Collect personal belongings.			19.
20. Put on coat.			20.
21. Exit recreation center.			21.
22.			22.
23.			23.
24.			24.
25.			25.

recorded next to the step in the middle column; if he or she is unable to perform the step independently, a − is recorded. The participant should be given at least two trials to perform the task in order to arrive at an accurate reading of his or her abilities. For every step that receives a minus, the right-hand column is used to note adaptations, teaching procedures, or strategies for participation.

Adapting Activities for Maximum Participation

To encourage active involvement in recreation activities by adolescents with Down syndrome, adaptations to activities may often be necessary. When planning adaptations, it is important to remember three guidelines:

1. *Provide adaptations to meet individual needs.* As noted previously, individualization is essential in recreation programming. No two people are alike, and even though one young person with Down syndrome may require a particular programmatic adaptation, such as one-to-one assistance from a peer to participate in a karate class, it cannot be assumed that all youth with Down syndrome will need the same intervention.
2. *Provide adaptations only when necessary.* Before committing to provide an adaptation, such as a flotation device during swimming lessons, consider whether the adaptation is absolutely necessary to promote the person's successful participation and enjoyment.
3. *View any changes or adaptations as temporary.* The ultimate goal of leisure skill instruction is for the participant to perform the activity independently, as a peer without a disability would perform it, in its original, nonmodified state. Sometimes, though, adaptations are needed.

There are at least four areas in which programmatic adaptations may be made. First, recreation *materials or equipment* may be modified—for example, the handle of a paint brush may be built up with foam and tape to facilitate its manipulation. Alternatively, the *rules* of a game may be modified—a participant in a basketball league may be allowed to travel three or more steps down the court without dribbling (over time, the number of steps permitted would be gradually reduced until no steps would be allowed). In addition, *lead-up activities* may be used to prepare a participant to learn increasingly complex recreation skills. For example, prior to engagement in a fast-paced, competitive volleyball game, the cooperative game of Newcomb (an adapted version of volleyball that requires the players to merely catch the ball and toss it over the net) could be taught. Furthermore, *skill sequences* may be rearranged or abridged in order to promote efficiency or enhance safety. For instance, instead of using a preheated oven, a teenager learning to bake brownies can wait to turn on the oven until *after* the pan of batter is placed on the oven rack. One should also take advantage of and/or advocate for environmental adaptations that can be made to improve architectural accessibility and ease of movement. Such adaptations could include curb cuts, ramps, handrails, elevators, accessible drinking fountains, widened doorways, and paved trailways.

Behavioral Teaching Methods to Promote Learning

Like adaptations, behavioral teaching methods can contribute greatly to the development of recreation competencies for young people with Down syndrome. In fact, they can make the difference between an adolescent learning a new recreation activity or losing interest in it. In our experience, particularly useful behavioral teaching techniques in recreation include 1) an instructional cue hierarchy and prompting system, 2) shaping and chaining, and 3) providing positive reinforcement for successfully performed skills.

An *instructional cue hierarchy and prompting system* provides a leisure educator with an ordered procedure for offering prompts to a participant, if needed, to encourage him or her to perform the steps in an environmental or task analysis. A participant should always be given an opportunity to self-initiate performance of a task or sequence before a prompt is offered. If, after waiting up to 10 seconds for a response, the participant does nothing, looks puzzled, or begins to lose interest, then a prompt is required. Prompts vary in their levels of intrusiveness; as a rule of thumb, one should offer the least-intrusive prompt first. The accepted order for providing prompts, from least to most intrusive, is verbal instruction, orienting gestures, modeling appropriate performance, and physical assistance and guidance (Wehman & Schleien, 1981). Similar to adaptations, as the learner acquires the skill, prompts should be withdrawn, or faded, to encourage the participant to draw cues from the natural setting and materials.

Although an instructional cue hierarchy is highly effective, one should bear in mind that people differ in the ways they respond to and tolerate different prompts. For instance, some people may react defensively to being touched by disengaging or pulling away. Others may respond most positively to verbal cues; still others may acquire information best through gestures, modeling, and demonstration. Therefore, when choosing an appropriate instructional cue, it is also important to be familiar with the participant's preferred learning mode.

Shaping is an instructional procedure that reflects the idea that learning and behavior change tend to occur in small increments. Thus, to shape a behavior means to reinforce the small approximations of change that lead to a final desired behavior. For example, if an adolescent with Down syndrome is enrolled in an aerobics class and needs to locate the gymnasium (housed in a community recreation center) from a bus stop outside the recreation center, a shaping procedure would call for reinforcing all of the successfully performed steps that lead him or her to the gymnasium. Thus, the teen would receive instruction and reinforcement for successfully locating the door to the community center, entering the facility, greeting the receptionist, asking for directions, identifying the correct hallway, and so forth, until the gymnasium was finally located. As the participant gains accuracy in his or her responses, rewarding small steps would be faded until only the final response, locating the gymnasium, would be reinforced (ideally, contextually, by the aerobics instructor greeting the participant by name).

Chaining refers to the order in which the steps on the environmental or task analysis are taught to a participant. Most skills are taught using a forward chain, which follows the usual order in which people perform the task, from start to finish. Sometimes, however, it is advantageous to use a backward chain, particularly if the most reinforcing portion of the activity is among the final steps on the task analysis, such as when operating a vending machine. In this instance, retrieving and eating the snack would be the most motivating steps on the task analysis and, consequently, the first steps that would be taught. Once those steps are mastered, the next time the task is taught, instruction would continue in reverse order, one step at a time, always including the previously taught step in the instructional sequence, until the participant can operate the vending machine in its usual sequence.

Positive reinforcement can be a powerful motivation for learning. By definition, reinforcers are those situational events that follow a participant's behavior and that increase the likelihood that the behavior will recur. Reinforcers may take the form of verbal praise and encouragement; sensory feedback such as flashing lights, music, or electronic sounds; or a "high five," snack, or special privilege. Reinforcement should be given only contingently on accurate performance of the desired behavior. Again, individual learners will vary in their reactions to different forms of reinforcers, so one must be aware of which reinforcer will motivate the learner most effectively.

Evaluation

Evaluation not only determines whether participant goals and objectives are being met but also measures the effectiveness of one's teaching, indicates where programmatic or procedural changes are needed, enhances documentation and accountability to administrators, and is useful for convincing potential funding sources to support program maintenance and expansion (Schleien et al., 1997). Evaluation of a recreation program should be accomplished in two ways: 1) ongoing monitoring of a participant's progress and 2) summative evaluation upon completion of the program.

Evaluation is a dynamic process designed to continually improve instruction for the benefit of participants. An evaluation process usually contains the following components (Heyne & Schleien, 1994):

1. Assess the need for participation in the recreation program.
2. Formulate individual instructional goals and objectives.
3. Determine instructional procedures.
4. Select instruments to measure attainment of participant goals and objectives.
5. Implement the recreation program.
6. Gather data on the participant's performance.
7. Analyze the data in an ongoing manner.
8. Incorporate necessary revisions into the program.
9. Conclude the program and analyze the data summarily.
10. Develop program revisions and recommendations, and submit these to administrators, advisory councils, participants, parents, and other interested individuals.
11. Begin a new program, implementing revised instructional procedures.

The Recreation Inventory for Inclusive Participation (see Figure 23.2) provides a useful format for efficiently tracking the participant's progress from week to week, from the beginning to the end of the program. That is, every time leisure instruction is provided, the instructor records the participant's independent performance of steps on the task analysis. The total number of independently performed steps is tallied and then compared across the duration of the program. This tracking system allows one to identify formative stumbling blocks to performance as they occur, in addition to documenting successful summary gains in leisure skill acquisition on completion of instruction.

CASE EXAMPLES

Today's individuals with Down syndrome are a new generation growing up in communities that typically offer them a wide variety of recreation services and supports. Hence, a number of today's adolescents with Down syndrome are, in contemporary jargon, pushing the envelope of community recreation accomplishment. Some of these individuals are presented in the case examples that follow. These case examples relate the stories of four young people with Down syndrome who have participated successfully in a wide variety of self-selected, age-appropriate recreation and sports activities that have taught them new skills, capitalized on their strengths, and contributed to their quality of life. The first three individuals participated in a range of activities, both specialized and integrated, through Project EDGE (Expanding Developmental Growth through Education).[1] Originally an experimental early intervention project, Project EDGE (Rynders & Horrobin, 1995) continued to follow project participants and their families through the teenage years and into adulthood, encouraging participants' use of the community for recreation purposes. The fourth case example highlights a young man's growth through participation in community recreation programming, almost all of which was inclusive.

Ronald: Pushing the Envelope in Body Building

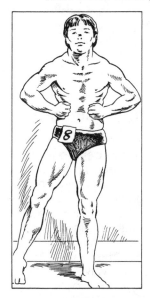

As an adolescent, Ron[2] became interested in lifting weights while accompanying his parents to their health club, where he enjoyed working out. As his physical ability developed, his parents were delighted to see his self-confidence improve too, and looked for additional outlets for his growing athletic interests and skills.

At the health club one day, Ron and his parents happened to run into the coach of the regular body-building club in their community who had heard about Ron's athletic accomplishments. The coach invited Ron to join his club. Ron's parents, apprehensive that his self-confidence could be shattered by his being matched up with peers without disabilities, decided nonetheless that the opportunity was too good to pass up. (Besides, Ron was continuing to be highly successful in traditional Special Olympics equestrian competition. Hence, Special Olympics accomplishment could, if necessary,

---

[1]The early intervention portion of Project EDGE was funded through grant OEG-09-332189-4533(032) from the U.S. Office of Special Education Programs and was directed by John Rynders and Margaret Horrobin. Portions of the follow-up phase are funded by the Rehabilitation Research and Training Center on Improving Community Integration for Persons with Mental Retardation, U.S. Department of Education (grant H133830072), National Institute on Disability and Rehabilitation Research.
[2]Project EDGE names used throughout are pseudonyms, but accounts are factual.

counterbalance any potentially negative experience in the regular body-building club.)

After months of training at the club, and with encouragement from club members without disabilities (who the coach had prepared to be supportive of Ron), Ron entered body-building competition. In his first competition with peers without disabilities, he did not place. At the second competition, he placed fifth against peers without disabilities. At his third competition, he received the Outstanding Teenager Award—and a standing ovation from the audience of more than 1,000 people.

At age 26, Ron continued to live at home while working at a restaurant as a dish washer, food preparer, and dining room busperson. Ron continued to compete in the inclusive body-building activities until the club closed when he was 16 years old. Consequently, Ron continued to compete in the Special Olympics while pursuing his long-standing interest in motorbiking and new interests in softball and basketball in the local community.

Helen: Pushing the Envelope in Figure Skating

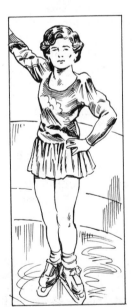

Anyone who has tried competitive figure skating knows how difficult and demanding it is. As an 8-year-old, Helen became fascinated with the idea of figure skating. Cultivating this interest, her parents enrolled her in an ice-skating program at the community ice arena, where she was paired with an older peer volunteer without disabilities who served as both a tutor and friend. For the next 2 years, she and her tutor-friend worked together, meeting twice a week to practice—and practice—and practice. During her adolescent years, Helen became interested in Special Olympics ice-skating competition, eventually becoming a state champion in figure skating in this program. At age 17, she competed at the International Special Olympics games, winning a silver medal.

From ages 17 to 21, Helen attended a regular high school, where she was mainstreamed in several curricular areas. She was popular with her classmates without disabilities, and when she soloed at the regular community ice-skating club show, a group of her friends created a large congratulatory banner to hang outside the school building.

At 26 years old, Helen experienced difficulty in finding convenient transportation (and enough time) to continue serious skating practice. Living independently (her choice) in an apartment that was a considerable distance from the ice arena, she filled her after-work hours (she was competitively employed in the food preparation area of a local restaurant) with taking care of her apartment, preparing her own meals, and visiting with friends in the apartment complex. (The apartment caters to adults with mild disabilities who need only occasional help from the building caretaker.) Helen also maintained regular contact with several friends, some of whom are in Project EDGE, who belong to an adult social club. They liked to go out to eat, to go bowling, attend movies, hang out together, and, occasionally, to go ice skating.

Ed: Pushing the Envelope in Performing Arts

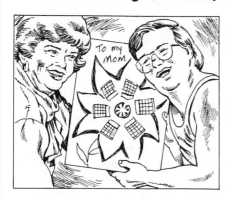

As a child, Ed participated in Special Olympics events such as track. But his passion was for "hamming it up" (one of his favorite phrases). In a regular high school, he earned small roles in several school plays, developing a sizable range of acting types.

As in Helen's and Ron's situations, Ed's parents were concerned that his abilities, when pitted against those of his peers without disabilities, would not fare well by comparison, and that Ed's self-concept would plummet. However, as was also the case with Helen and Ron, Ed's parents realized that a golden opportunity to promote Ed's acting gift was too good to ignore. The opportunity appeared as follows.

Shortly after Ed graduated from high school, his parents noticed an ad in a newsletter of The Arc (formerly the Association for Retarded Citizens of the United States) advertising the fact that a small group of actresses and actors without disabilities were attempting to establish an integrated theater group. The group, Interact Theater, was holding open auditions for people with and without disabilities who had acting ability. Ed was one of 95 people who auditioned, and he was selected (as were 9 others, 4 of whom had a disability). For more than 7 years, Ed held a number of acting roles (one of them a starring role). As this book was being written, he was pursuing his acting interests while continuing his cleaning job at a local fabric store, working half-time at each. Interact Theater has received a federal grant to establish a center on the visual and performing arts. If all goes well, Ed may eventually become employed as a full-time actor.

Kevin: Pushing the Envelope of Community Inclusion

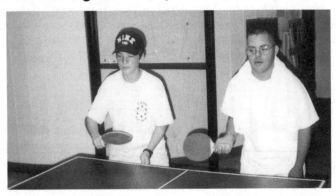

Similar to most young children, Kevin's early recreation opportunities occurred within the context of his family life.[3] When he reached age 5, his parents, Pat and Tom, began to seek community recreation opportunities for Kevin. Influenced heavily by the specialized education services that Kevin had received, his parents at first believed that "specialization meant better." Consequently, Pat registered Kevin for several adaptive recreation programs offered through the local city recreation and park program. As Kevin participated in adapted activities, however, Tom and Pat began to feel increasingly dissatisfied. Adaptive recreation classes were offered in recreation centers that were scattered about the city—none of which took place at the family's neighborhood community center. Kevin, the youngest of the participants (who ranged in age from 5 to 60 years), had no peer models with whom to play. In addition, to accommodate working participants' (or adults') schedules, special classes were held in the evening. Kevin, being very young and needing to rise early to attend school, was tired by 7 P.M. Often he fell asleep even before he arrived at his class.

---

[3]The authors thank Kevin Tommet and his parents, Patricia and Thomas Tommet, for contributing their thoughts and experiences to this story. We are indebted to the Jewish Community Center of the Greater St. Paul Area (Minnesota) for providing inclusive practices since the 1980s. Names used in Kevin's story are actual.

When Kevin turned 10 years old, Pat and Tom became concerned that he was beginning to show signs of self-stimulatory behavior during his child care program. While looking for new child care services, Pat came across an article advertising an inclusive recreation program at the local Jewish Community Center (JCC). When she inquired about involving Kevin in the JCC's program, she learned that the JCC provided all of the necessary specialized supports a child with Down syndrome might need, but within the context of regular recreation activities alongside peers without disabilities.

The first day that Kevin attended the child care program at the JCC, arrangements were made for Pat to provide an orientation about Kevin's needs and abilities to the youngsters without disabilities. She introduced Kevin to the children, described his preferences and interests, shared a video about Down syndrome, and answered the children's questions. To support Kevin in the new environment, the JCC provided a ''trainer advocate'' who gave him one-to-one assistance when he needed it. This support was offered as long as Kevin required it and was gradually faded out as he gained greater competence and confidence. Eventually, the trainer advocate was totally withdrawn, and Kevin was supported by the child care teacher only, in much the same way that she provided support to all the children. Kevin's initial positive experiences in child care motivated his parents to enroll him in other JCC programs. Throughout his adolescence, Kevin participated in numerous inclusive programs, including swimming, basketball, youth theater, racquetball, summer day camp, soccer, wrestling, and track. During his junior and senior years in high school, Kevin was employed by the JCC as a camp counselor, as was the custom for qualified teens without disabilities who grew up as participants in the program.

Tom and Pat noticed tremendous growth in Kevin throughout his years participating in inclusive recreation programs at the JCC, particularly in the areas of skill acquisition, socialization, and self-esteem. They believe that the skills that Kevin learned at the JCC far exceeded any learning that had occurred previously in adaptive recreation programs. His body strength and physical fitness increased significantly, as did his problem solving, risk taking, and social competencies. In addition, through his participation in inclusive recreation activities, Kevin accomplished one of the most important developmental tasks of adolescence—he became prepared to live independently in the community.

Kevin's parents grew also from their son's experiences. They learned that they were just like other families at the JCC, except that they happened to have a child with Down syndrome. They learned advocacy skills, in that Kevin's positive inclusion experiences in recreation gave Pat and Tom the confidence to seek inclusive services for him at the neighborhood high school. Most important, Pat and Tom learned that ''it is Kevin's vision that counts.'' Others in society may try to limit his growth, but ultimately it is Kevin's own hopes and dreams—and abilities—that will dictate his future.

CONCLUSIONS

This chapter has provided an overview of the ways in which recreation can enhance the lives of adolescents with Down syndrome; it has outlined practical strategies to promote leisure instruction and participation in inclusive recreation activities; and it has offered case examples of adolescents with Down syndrome whose lives have been changed significantly owing to recreation participation.

Societal barriers that would restrict the participation and accomplishments of individuals with disabilities are beginning to disappear. Indeed, the future has never looked more promising for young people with Down syndrome. If we as parents, family members, advocates, and leisure educators continue to listen to the needs and preferences of young people with Down syndrome; if we continue to build upon their strengths, abilities, and contributions; and, if we cultivate the development of community groups that are truly inclusive, adolescents with Down syndrome will prosper in areas of recreation and sport that formerly appeared out of their reach. In the future, we can expect to see individuals with Down syndrome participating in a full range of meaningful recreation and sport activities across the life span—activities that are self-selected and age-appropriate, and that enrich the quality of life of both the participants and their communities.

REFERENCES

Americans with Disabilities Act (ADA) of 1990, PL 101-336, 42 U.S.C. §§ 12101 et seq.

Ashton-Schaeffer, C., Bullock, C., Shelton, M., & Stone, C. (1995). *Summit on therapeutic recreation as a related service.* Chapel Hill, NC: Center for Recreation and Disability Studies.

Brown, L., Branston, M., Hamre-Nietupski, S., Pumpian, I., Certo, N., & Gruenewald, L. (1979). A strategy for developing chronological age-appropriate and functional curricular content for severely handicapped adolescents and young adults. *Journal of Special Education, 13*(1), 81–90.

Bruininks, R.H. (1974). Physical and motor development of retarded persons. In N.R. Ellis (Ed.), *International Review of Research in Mental Retardation* (pp. 209–261). New York: Academic Press.

Certo, N., Schleien, S., & Hunter, D. (1983). An ecological assessment inventory to facilitate community recreation participation by severely disabled individuals. *Therapeutic Recreation Journal, 17*(3), 29–38.

Dattilo, J., & Barnett, L.A. (1985). Therapeutic recreation for individuals with severe handicaps: An analysis of the relationship between choice and pleasure. *Therapeutic Recreation Journal, 19*(3), 79–91.

Dattilo, J., & Mirenda, P. (1987). The application of a leisure preference assessment protocol for persons with severe handicaps. *Journal of The Association for Persons with Severe Handicaps, 12*(4), 306–311.

Education for All Handicapped Children Act of 1975, PL 94-142, 20 U.S.C. §§ 1400 *et seq.*

Gaylord-Ross, R. (1980). A decision model for the treatment of aberrant behavior in applied settings. In W. Sailor, B. Wilcox, & L. Brown (Eds.), *Methods of instruction for severely handicapped students* (pp. 135–158). Baltimore: Paul H. Brookes Publishing Co.

Green, F., & Schleien, S. (1991). Understanding friendship and recreation: A theoretical sampling. *Therapeutic Recreation Journal, 25*(4), 29–40.

Heyne, L., & Schleien, S. (1994). Leisure and recreation programming to enhance quality of life. In E. Cipani & F. Spooner (Eds.), *Curricular and instructional approaches for persons with severe disabilities* (pp. 213–240). Boston: Allyn & Bacon.

Individuals with Disabilities Education Act (IDEA) of 1990, PL 101-476, 20 U.S.C. §§ 1400 *et seq.*

Kazdin, A., & Erickson, L. (1975). Developing responsiveness to instructions in severely and profoundly retarded residents. *Journal of Behavior Therapy and Experimental Psychiatry, 6,* 17–21.

Kissel, R., & Whitman, T. (1977). An examination of the direct and generalized effects of a play-training and overcorrection procedure upon the self-stimulatory behavior of a profoundly retarded boy. *AAESPH Review, 2,* 131–146.

Matthews, P. (1980). Why the mentally retarded do not participate in certain types of recreational activities. *Therapeutic Recreation Journal, 14*(1), 44–50.

Paloutzian, R.F., Hasazi, J., Streifel, J., & Edgar, C. (1971). Promotion of positive interaction in severely retarded young children. *American Journal of Mental Deficiency, 75*(4), 519–524.

Putnam, J.W., Werder, J.K., & Schleien, S.J. (1985). Leisure and recreation services for handicapped persons. In K.C. Lakin & R.H. Bruininks (Eds.), *Strategies for achieving community integration of developmentally disabled citizens* (pp. 253–274). Baltimore: Paul H. Brookes Publishing Co.

Rynders, J., & Horrobin, J.M. (1995). *Down syndrome, birth to adulthood: Giving families an EDGE.* Denver: Love Publishing Co.

Rynders, J., & Schleien, S. (1988). Recreation: A promising vehicle for promoting the community integration of young adults with Down syndrome. In C. Tingey (Ed.), *Down syndrome: A resource handbook* (pp. 182–198). Boston: College-Hill Press.

Schleien, S., Certo, N., & Muccino, A. (1984). Acquisition of leisure skills by a severely handicapped adolescent. *Education and Training of the Mentally Retarded, 19*(4), 297–305.

Schleien, S., & Larson, A. (1986). Adult leisure education for the independent use of a community recreation center. *Journal of The Association for Persons with Severe Handicaps, 11*(1), 39–44.

Schleien, S., Light, C., McAvoy, L., & Baldwin, C. (1989). Best professional practices: Serving persons with severe multiple disabilities. *Therapeutic Recreation Journal, 23*(3), 27–40.

Schleien, S.J., & Meyer, L.H. (1988). Community-based recreation programs for persons with severe developmental disabilities. In M.D. Powers (Ed.), *Expanding systems of service delivery for persons with developmental disabilities* (pp. 93–112). Baltimore: Paul H. Brookes Publishing Co.

Schleien, S.J., Meyer, L.H., Heyne, L.A., & Brandt, B.B. (1995). *Lifelong leisure skills and lifestyles for persons with developmental disabilities.* Baltimore: Paul H. Brookes Publishing Co.

Schleien, S.J., Ray, M.T., & Green, F.P. (1997). *Community recreation and people with disabilities: Strategies for inclusion* (2nd ed.). Baltimore: Paul H. Brookes Publishing Co.

Schleien, S., & Werder, J. (1985). Perceived responsibilities of special recreation services in Minnesota. *Therapeutic Recreation Journal, 19*(3), 51–62.

Strain, P. S. (1975). Increasing social play of severely retarded preschoolers through sociodramatic activities. *Mental Retardation, 13,* 7–9.

Wehman, P. (1977). *Helping the mentally retarded acquire play skills: A behavioral approach.* Springfield, IL: Charles C Thomas.

Wehman, P., Renzaglia, A., Berry, G., Schutz, R., & Karan, O. (1978). Developing a leisure skill repertoire in severely and profoundly handicapped adolescents and adults. *AAESPH Review, 3*(3), 162–172.

Wehman, P., & Schleien, S. (1981). *Leisure programs for handicapped persons: Adaptations, techniques, and curriculum.* Austin, TX: PRO-ED.

West, P. (1981). *Vestiges of a cage: Social barriers to participation in outdoor recreation by the mentally and physically handicapped (Monograph #1).* Ann Arbor: University of Michigan, Natural Resources Sociology Research Lab.

Whitman, T.L., Mercurio, J. R., & Caponigri, V. (1970). Development of social responses in two severely retarded children. *Journal of Applied Behavior Analysis, 3,* 133–138.

24

Special Olympics and Athletes with Down Syndrome

Thomas B. Songster
George Smith
Michelle Evans
Dawn Munson
David Behen

Special Olympics is the world's largest program of sports training and athletic competition for children and adults with mental retardation. Almost 2 million Special Olympics athletes in more than 20,000 communities, in every state in the United States, and in more than 150 countries take part in year-round training and competition in 24 Olympic-type individual and team sports (Special Olympics International [SOI], Public Relations, 1995). These athletes are trained, coached, encouraged, and cheered by more than half a million family members and volunteers worldwide who work intensively to further the Special Olympics cause, from fundraising to administration, from providing transportation to coaching athletes and officiating at Special Olympics Games. Throughout the world, Special Olympics is widely recognized as the program that most nearly fulfills the Olympic ideal of sports—competition not for money, victory, endorsements, personal glory, or national pride, but for the sheer joy of taking part.

When Eunice Kennedy Shriver founded Special Olympics in 1966, she was convinced that the lessons learned through sports would translate into new competence and success in school, in the workplace, and in the community. Above all, she wanted the families and neighbors of children with mental retardation to see what these athletes could accomplish, to take pride in their efforts, and to rejoice in their victories. Once ignored

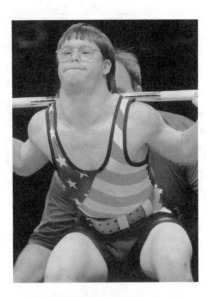

Research shows improved self-esteem in
Special Olympics powerlifters.

and neglected, hidden at home or isolated from their communities, children
with mental retardation are now gaining respect and acceptance often
largely through Special Olympics, where they have been able to reveal
their virtues and display their gifts. For many families with a child with
mental retardation, Special Olympics has become a symbol of hope. For
the athletes involved in Special Olympics, the program offers a lifetime of
active participation in sports. For volunteers and the public, the program
uplifts the spirit and touches the heart, emphasizing people's common
humanity.

EXPANDING SPORTS TRAINING
AND COMPETITION OPPORTUNITIES

The central purpose of Special Olympics is embodied in its program of
sports training and competition. At the time of its founding, the Special
Olympics Organizing Committee surveyed schools and institutional facilities and determined that fewer than 10% of people with mental retardation
spent as much as 1 hour per week participating in physical activities (SOI,
Public Relations, 1995). Most spent no time at all in such activities, because there were no opportunities anywhere for sports training or athletic
competition.

Why? Because the conventional wisdom said that intelligence is a
fixed and permanent measurement of ability; that the IQ could not be
enhanced; that people with mental retardation were like children who did

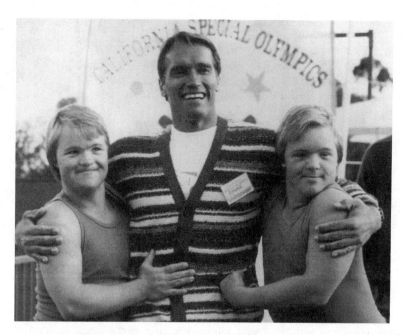

Long-time volunteer Arnold Schwarzenegger encourages Special Olympics athletes in powerlifting.

not have the physical, emotional, or intellectual capacity for the rigors of competitive sports.

Today, with its competitors ranging in age from 8 to 80 and above, Special Olympics has an obligation to provide a full, year-round menu of sports training and competition for all its athletes and to greatly expand its outreach to young people with mental retardation who are not yet taking part.

SPECIAL OLYMPICS WORLD GAMES

Special Olympics World Games are held as alternating winter and summer events biannually. The 1995 Special Olympics World Games were held in New Haven, Connecticut, with 7,000 athletes from more than 140 countries competing in aquatics, athletics, basketball, bowling, cycling, equestrian sports, football (soccer), gymnastics, roller skating, softball, tennis, volleyball, badminton, bocce, golf, powerlifting, sailing, table tennis, and team handball (SOI, Games Committee, 1995). Athletes with mental retardation competed at all ability levels, from the 25-meter assisted walk race to the full-length 26-mile, 385-yard marathon (SOI, Games Committee, 1995).

Of the 70 staff members who organized these Games, 10% had mental retardation and worked full-time along with their peers. As employees of the Games Organizing Committee, these Special Olympics athletes served

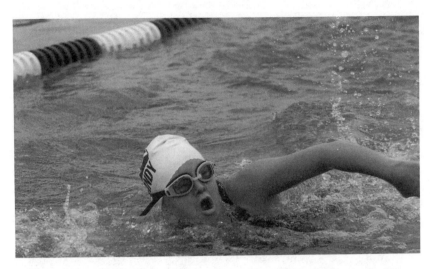

Special Olympics athletes participate in a variety of events ranging from the 10-meter assisted swim to the 200-meter butterfly, depending on their ability.

as members of the Games committees, worked in the Games office, gave public speeches and television interviews, and participated in training of staff and volunteers.

More than 15% of the Special Olympics athletes attending the Games participated in Unified Sports, which involves training and competing on teams with peers without mental retardation. For the first time, Special Olympics athletes participated as Games Officials. Forty-six individuals with mental retardation became certified officials through sports governing bodies and joined with a mentor official to officiate their favorite sport at the Games.

Special Olympics athletes have become advocates for their own needs and causes. Many have been trained as speakers and travel to schools, civic organizations, government and policy hearings, and to other Special Olympics events to speak about various issues related to disability and to convey their Special Olympics experiences. Throughout Special Olympics programs worldwide, athletes with disabilities are taking greater roles on the playing fields as coaches and in boardrooms as members of policy-making groups.

SPECIAL OLYMPICS ATHLETES ATTENDING GAMES

Special Olympics programs provide a unique opportunity to bring together a cross-section of children with mental retardation, including those with Down syndrome. Athletes join Special Olympics by contacting their local Special Olympics group, meeting established criteria for eligibility, obtaining a medical and parental release, and participating in an 8-week training program in the sport of their choice. They then have the opportunity to participate at the next higher level of competition—the state or regional level. Participants in the World Games are randomly selected from athletes who participate in Special Olympics games at lower levels of competition. To be eligible for World Games, athletes have won a gold medal in one of the many ability groupings at the next lower level of competition (state or regional) in their sport.

The following medical, age, and sports participation data relate to Special Olympics athletes with Down syndrome who participated in the 1991, 1993, and 1995 World Games (see also Tables 24.1–24.3):

- Approximately 13.39% of all athletes participating in Special Olympics World Games have Down syndrome.
- Athletes with Down syndrome have fewer medical problems than athletes without Down syndrome, especially in the categories of heart problems, seizure disorders, and hearing and vision problems. For instance, almost 8% of the athletes without Down syndrome had seizures, whereas only 0.31% of athletes with Down syndrome reported seizure disorders. In addition, Special Olympics athletes with Down syndrome had less than half as many vision and hearing problems as athletes without Down syndrome.
- Athletes with Down syndrome at World Games reported a significantly lower percentage of emotional problems, asthma, and bone/joint problems. In each of these categories, less than 0.05% of athletes with Down

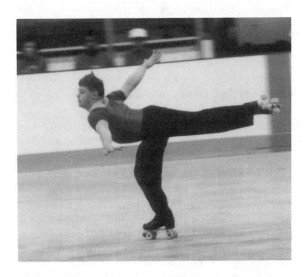

Figure skating is one of the official Special Olympics winter sports.

Table 24.1.   Special Olympics International World Games medical statistics

Disability	Athletes with Down syndrome (%)	Athletes without Down syndrome (%)
Down syndrome	13.39	-0-
Atlantoaxial instability	1.02	.77
Diabetes	.10	.81
Hearing aid problems	.80	3.57
Heart / blood pressure problems	1.13	2.45
Motor impairment	.03	.58
Seizures	.31	7.99
Special diet needs	.57	2.38
Vision problems	2.41	7.97
Wheelchair	.04	.64
Other	.95	7.36
Allergies to food / bug bites[a]	.40	3.62
Asthma[a]	.15	3.36
Bleeding[a]	.04	.41
Bone / joint problems[a]	.40	3.18
Emotional problems[a]	.33	6.08
Fainting[a]	.21	.93
Head injury / history of concussion[a]	.01	1.83
Heat stroke / exhaustion[a]	.18	.64
Hernia or absence of one testicle[a]	.24	1.21
Kidney problems[a]	.04	.56
Recent contagious disease or hepatitis[a]	.12	.31

Data from Special Olympics International World Games (1991, 1993, 1995).

Notes: Statistics are based on number of athletes with Down syndrome only (1,878) and number of athletes without Down syndrome only (12,144).

[a]Only 1995 statistics available.

syndrome reported problems, compared to 3%–6% of athletes without Down syndrome.

- Athletes with Down syndrome at World Games participated in all of the Special Olympics sports activities alongside athletes without Down syndrome. Athletes with Down syndrome had markedly higher participation rates in aquatics, gymnastics, bowling, powerlifting, and equestrian sports than athletes without Down syndrome.
- In complex sports such as golf, gymnastics, and figure skating the percentage of athletes with Down syndrome participating far exceeded the percentage of athletes without Down syndrome.

The data highlighted here and in Tables 24.1–24.3 are remarkable in terms of the health and sport participation of people with Down syndrome. In each of the 22 medical categories cited in Table 24.1 (Down syndrome

Table 24.2. Special Olympics International World Games age statistics

Age breakdown	Athletes with Down syndrome (%)	Athletes without Down syndrome (%)
8–15 years	8.15	12.14
16–25	55.22	57.30
26–35	27.96	21.06
36–50	7.93	8.20
51 years and older	.64	1.27
Unknown	.11	.03

Data from Special Olympics International World Games (1991, 1993, 1995).

Notes: Statistics are based on number of athletes with Down syndrome only (1,878) and number of athletes without Down syndrome only (12,144). Each separate category should add up to 100%.

and atlantoaxial instability), athletes with Down syndrome had a lower percentage of health problems than the other participating Special Olympics athletes. Moreover, the percentage of Special Olympics athletes with Down syndrome participating in many sport events offered at the World Summer and Winter Games was equal to or higher than the percentage of Special Olympics athletes without Down syndrome. This unique comparison includes sports such as gymnastics, powerlifting, distance running, swimming, badminton, and tennis that in 1985 would not have been considered possible (SOI, Games Committee, 1996).

SPECIAL OLYMPICS RESEARCH AND EVALUATION

Although Special Olympics has routinely assessed its sports and training mission, researchers have not extensively evaluated Special Olympics goals in terms of the social and emotional realms. As described here, preliminary work suggests some effect of Special Olympics on self-esteem, and many parents have anecdotally reported that their child's self-esteem has improved as a result of his or her involvement in Special Olympics (Klein, Gilman, & Zigler, 1993). Although increased self-esteem has previously been reported in Special Olympics relative to non–Special Olympics athletes, this has not always been a consistent finding (Bell, Kozar, & Martin, 1990; Edmiston, 1990; Wright & Cowden, 1990).

In 1996, two researchers at the Yale Child Study Center published results of a study whose objective was to evaluate the social and emotional goals of Special Olympics International, specifically in terms of whether it facilitates social competence and self-esteem in children with mental retardation (Dykens & Cohen, 1996). The findings were triangulated across three studies on the social competence, adaptation, and self-perceptions of 104 athletes (mean IQ, 59). Study 1 related behavior to athletes' length of time in Special Olympics; Study 2 compared Special Olympics Team USA

Table 24.3.   Special Olympics International World Games sport statistics

Sports	Athletes with Down syndrome (%)	Athletes without Down syndrome (%)
Alpine skiing	2.13	2.11
Aquatics	17.41	7.22
Athletics	13.84	18.38
Badminton	.21	.31
Basketball	3.35	8.31
Bocce	2.50	1.05
Bowling	10.22	5.89
Cross-country skiing	2.34	2.36
Cycling	1.76	2.11
Equestrian	3.46	2.05
Figure skating	1.33	.87
Floor hockey	2.13	4.06
Football	5.86	14.55
Golf	1.44	.90
Gymnastics	15.02	3.33
Powerlifting	5.38	2.55
Roller skating	1.33	1.90
Sailing	.48	.68
Softball	1.65	6.32
Speed skating	.59	1.35
Table tennis	1.70	1.80
Team handball	1.22	2.55
Tennis	2.45	1.80
Volleyball	2.18	7.56

Data from Special Olympics International World Games (1991, 1993, 1995).

Notes: Statistics are based on number of athletes with Down syndrome only (1,878) and number of athletes without Down syndrome only (12,144). Each separate category should add up to 100%.

to an appropriately matched group of non–Special Olympics athletes; and Study 3 assessed Team USA before and 4 months after their participation in the World Games in Salzburg, Austria.

Relative to IQ, Dykens and Cohen (1996) found length of time in Special Olympics to be the most powerful predictor of social competence. Special Olympics athletes had higher social competence scores and more positive self-perceptions than the comparison group of matched children with mental retardation who had never participated in Special Olympics.

Other Special Olympics International research has focused on the following areas: 1) making a maximum contribution to each person with mental retardation to develop healthy lifestyles through training and competitive activities; 2) making Special Olympics more efficient to maximize all opportunities for athletes; 3) making the Special Olympics program as cost-effective as possible; 4) developing sports training programs that offer equal opportunities for people at all levels of ability to participate and derive benefits; and 5) making volunteer work more rewarding to individuals.

Emphasis has also been placed on completing research that can be generalized to other countries. For example, the Dykens and Cohen (1996) study has been replicated in five other countries (Chile, Canada, Kenya, Russia, and the Czech Republic) to determine if these universal benefits accrue to all Special Olympics athletes.

Does this mean that Special Olympics athletes with Down syndrome have better health and are able to accomplish more than experts previously thought possible? It certainly would appear that the myth of children with Down syndrome having more health problems and accomplishing less in comparison to other children with mental retardation is invalid. What is more, most experts have assumed that Special Olympics athletes with Down syndrome are probably lower skilled in comparison with other Special Olympics athletes. This is simply not true. Athletes with Down syndrome, when provided proper training, ample competition opportunities, and good coaching, continue to expand the limits (implying a traditional stigma) that have been associated with the disorder. In fact, no limits are appropriate at all.

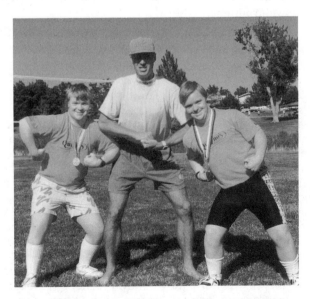

World champion athletes such as Karch Kiraly teach sports skills and learn life lessons from Special Olympics athletes.

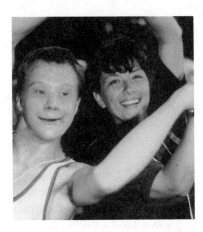

Beyond sports and competition, the Special Olympics provides opportunities for sharing and friendship.

SPECIAL OLYMPICS ATHLETE AND FAMILY PROFILES

Many Special Olympics athletes with Down syndrome have shown enormous strength of character, varied skills, and the ability to share unique insights with others. The many successes of these individuals transcend training and competition and influence others in our world. The following case examples describe some accomplishments of Special Olympics athletes with Down syndrome.

Nicholas R. Del Bueno, Parent of Special Olympics Athlete Terresa Del Bueno

As a parent of a daughter with Down syndrome, I want to explain what Special Olympics means to me. It means education, first and foremost; an opportunity to tell people—and specifically parents of Down syndrome children—why physical activity is so very important, and making people understand what Down syndrome children can do from day to day. Other than participation, the biggest boost the kids receive from Special Olympics isn't just the applause from the volunteers, coaches, and onlookers—the biggest boost they receive is from their parents. What a tremendous difference in those kids who are alone versus those with family support! I'm not a psychologist or a psychiatrist. I'm just a parent trying to get the best break for my daughter.

We've come a long way from the days of locking children away and forgetting about them. They're now in school, in sheltered workshops, and some are holding full-time jobs. Special Olympics has helped to make this happen.

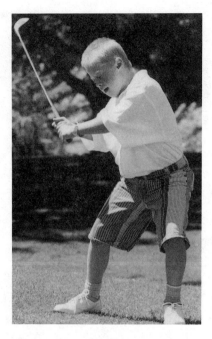

Golf has been added to the official sport category in the Special Olympics.

Anthony Martinez, Texas Special Olympics Athlete in Golf

Anthony loves golf and imitates his hero Chi Chi Rodriquez by doing his ''Zorro'' impression after sinking a putt. Although Anthony has been successful in Special Olympics competition since the age of 8, his greatest and most recent accomplishment was participating with his father as a Unified Sports golf team at the 1995 World Summer Games in New Haven, Connecticut.

Anthony lives in Texas with his parents and two brothers. Having graduated from Gregory Portland High School from his mainstreamed program and acting as manager of the football team, Anthony is now looking ahead to full-time employment. While working on this major project, he spends his time on hobbies, cleans house, and plays golf.

Anthony's father believes that his participation in Special Olympics has not only given Anthony health and self-esteem benefits but has brought father and son closer together. As a testament to Anthony's achievements, he was elected the Pan American Golf Association golf athlete of the year (Pan American Golf Association, 1995).

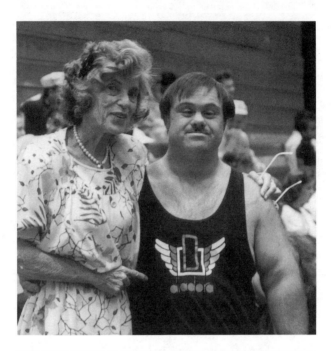

Eunice Kennedy Shriver congratulates Donald Pyskaty, Special Olympics athlete from New Jersey.

Donald Pyskaty, New Jersey
Special Olympics Athlete in Powerlifting

Before becoming a Special Olympics powerlifter, Donald Pyskaty weighed well over 300 pounds and was not in the "good shape" in which he can now claim to be. After years of training with Special Olympics powerlifting coach Tony Tierno, Don won four gold medals at the 1991 Special Olympics World Games and four more at the 1995 Special Olympics World Games. Donald is now 272 solid pounds with 17% body fat. At the 1995 World Games, he did a combined lift of 1,024 pounds for his gold medal (SOI, Games Committee, 1995).

Don considers his mom, Helen, his biggest motivator, although his six brothers and sisters are also very proud of his accomplishments. He lives in Fairview, New Jersey, and works as a forklift driver at his family's business. In his spare time, between work and powerlifting, Don works at his computer on various science projects. Twice he has helped to raise $11,000 for his Special Olympics local program in a lift-a-thon, and he has started to coach younger athletes in powerlifting.

Chris Burke, Television Personality and Massachusetts Special Olympics Athlete

Life goes on for Chris Burke, even after his performance in the TV series *Life Goes On.* His guest acting roles have included the made-for-TV movie *Jonathan, the Boy Nobody Wanted,* the television series *Commish,* and the miniseries *Heaven and Hell.* He also keeps a busy schedule making special appearances at schools and Special Olympics events worldwide.

Chris credits his parents, two sisters, and brother for his success. His experiences in Special Olympics have covered many areas from athlete to celebrity. He began his involvement in Special Olympics in Massachusetts, competing in the long jump, the 50-meter and 100-meter dash, and the softball throw.

Chris is an extraordinary example of the success that a person with Down syndrome can have from competing in sports, to acting, to serving as a volunteer aide for children with multiple disabilities. He continues to hurdle stigmatic boundaries with the publication of his biography, *A Special Kind of Hero* (1995), and has also coproduced a compact disc entitled ''Singer with the Band.''

Eresi Yarney, Wisconsin Special Olympics Athlete in Gymnastics

Eresi Yarney lives in Grafton, Wisconsin, and has participated in Special Olympics since she was 8 years old. Besides being a member of the U.S. Group Rhythmic Gymnastics Team and multiple-medal winner at the 1995 Special Olympics World Games, Eresi is a concerned citizen and activist with special interest in health care and gun control. She is regularly involved in her community as a volunteer.

Eresi lives with her parents and three sisters and attends Grafton High School, where her classmates call her the ''Gold Medal Girl'' in recognition of her gymnastic accomplishments. She dreams of becoming a rock singer and of someday making her own albums. Eresi is extremely interested in raising money for children in Rwanda; she dedicated one of her gold medals to the children of Rwanda at the 1995 World Summer Games. She is also writing a book about her life.

Mike and Mark Hembd, Colorado
Special Olympics Unified Sports Athletes

According to the parents of Mike and Mark, twin boys with Down syndrome, Special Olympics has been the adhesive that has kept the family strong physically and mentally. Mike and Mark, now 25, have competed since they were 8 years of age, and they share a room full of medals earned from various sports competitions. Both are members of their Unified Sports softball team. In addition to the benefit of exercise that Special Olympics has afforded and their coaches' emphasis on good nutrition, Special Olympics has assisted in the overall mental health of Mike after he was diagnosed with post-traumatic stress syndrome as a result of a severe car accident. During this time, Mike stopped eating, talking, and walking. He regained his former vitality, however; a recovery that his family credits to Special Olympics and to the friendship of Kordell Stewart, of the Pittsburgh Steelers. Mike's parents feel that Special Olympics saved Mike's future by offering him activities that would build his self-esteem and allow him to work through his trauma.

Mike and Mark now ride the bus to the YMCA every day to work out. Their parents feel that Special Olympics has helped to improve their physical health, self-esteem, motivation, and self-discipline.

ATHLETES WITH DOWN SYNDROME IN THE 21ST CENTURY

As the 21st century approaches, Special Olympics is challenged to continue to provide relevant recreation choices for youngsters with Down syndrome. Critical social, philosophical, health, and medical considerations will play important roles in providing high-quality and meaningful opportunities for these youngsters.

Consistent with U.S. society in general, there will be a "graying of Special Olympics." Medical advances and healthier lifestyles will mean that people, including those with Down syndrome, will live longer. Many of these older individuals with Down syndrome will want to continue participating in Special Olympics programs beyond adolescence. Special Olympics will thus need to expand both the availability and types of sports programs offered to other athletes. Sports like bocce, bowling, shuffleboard, sailing, walking, cross-country skiing, and tennis are already being incorporated into Special Olympics. More of these activities, conducted in settings and competitive atmospheres that will appeal to older athletes, are being organized.

Another area that Special Olympics will need to consider is early intervention with young parents who have a child with Down syndrome.

Like any parent, parents of a child with Down syndrome are eager to provide sports opportunities for their son or daughter. Programs are needed for very young children with Down syndrome that focus on developing locomotor skills, hand–eye coordination, and basic fitness. Programs must be offered that allow children with Down syndrome to participate in the sports and activities that their peers without Down syndrome also prefer. Sports like soccer, in-line skating, swimming, alpine skiing, and cycling, which can be learned through Special Olympics, will open the door to additional sports and recreation opportunities outside of the organized program.

Current research shows that the fitness level of American adolescents is decreasing. The U.S. population has become much more sedentary. Special Olympics will need to increasingly emphasize the fitness component of the program in order to meet and stay consistent with public health initiatives. For instance, athletes will have more formal year-round training grounded in strength and cardiovascular conditioning as well as sports skills development. Special Olympics will have to contribute to the overall fitness of this segment of the population. It is hoped that this effort will be part of a wider effort on behalf of the individual, his or her family, the school, and community sports organizations to promote healthy and active lifestyles.

In 1987, the Unified Sports program was introduced by Special Olympics. In this program, Special Olympics athletes and their peers without mental retardation are placed on teams to train and compete against other Unified Sports teams (SOI, Unified Sports Committee, 1995). The program has given Special Olympics athletes the opportunity to play side by side as equals, often for the first time, with their peers without disabilities. Other Special Olympics programs such as Partners Club, a peer coaching program, and Sports Partnership, which integrates Special Olympics teams and school varsity teams, are being expanded. There will be a strong emphasis on bringing members of the broader community into Special Olympics as participants, coaches, and volunteers in other capacities, leading to increased opportunities for interaction between people with and without disabilities.

Special Olympics will furthermore need to continue to reach out to athletes with Down syndrome who are in settings currently underserved in the program. Participants in urban and rural settings and those from low socioeconomic status areas will be targeted, as will athletes from single-parent families. A major outreach to underdeveloped countries will also continue.

In order to maintain and expand Special Olympics services, collaboration and partnership between Special Olympics and other organizations and agencies is becoming essential. Special Olympics hopes to be a leader in the effort to connect community-based resources so that services will not only continue but can be enlarged and improved. Specific partnerships with the schools will assist in providing additional and complementary programs through Special Olympics.

In the coming years, more and more individuals with Down syndrome will be employed or seeking employment in the public and private sectors. Special Olympics will need to extend its efforts into the workplace in order to provide opportunities for Special Olympics athletes. Through programs like Unified Sports, co-workers will also be able to enjoy the benefits of participation in Special Olympics.

CONCLUSIONS

Special Olympics believes that consistent training and sports competition are essential to the physical, mental, and social development of young people with mental retardation. For participants, the benefits of such training and competition go beyond the important outcomes of learning functional sports skills and improving health and fitness and include stimulating self-confidence and promoting acceptance by society.

By offering sport in its purest form, Special Olympics has been a catalyst in bringing people with mental retardation out of the shadows of neglect and into the mainstream of life. The enhanced well-being and quality of life of those athletes have encouraged families to recognize the gifts and abilities of their loved ones with disabilities; indeed, individuals from all walks of life have been inspired to celebrate the unlimited potential of the human spirit by sharing the skill, courage, and joy expressed in the lives of Special Olympics athletes.

Eunice Kennedy Shriver summarized the meaning of Special Olympics in a speech during the opening ceremonies of the 1995 World Summer Games:

> In a world where poverty, war, and oppression have often dimmed people's hopes, Special Olympics athletes rekindle that hope with their spiritual strength, their moral excellence, and their physical achievements. As we hope for the best in them, hope is reborn in us.

REFERENCES

Bell, N., Kozar, W., & Martin, A. (1990). Impact of Special Olympics on participants. *Special Olympics International, Inc., Research Monographs, 1*, 20–24.

Dykens, E.M., & Cohen, D.J. (1996). Effects of Special Olympics International on social competence in persons with mental retardation. *Journal of the American Academy of Child and Adolescent Psychiatry, 35*, 223–229.

Edmiston, P.A. (1990). The influence of participation in a sports training program on the self-concepts of the educable mentally retarded attending a one-week Special Olympics sports camp. *Special Olympics International, Inc., Research Monographs, 1*, 25–29.

Klein, T., Gilman, E., & Zigler, E. (1993). Impact of Special Olympics on participants. *Mental Retardation, 31*(1), 15–23.

Pan American Golf Association. (1995, December). *44th Annual Trophy Presentation,* Corpus Christi, TX.

Shriver, E.K. (1995). *You have the right* [Opening ceremonies speech]. Washington, DC: Special Olympics International.

Special Olympics International, Games Committee. (1995). *Special Olympics International World Games Results.* Report no. 1. Washington, DC: Author.

Special Olympics International, Games Committee. (1996). *Special Olympics International World Games Age and Sports Participation Statistics.* Report no. 4. Washington, DC: Author.

Special Olympics International, Medical Committee. (1996). *Special Olympics World Games Medical Statistics.* Report no. 1. Washington, DC: Author.

Special Olympics International, Public Relations. (1995). *Special Olympics International World Games Factsheet.* Report no. 1. Washington, DC: Author.

Special Olympics International, Unified Sports Committee. (1995). *Special Olympics International Unified Sports Program.* Report no. 1. Washington, DC: Author.

Special Olympics International World Games. (1991). *1991 Special Olympics International World Games medical report.* Washington, DC: Author.

Special Olympics International World Games. (1993). *1993 Special Olympics International World Games medical report.* Washington, DC: Author.

Special Olympics International World Games. (1995). *1995 Special Olympics International World Games medical report* (Report no. 1). Washington, DC: Author.

Wright, J., & Cowden, J.E. (1990). Changes in self-concept and cardiovascular endurance of mentally retarded youths in a Special Olympics swim training program. *Special Olympics International, Inc., Research Monographs, 1,* 30–34.

25

Youth and Community Life

Expanding Options and Choices

Julie Ann Racino

A shift is occurring in the United States away from traditional, professionally controlled services and toward a focus on support and personal assistance that encourages personal autonomy and community membership (Bradley, Ashbaugh, & Blaney, 1994; Lakin, Hayden, & Abery, 1994; Roberts & O'Brien, 1993). Policy institutes have brought together leaders in the United States to create philosophical and policy statements supporting children and adults (reprinted in Racino, 1992; Taylor, Racino, & Walker, 1995). Yet, adolescents with mental retardation, including those with Down syndrome, have remained relatively unrepresented in the movement away from a continuum of residential, vocational, and educational facilities to more flexible, consumer-responsive approaches. Although youngsters with mental retardation are supported to remain with their families, attend reg-

This chapter was supported in part by the National Institute on Disability and Rehabilitation Research (NIDRR) under grant H13340005-95, Office of Special Education Programs, U.S. Department of Education, with a subcontract from the World Institute on Disability, Research and Training Center on Personal Assistance Services to Community and Policy Studies. The content does not necessarily represent the views of the NIDRR or the federal government. The author thanks Ellie Macklin, previously from the Cornell University School of Human Development and Family Studies, College of Human Ecology, for her work and perspectives on youth.

This chapter is adapted in part from an edited collection of five reports on personal assistance services (PAS) primarily for, by, and with people with mental retardation, psychiatric disabilities or survivors, and physical disabilities, as well as youth with disabilities, prepared for the World Institute on Disability (see in particular Racino, 1995b, 1995c). For an article on PAS (cross-disability), see Racino (1995a); with respect to mental retardation, see Racino (1991).

ular schools, and participate in community life, their transition to adulthood has remained largely separated from the growth and development of youth without disabilities.

With adults and adolescents with mild disabilities, expectations may remain low for career advancement (outside of sheltered workshop or day habilitation settings), control of their own services (e.g., money decisions), marriage and the raising of families (e.g., sterilization), friendships, and decisions about their own health and well-being. Adults with disabilities, for example, may be excluded from access to legal and support services when disagreements occur with family or professionals (i.e., people with disabilities are often at risk for being declared incompetent to make decisions).

This chapter provides an overview of public policy frameworks that have been established or are being developed in relation to support and personal assistance for people with disabilities (see Table 25.1 for working definitions in this regard). The chapter highlights the relationship between personal assistance and lifestyles, self-advocacy, and transition; describes the status of developments in housing, education, employment, and recreation; delineates a context for youth decision making vis-à-vis personal assistants; and briefly outlines emerging issues in support systems and suggested approaches for future change.

FRAMEWORKS FOR YOUTH DEVELOPMENT:
POLICY OPTIONS AND PERSONAL ASSISTANCE SERVICES

Seven public policy frameworks are presented in this section: youth development as public policy framework; a "capability-autonomy" public policy perspective; personal assistance services (PAS); the Americans with Disabilities Act (ADA) of 1990 (PL 101-336) (legal advocacy); PAS as a prevention approach (as contrasted with a health and wellness approach); family support and PAS; assistance as a natural part of the environment; and PAS and community support.

Youth Development as Public Policy Framework

Youth development is one of the frameworks described by Jackson, Felner, Millstein, Pittman, and Selden (1993), who considered it a "process in which youth are engaged" (p. 14). Like housing and support (Racino, Walker, O'Connor, & Taylor, 1993), youth development is not a prevention, problem-focused program. As emphasized by Jackson et al. (1993):

> Youth development goes on whether or not we have supports. It is precisely because of this that we have a responsibility to offer supports, opportunities or services that help young people find socially positive and constructive ways to meet their needs and to develop and use a broad array of competencies. (p. 187)

Table 25.1.   Community support and services

A new language regarding community support and support services for, by, or with people with disabilities has been developing in the disability field. In the context of a service framework, these overlapping categories include the following (the definitions of which tend to change based on research in the field):

Person-centered planning

New approaches to individual planning such as personal futures planning (Mount & Zwernik, 1988), MAPS (Vandercook, York, & Forest, 1989), and essential lifestyle planning (Smull & Harrison, 1992) have assisted in changing both the way people think about and plan for support services for and with people with disabilities. These reflect a different way of thinking about assessment and planning, with a focus on valued life outcomes such as community presence, personal choices, respect, competencies, and community participation.

Personal supports / flexible and individualized supports

Personal supports and individualized and flexible supports are terms that describe support (Racino & O'Connor, 1994) and support services that are person-centered across environments (e.g., home, work, school, recreation) including relationships, services, training, adaptations, communication, accommodations, and income supports. Personal supports are part of a movement to reconceptualize human services and are an outgrowth from the mental retardation field. In a broadened sense, personal assistance can have a similar meaning, but with a stronger emphasis on self-determination.

Personal assistance

Personal assistance has been defined as a person performing activities for another person with a disability that the latter person would typically do for himself or herself were it not for the disability (Litvak, Zukas, & Brown, 1991). Personal assistance can take many forms, including "assistance with such tasks as dressing, bathing, getting in and out of bed or one's wheelchair, toileting, eating, cooking, cleaning house, and on-the-job support. It also includes assistance from another person with cognitive tasks like handling money and planning one's day or fostering communication access through interpreting and reading services" (Consortium of Citizens with Disabilities, 1992, p. 1). Personal assistance can occur across sites—home, work, school, recreation—and in the community.

Supported or assisted living

Supported living represents a movement within the developmental disabilities field to provide support services in regular housing to adults with disabilities. Direct support services can be provided by paid staff, including live-in roommates or boarders, paid neighbors, a person hired as an attendant, a support worker or personal assistant, as well as more traditional agency and shift staffing. Professionals, friends, families, and other "informal supports" can also assist people to live in their own homes (Racino et al., 1993; Smith, 1990). Supported living may be joined with a movement toward decent, affordable, accessible housing.

Family supports and supported parenting

Sometimes the kinds of supports and services that are needed or wanted are family support. This may be the case when a person with a disability heads a household, when a child with a disability is involved, or at times when family members are the caregivers. Family support strategies can include family subsidies; family-centered services such as support workers, support groups, chore assistance, and in-home training to deal with crises and behaviors; and the provision of durable goods that may be related to medical condition or family need (Knoll et al., 1990). Supported parenting represents a combination of supported living and family supports.

(continued)

Table 25.1. *(continued)*

Community supports

Community supports refers to efforts to work within the community and ``generic'' services to ensure access by all people, including those with disabilities. These support strategies can include situations where a disability agency provides funding to a community agency to expand its staffing to include people with greater needs in its regular services, errand services open to the community-at-large, accessible transportation, or community emergency systems available to all citizens.

Assistive technology

Both high- and low-technology devices have been a significant factor in allowing people with disabilities to live in typical housing, work at regular jobs, and participate in all aspects of the community. These devices include advances in communication technology, whereby people can now more readily express their needs and opinions; emergency systems (medic alert, lifelines, intercoms); and adaptive devices that can substitute for paid staff (timers, tape recorders). Assistive technology also includes durable medical equipment, from inexpensive eating aids to environmental control devices, wheelchairs, and ventilators.

Case management / service coordination

Service coordination is an essential feature of practical assistance, since the management tasks involved in working with systems that are fragmented, diverse, and, in some cases, have only limited expertise mean that ``assistance can be difficult to locate, coordinate and manage, and in some cases, must be created'' (Johnson, 1985). Systems that promote choice and flexibility include personal selection, hiring, and management of the service coordinator, if so desired, by the person with a disability. Some people have argued that case management and service coordination can be replaced by user-directed personal assistance.

Advocacy services

Access to advocacy services that are independent of any service provider is an important aspect of any system of supports. People with disabilities will still face discrimination as well as acceptance by diverse sectors in society. They need access to advocacy services to address their needs and to ensure that their rights and viewpoints are represented.

From Racino, J.A. *Living in the community: Toward supportive policies in housing and community services.* (1993b, December). Report prepared by Community and Policy Studies for the New York State Department of Health; adapted by permission.

Youth development, as distinguished from youth programs, offers an approach to integrating the health, education, and community sectors, and to developing service and policy for, by, and with youth with diverse disabilities (including Down syndrome),[1] ethnicities, cultural background, status, and income.

A "Capability-Autonomy" Public Policy Perspective

The basic frameworks governing disability public policy have tended to be based on a disability perspective (i.e., people are provided services as a

---

[1]*Youth with diverse disabilities* includes youth with significant and multiple disabilities, as well as youth with mild disabilities; in this chapter, adolescents with Down syndrome are specifically included in this definition.

special interest group) (e.g., Individuals with Disabilities Education Act [IDEA] of 1990, PL 101-476). A "capability-autonomy" perspective (Rubin & Millard, 1991) rests on the concepts of social justice and personal autonomy, not paternalism (which is prevalent in the field of mental retardation), and contrasts with a "minority group" model whereby people are viewed as disenfranchised and entitled to special interest group accommodations.

PAS and the ADA

Within the framework of the ADA, children and youth with disabilities have access to the same opportunities as other youngsters (e.g., walking down a store aisle to look for toys, making telephone calls to a close relative without special assistance to do so—instead, simply as a matter of course). The ADA is the missing link in children's civil rights laws, with its greatest potential impact being that of creating hope for the future, including opportunities for careers (Chaikind, 1992).

Personal Assistance as a Prevention Approach

Youth with disabilities are considered one of four major "at-risk youth" groups (together with adolescents in rural areas, adolescents in inner-city high-poverty neighborhoods, and homeless youth). Personal assistance can be conceptualized within a prevention framework as a way for children, youth, and their families to maintain healthy individual and family lifestyles of their own choosing. A prevention framework (Crocker, 1992) contrasts with a health and wellness approach (Marshall, Johnson, Martin, & Saravanhabhaven, 1992) in being less community-based and more intervention-based.

Prevention can be a viable framework for "service system" forms of personal assistance (as distinguished from community forms of personal assistance services) or for approaching personal assistance in the context of health care reform. However, it would be necessary to examine and reframe basic assumptions (e.g., What is at risk and what is to be prevented?), the definition of prevention, the outcomes of prevention, "innovative programs," evaluative approaches, and frameworks for understanding public policy (see annotated bibliography on PAS regarding preventive services in mental health).

Family Support and PAS

Family support can be considered "a right of all parents" (Schleifer, 1989) and their families, with each family member sharing different perspectives on what *support* means. What children and youth know and how they feel (in contrast to a strictly "parents know what is best" approach) has not received as much attention within the national family support movements. Five family support movements (as distinguished from children's rights movements) that influence public policies are the family resource coalitions, state family support programs, family-centered health practices (Johnson, 1990) (e.g., Association for the Care of Children's Health), family-focused early interventions, and family support programs for people with developmental disabilities (Dunst, Trivette, Starnes, Hamby, & Gordon, 1993). Family support is often considered as distinct from family preservation movements of all families in society, child welfare practices with families, and permanency planning (e.g., stable relationships and a home for the child) as a philosophy and practice (Taylor & Racino, 1987).

Assistance as Natural Part of Environment

Personal assistance has become equated with service and funding models. However, another way to consider assistance is as a natural aspect (see Racino, 1994) of the ways people relate to one another, and as a natural part of environments, whether work; school; home; recreation; or political, economic, community, or spiritual life ("as available as air"). This type of approach means examining the societal and community contexts into which personal assistance services are built: medical care, technology, housing, environmental accessibility, transportation, education, employment, pension, and advocacy (Nosek, 1989).

Personal Assistance and Community Support

Youth with significant disabilities have been excluded from regular opportunities in the community, partly as a result of the legal principle of LRE (least restrictive environment), which ties level of disability to type of setting (i.e., home, school, work) and to restrictions of rights (Taylor, 1988; Taylor, Racino, Knoll, & Lutfiyya, 1987). Supporting youth with disabilities to live their own lives as contributing members of society means moving away from continuum and facility-based services as frameworks for service and policy designs (Racino & Knoll, 1986).

Community approaches to personal assistance are sometimes considered in terms of access to the community and opening doors to give people a chance. Another way to approach community access is as social, participatory, and leadership access (i.e., more than changing physical access in the ways that cities and communities approach areas such as streets and traffic lights) (see also Racino, 1995a).

LIFESTYLES OF YOUTH WITH DISABILITIES

A key objective of personal assistance is to assist youth to live lifestyles of their own choosing and to support the creation of better and more diverse options (see also Racino, 1995a, for another separate line of research [e.g., recreation and interest development] and field development). Personal assistance can be a means to "afford all people with disabilities the opportunity to live, work, go to school and be [with] friends and family" in communities (Stewart, 1991, p. 71). The lifestyles of young people go beyond the day-to-day aspects of home and family life, extending to school; friendships and social life; recreation; careers; jobs and business; and ethical, spiritual, and political development.

Adolescent "programs" and "interventions" have tended to emphasize disability more than the "normal" growth and development of adolescents (e.g., relationships, sexual development, freedom from adult supervision). Adolescents are starting to define "who they are and what they'll become as adults" (Schleiper, 1990). They are exploring their feelings and values, trying to determine what a "good" adult life will mean, and are beginning to "criticize their parents' weaknesses." Healthy development of youth with or without disabilities includes: how to choose among goals, how to persevere, how to have patience, how to recognize the challenges of life and enjoy meeting them (Moreillon, 1992), and to develop a sense of "independence of spirit" (Deegan, 1992) and of community.

People First

One way people with mental retardation have come together is in self-advocacy groups, which are run by people with disabilities so that people will have opportunities to learn to speak up for ourselves and to work on issues such as transportation, personal attendants, and a circle of friends. Self-advocacy groups are organized on the local, state, national, and international levels with the international conference held in Canada and the national conference held in Virginia in 1994.

Several of the concerns expressed by people involved in self-advocacy are the use of the term *mental retardation* as a label that reflects negatively on the person and his or her capacities and opportunities, abuse and the failure to take reports of it seriously, lack of staff support for activities that the individual wants to participate in, lack of freedom to come and go, individualized service plans that are broken promises, the loss of benefits when working, lack of money for clothes and equipment (e.g., communication devices, computers), and the lack of affordable and available transportation for work and recreation. Homes, careers, jobs, marriage, and families (including adoption) are also on some self-advocacy agendas (e.g., Racino, 1993a).

Transition to Adulthood

Personal assistance can be framed in the context of everyday life and the transition of youth to the complexities of adulthood (for adult living roles, see Frey & Nieuwenhuijsen, 1992). Transition of and/or by adolescents with disabilities in both rehabilitation and education has emphasized the movement from school to adult services, and especially employment and interagency coordination. Adolescent health care focuses on personal transitions (e.g., self-determination) and transition from pediatric to adult health care (Blum et al., 1993). This section briefly highlights transitions from personal perspectives (versus institutional or organizational transitions).

Home and School Life   At home and in school, adolescents may or may not be asked how they feel about their lives. They may or may not have opportunities to develop their own ideas about where they want to live or with whom they want to work as they grow older. Parents may also be expected to provide assistance to their children, including when they participate in activities with teen-age peers. Youth may be exploring what adulthood means within the school context, with assistants often responsible to teachers instead of to the students.

Work, Careers, and Politics   Adolescents are investigating the world of work (career development) through membership in clubs and other organizations; sports; enrolling (often forms of team approaches in the business sector) in courses that enlarge their knowledge of various occupations and/or of life; and, for young women, learning about nontraditional careers. Adolescents may also be learning good work habits and handling an allowance at home; gaining entrepreneurial skills for future success (Jones, 1995); becoming involved with political issues such as poverty, taxes, and education (Tabitha, 1995); and dealing with comparisons to their peers without disabilities.

Parenting, Sexuality, and Marriage   Youth with and without disabilities are also exploring their sexuality; developing gendered, ethnic, and cultural identities; and considering starting families of their own. One of the greatest barriers that parents with mental retardation face is societal prejudice regarding their capacity to raise their children (Hayman, 1990). Youth are learning that adults with disabilities can and do raise their own children, sometimes without formal services but with assistance from families or friends; and at other times with the aid of agency support services (Peter, 1991; Ulmer, Webster, & McManus, 1991).

Recreation and Social Life   Adolescence is a time for developing an independent social life with other youth (i.e., having fun) and often expanding interests into unexplored areas. Youth may learn to drive (with implications for peer relationships); they may develop private and shared activities (e.g., music, art) that may be lifelong; they may begin to form social habits (e.g., social drinking [Susser, 1995]); and they may participate in extracurricular activities after school (e.g., drama, science clubs, nursing, youth interest groups) and in community organizations (e.g., YMCA/YWCA).

Options for Housing, Recreation, Education, and Employment

Developments in the mental retardation and developmental disabilities fields have proceeded along separate pathways in the areas of housing, recreation, education, and employment. Typically, the emphasis has been on development of supportive program models such as supported living (e.g., Smith, 1990) and supported housing (Carling, 1993), and supported employment (Wehman et al., 1991). These approaches are inclusive of people with significant disabilities such as mental retardation, physical and sensory disabilities, technological needs, and secondary disabilities (e.g., substance abuse, psychiatric disturbances).

Housing

This is my own pad. I have my own keys and I come and go as I please. . . . I come home and sit if I want to. (Racino, 1993b)[2]

In the 1990s, principles based on community membership and personal autonomy framed new housing and support options (Ostroff & Racino, 1991) for diverse groups of people with disabilities (e.g., Research and Training Center on Accessible Housing, 1993; Research and Training Center on Community Integration, 1990). This movement toward regular housing with support has included people who were previously confined to institutions (e.g., nursing homes, intermediate care facilities, state institutions) or facility-based services (e.g., group homes or supervised apartments) and were considered to be "too disabled" to live in their own homes with support services. The Research and Training Center on Accessible Housing has prepared a set of "Principles for the Creation of Housing and Support," as follows[3]:

1. **Increased personal autonomy of people with disabilities in their choice of housing and support.**
    People with disabilities, like other citizens (and families), should have an opportunity to choose from a variety of options in housing types, locations, living arrangements, and support resources.
2. **Community inclusion of people with disabilities to increase full participation in all aspects of home, neighborhood and community life.**
    Self-management of cooperative living arrangements and involvement in

---

[2]The quotations from Racino (1993b) in this chapter are from adults with disabilities.

[3]These principles appear in Research and Training Center on Accessible Housing (1993). *Application to NIDRR for a National Housing and Support Coalition*, North Carolina State University; and a New York State policy paper prepared for the Department of Health, *Living in the Community: Toward Supportive Policies in Housing and Community Services*.

neighborhood associations and other support networks are promising methods for inclusion of people with disabilities (and families with children and
adolescents with disabilities).[4]

3. **Development of personalized and community support resources ranging
from natural supports (families, friends, and neighbors) to personal
assistance.**
Every person should have access to the support and assistance appropriate
to [his or her] needs and interests. Resources and delivery methods need to
maximize the personalization of support and the use of both natural and fee-
based supports generically available in the community.

4. **Reliance on generic (vs. specialized), affordable, and accessible (new construction and rehabilitation) housing integrated within communities and
neighborhoods.**
Housing needs to be focused on as a housing, not a disability, issue. Generic
housing options need to be accessible to all, provide a basic level of accessibility where feasible, and integrated in diverse neighborhoods. This should
include home modifications that permit young children (and adolescents)
with disabilities to remain in their family home rather than reside in a specialized care environment.

5. **Promotion of home ownership, universal design, and other approaches
and concepts which advance the inclusion of people with disabilities as
part of the normal fabric of community life.**
A full range of lease and home ownership options should be available, including single-family homes, condominiums, cooperative housing, and individual apartments. Universal design (Mace, Hardie, & Place, 1991) will be
encouraged for any new housing.

6. **Separation and coordination of housing and support services—and
financing of housing and support—at the individual, local and state level.**
The need for support should not determine the choice of home or the housing
type (e.g., skilled nursing facility). Similarly, funding for a particular facility
should not be tied to a particular facility or to funding for housing. Yet,
concerted efforts must also be made to coordinate housing and support resources. (Research and Training Center on Accessible Housing, 1993, pp.
6–8)

Adolescents will generally still be residing with their families in housing
in the community (e.g., single-family homes, condominiums, apartments,
cooperatives, mobile homes, duplexes, multifamily houses). However, in
some instances, older adolescents may have moved from family situations
(e.g., because of abuse), and in these instances, they may be living with
relatives, friends, extended family, roommates, or another family, with or
without supportive services. Adolescents may also be preparing to move
to their own places or other arrangements (e.g., shared apartments, another
family) and may have opportunities to explore other housing options in the
communities where they wish to reside.

---

[4]The author supports mixed-income, intergenerational housing associations;
these differ, for example, from segregated housing associations that have developed
in the United Kingdom (e.g., Racino et al., 1993).

Recreation

I can't imagine a first date and you're wondering about taking a personal assistant with you. (Racino, 1993b)

Recreation integration has been developed along three major lines: reverse mainstreaming (bringing youth without disabilities into activities and programs developed and funded for youth who have disabilities); inclusion of individuals with disabilities into community programs; and joint planning of programs between therapeutic recreation (or disability specialists) and generic recreation leaders (Schleien, Rynders, & Green, 1994). More recent innovations have focused on changing the nature and constraints of recreation places, and on mutual forms of community development. Recreation and community connections in the disability field have also been used as substitutes for the lack of paid employment (e.g., day treatment, habilitation).

Recreation can be considered part of the right to a normal life. Accordingly, community recreation may be accessible, affordable, and open to youth with disabilities. Youth with disabilities can be offered opportunities to develop their own interests (e.g., active sports like sailing, aerobics, fitness, swimming and skateboarding, dances and parties) and relationships outside the family. At the same time, the family may also have a natural opportunity to pursue their own activities and the things that need to get done (e.g., shopping).

Education

[The law] is very unfair to people like me who have been denied a good foundation, a basic elementary and high school education, against our will. (Racino, 1993b)

Three important concepts related to educational opportunities for *all* youth include approaches to inclusive schools for all children (Stainback & Stainback, 1990); a lifelong approach to learning; and reinterpretation of supports from the perspectives of children's interactions with each other and with "grownups" (Ferguson, Meyer, Jeanchild, Juniper, & Zingo, 1992). The latter discusses the role of the "inclusion facilitator," the development of collaborative and consultative relationships, and the theme of "effective inclusion depends on figuring out what to do with grownups." Transition to adult education, particularly for people who feel they have been denied basic education as children (e.g., through institutionalization), is also an expressed need.

Employment

I didn't have money and I didn't have a job either. At that time, it was hard to find jobs because there aren't that many out there . . . not many good jobs out there. (Racino, 1993b)

The primary approaches to employment outside of workshops have been the job coach model(s) of transitional and long-term supports (supported employment), the use of "natural supports" in the workplace, the changing of environments either in line with principles of quality management or of accepting workplaces that promote and/or practice social acceptance, and, more recently, the use of routine employer supports (e.g., employee assistance, child care, work at home) for employees with disabilities. The broadening of the roles of the job coach into social service areas on and off the job, increased choice in employment and addressing the systems barriers to choice, and the emphasis on "valued jobs" (Test, Keul, & Howell, 1993) and careers, and the implementation of the Americans with Disabilities Act (e.g., reasonable accommodations) (Mancuso, 1990) reflect changes occurring in the disability field, and to some extent, in the business sector.

SUPPORTS: WHEREVER YOUTH
LIVE, GO TO SCHOOL, WORK, AND PLAY
The multidimensional concept of support (e.g., actions, attitudes, values, personal experiences, relationship descriptor, standards and expectations, goals and accomplishments) (Racino & O'Connor, 1994) is reflected in the definition of *mental retardation* as described by the American Association on Mental Retardation (Luckasson et al., 1992). Community supports and services in the mental retardation and developmental disabilities fields are described in Table 25.1. Other ways of referring to supports are as social and informal supports, emotional and behavioral supports (Horner et al., 1990; Smull & Harrison, 1992), consumer-initiated supports, community supports, and cognitive supports. The term *personal assistance services* has also taken on broader meaning in political, social, economic, spiritual, and community life.

Personal Assistance Services for All: Youth at Risk
Personal assistance services (Litvak, Zukas, & Heumann, 1991) have been described as being for people of all ages, disabilities, ethnicities, cultures, and income levels. This includes families at risk; people with "dual diagnoses" (e.g., mental retardation and psychiatric disabilities); and youth with technological, communication, speech, medical, and hearing needs. Personal assistance can have a variety of meanings since "everyone has their own way of thinking about what personal assistance is all about" (Racino, 1996).

The concept of universal access is based, in part, on beliefs about the relationship of human beings to society, and about the ways in which societal acceptance and "rights" are understood. Universal access refers to how "everyone" should be treated. Both youth with disabilities and their families, as well as the organizations that support them, have been undervalued and underfunded (e.g., Jackson et al., 1993). (For instance, youth with Down syndrome may not be included in youth programs, or they may be included only with support services from disability agencies.)

On an individual level, personal assistance can enable youth, for example, to get involved in the community, to participate in youth activities independent of their families, to develop relationships with other teens (and people of diverse ages), to plan a career (and future lifestyle), to locate a job and attend school, to feel emotionally supported, to move away from abusive family situations, and to reduce time spent on some tasks in order to make available more time for other more valued or necessary activities.

YOUTH DECISION MAKING AND PERSONAL ASSISTANTS

Parents and caregivers vary in how they raise their children, in how decisions are made within the family structure, and in how outsiders (including paid and nonpaid professionals and volunteers) are invited into the home or to share other aspects of family and community life. The dynamics affect how support is offered (e.g., nature of who decides and how these tasks are accomplished) in the home, as well as in special recreational, employment, religious, and political areas of life for the youth and his or her family.

It is the nature of people—whether children, youth, or adults—to make mistakes, and parents retain some ethical, social, and legal responsibilities for the mistakes of their children. Adults with disabilities are at risk of being deemed incompetent or of being unfairly punished whenever a human mistake or problem occurs. This pattern begins in childhood, when an error made by the youth with a disability or expression of a difference in opinion may be ascribed to the disability. Addressing this prejudice is often complicated by the fact that youth with mental retardation may need assistance and support with decision making and communication.

Decision making can be considered a right in an individual's life, a recognition of his or her human dignity as central to happiness and freedom from coercion. One young adult, who identified herself as a self-advocate, described what she wanted:

> Just to get an apartment and a roommate, and maybe down the line find someone to marry and maybe adopt a child. . . . I think I would be a good mother. (Racino, 1993, p. 5)

At times, adults with mental retardation are seeking to contest guardianship and competency actions, including actions taken by their parents or legal guardians (G. Dybwad, personal communication, 1988) that may affect their opportunities to decide where they live, to manage their money, to develop relationships, and to start families of their own.

Information Access: One Basis for Life Decisions

Parents and extended families have diverse ways of raising their children, with some retaining control over information access, deciding that it is in the best interests of their children to limit their "right to know." Yet, access to information can be considered a right regardless of age or ability. As one supporter of personal assistance information access as part of a national study on the perspectives of consumer experts on PAS stated: "The children have a right to gain that knowledge" (Racino, 1995b, p. 7).

Information access forms the basis for decision making and "being able to think freely" and, as such, is central to young people's development into adulthood. According to one informant, simply being aware of personal assistance options "is a really big thing." Information access is also a safeguard for youth with disabilities—for example, against a guardian taking advantage of a person ("Just because someone's a legal guardian doesn't mean that they are going to do everything in the best interest of the person" [Racino, 1995b, p. 8]).

PAS and Independent Living Centers

The "independent living" idea holds that a person controls his or her personal assistants and has responsibility for hiring and firing them. Independent living centers, developed by people with disabilities throughout the United States and worldwide, may offer referral and registry services for PAS, provide or offer training for personal assistants, and assist in negotiations with assistants, if desired by the person with a disability. To foster individually defined lifestyles, the independent living ideal has been described as limiting externally imposed sets of rules regarding how personal assistance services are provided. Support services may also assist in the decision-making process, with the ideal in independent living of having decision-making assistance separate from the providing organizations.

Personal Assistants: Relationships with Youth   People have different expectations regarding the nature of their relationship with their personal assistant(s) (i.e., the people who assist the individual, as well as others in their lives, if they so desire). Some people expect or prefer a friendship/ camaraderie or a family-type relationship with an assistant, whereas others may want solely an employee–employer relationship. Some assistant relationships may be paid services, whereas others may be offered freely or nurtured by the youth and their family and friends.

Some adolescents might prefer personal assistants who are similar to them in age because of the possibility of similar interests; more natural integration into relationships with other teens with or without disabilities; overcoming prejudice regarding the unreasonableness of teens (Figueroa et al., 1991); the possibility of developing less of a caregiving relationship; and the perception of greater freedom.

At the same time, adults may be valued as personal assistants by adolescents because adults can serve as mentors "to help transmit both skills and values" between generations (Moreillon, 1992). A mentoring approach may be preferred by teens who place more value on the wisdom of life experiences of people who may or may not also have disabilities. Personal assistants can assist youth to move to adult lives without the dependence on parents that financial and support systems often still require.

SYSTEMS OF SUPPORT

What is clear is that lack of information and awareness across (state level) agencies is the norm, not the exception, for agencies and programs in this crucial area concerning youth with chronic conditions. (National Center for Youth with Disabilities, 1993, p. 24)

Changing beliefs, policies, and practices about personal assistance and community support have influenced support systems and services. Services integration is reflected in the movements toward better quality education, housing, employment, transportation and recreation, as well as in other areas of disability services. Integrated services delivery for youth and adolescents (National Conference of State Legislators, 1988) and integrated community health delivery (Bearinger & McAnarney, 1988) are other forms of services integration (see also integrated services systems and personal assistance, Racino, 1995a).

Service and systems integration have often been based on an integrated approach to planning, community-wide analyses of populations, bringing services to client-citizen, client-centered education in self-help, unification of administration, integration of professional concepts, and an evaluation of effectiveness of holistic approaches versus components alone (Mikulecky, 1974). However, a 1991 review of 20 years of services integration efforts indicated that these efforts have met with little success, particularly in terms of major institutional reform (U.S. Department of Health and Human Services, 1991).

The processes of change in U.S. society involve multiple institutions and organizations, of which people are a part and shape and form. Many of these organizations are reflected in communities and localities, and changes in state and federal structures (e.g., in regard to personnel and financing) must be considered in terms of these localities. The following are four principles related to change:

Community development as a way of thinking A shift needs to occur toward community development for all people. Housing, schools, employment, recreation, and cultural organizations can be shaped to reflect all the people in the community. "Community service financing should be understood in terms of community development in which local needs and resources are carefully assessed" (Hemp & Hayden, 1992).

Capacity building as a goal Development is an ongoing process requiring the formation of local coalitions that can flexibly adapt as experience occurs, guiding the ongoing capacity-building process. These processes reflect personal, associational, organizational, and community development.

State's role as supporting local efforts The primary role of the state is to guide and support local efforts and provide supporting mechanisms, such as financing, to make these possible. In many ways, current reform efforts involve a breaking down of these structures, which have taken control away from people on the local level.

User-driven outcomes One central outcome must be the development of income and other supports and services, as well as education, housing, employment, culture, and recreation that people want and need in society, based on individual definitions of quality of life.

Suggested Approaches to Change

A framework for change includes several approaches based on different beliefs about people and communities. All of these approaches can be considered person-centered approaches (but with a stronger self-determination component), whereby changes occur from the lives of individuals and preferences (e.g., Mount & Zwernik, 1988; O'Brien, 1987; Vandercook, York, & Forest, 1989). Characteristics of these five major approaches (advocacy and diversion from personal assistance services; user-directed approaches; agency-based approaches; community change approaches; and systems change approaches) are as follows:

Advocacy and Diversion from Services

- Independent information and public education (with access to children, youth, and adults, including those who have legal guardians, conservatorships, or payees)
- Advocacy "access" (e.g., for or by children, youth, and adults who are in danger of being deemed incompetent)
- Optional deterrents to paid service involvement (as distinct from payors and providers of services with conflicting interests)
- Nongovernmental supported components, inclusive of "integrated" options

User-Directed Approaches

- Strategic inclusionary future planning within a human ethics framework
- Age-based access (e.g., with youth with and without disabilities)
- Self-determination in the context of collaborative decision making
- Access to services for hiring, training, negotiating with, or terminating personal care assistants (not case management or brokerage)

- Direct funding access for service purchase (if desired)
- Quality of life and the role of services as defined by each person

Agency-Based Approaches

- Generic health care (e.g., home care agency), reform of disability and community agencies (e.g., employment, recreation)
- Access to management, coordination, and/or "cognitive support" as distinct from "access services" and provider organizations
- User-determined roles of paid services (inclusive of roles with family and friends)
- Changed relationships between service users and agencies (based upon perspectives of "support") and between agencies and communities
- Changed ways of thinking about "agency functions" and "agency mission" (e.g., "eligibility," "terminations," "training," "service plans," "goals," "staffing")

Community Change Approaches

- Community assistance approaches (e.g., city access to PCAs)
- Community and human ethics approaches (i.e., justice, honesty, freedom from harm)
- Community support (e.g., natural approaches of supporting one another)
- Creation of community environments (e.g., noncompetitive, "porous boundaries")

Systems Change Approaches

- An integrated nondisability/disability framework for U.S. public policy
- Health care reform (e.g., revised frameworks for prevention, integration of mental health and generic health, community health)
- Cross-disability (integrated human services) reform as interim step toward public policy reform
- Financing reform supporting nondisability/disability public policies

PROMISE OF THE FUTURE

Youth hold the promise of the future. Today youth with disabilities have opportunities that were not viewed as possible or achievable even in the mid-1980s. Personal assistance and support are potential avenues to changing the ways in which programs and institutions interact with youth, thus contributing to societal and community change. As Jackson et al. (1993) concluded, "Changes will be needed in all of the institutions interacting with youth; not just the health and education sectors, but also community youth-serving agencies, religious organizations, private industry, and the research community" (p. 189). As described in this chapter, these changes would affect how our public policies are framed; the ways in which housing, education, recreation, and employment are pursued; the ways support is offered; and, most important, the expectations that youth with disabilities and others hold for our future in the coming decades.

REFERENCES

Americans with Disabilities Act (ADA) of 1990, PL 101-336, 42 U.S.C. §§ 12101 et seq.

Bearinger, L.N., & McAnarney, E.R. (1988). Integrated community health delivery for youth: Study group report. *Journal of Adolescent Health, 9*(Suppl.6), 365–405.

Blum, R.W., Garell, D., Hodgman, C., Jorrissen, T., Okinow, N., Orr, D., & Slap, G. (1993). Transitions from child-centered to adult health-care systems for adolescents with chronic conditions. *Journal of Adolescent Health, 14,* 570–576.

Bradley, V.J., Ashbaugh, J.W., & Blaney, B. (Eds.). (1994). *Creating individual supports for people with developmental disabilities: A mandate for change at many levels.* Baltimore: Paul H. Brookes Publishing Co.

Carling, P. (1993). Housing and supports for persons with mental illness: Emerging approaches to research and practice. *Hospital and Community Psychiatry, 44*(5), 439–449.

Chaikind, S. (1992). Children and the ADA: The promise of tomorrow. *Exceptional Parent, 22*(2), M8–M10.

Consortium of Citizens with Disabilities. (1992). *Recommended policy directions for personal assistance services for Americans with disabilities.* Washington, DC: Author.

Craig, R., & Wright, B. (1988). *Mental health financing and programming.* Denver, CO: National Council on State Legislators.

Crocker, A. (1992). Data collection for the evaluation of mental retardation prevention activities: The fateful forty-three. *Mental Retardation, 30*(6), 303–317.

Deegan, P. (1992). The independent living movement and people with psychiatric disabilities: Taking back control of our own lives. *Psychosocial Rehabilitation Journal, 15*(3), 3–19.

Dunst, C., Trivette, C., Starnes, A., Hamby, D., & Gordon, N. (1993). *Building and evaluating family support initiatives: A national study of programs for persons with developmental disabilities.* Baltimore: Paul H. Brookes Publishing Co.

Ferguson, D., Meyer, G., Jeanchild, L., Juniper, L., & Zingo, J. (1992). Figuring out what to do with grownups: How teachers make inclusion "work" for students with disabilities. *Journal of The Association for Persons with Severe Handicaps, 17*(4), 218–226.

Figueroa, E., Kolasa, K., Horner, R., Murphy, M., Dent, M., Ausherman, J., & Irons, T. (1991). Attitudes, knowledge, and training of medical residents regarding adolescent health issues. *Journal of Adolescent Health, 12*(6), 443–449.

Frey, W., & Nieuwenhuijsen, E. (1992). *Nomenclature responsive to the goals of the Americans with Disabilities Act.* Lansing, MI: Disability Research Systems.

Hayman, R. (1990). Presumptions of justice, law, politics, and the mentally retarded parent. *Harvard Law Review, 103,* 1202–1271.

Hemp, R., & Hayden, M. (Eds.). (1992). Financing community services for persons with disabilities: State agency and community provider perspectives. *University of Minnesota Policy Research Brief, 4*(1).

Horner, R., Dunlap, G., Koegel, R., Carr, E., Sailor, W., Anderson, J., Albin, R., & O'Neil, R. (1990). Toward a technology of nonaversive behavioral support. *Journal of The Association for Persons with Severe Handicaps, 15*(3), 125–132.

Individuals with Disabilities Education Act (IDEA) of 1990, PL 101-476, 20 U.S.C. §§ 1400 *et seq.*

Jackson, A., Felner, R., Millstein, S., Pittman, K., & Selden, R. (1993). Adolescent development and educational policy: Strengths and weaknesses in the knowledge base. *Journal of Adolescent Health, 14*(3), 172–189.

Johnson, B. (1990). The changing roles of families in health care. *Children's Health Care, 19*(4), 234–241.

Johnson, T.Z. (1985). *Belonging to the community.* Madison, WI: Options in Community Living.

Jones, M. (1995). Smart cookies. *Working Woman, 91,* 50–52.

Knoll, J., Covert, S., Osuch, R., O'Connor, S., Agosta, J., & Blaney, B. (1990). *Family support services in the United States: An end of decade status report.* Cambridge, MA: Human Services Research Institute.

Lakin, C.K., Hayden, M.F., & Abery, B.H. (1994). An overview of the community living concept. In M.F. Hayden & B.H. Abery (Eds.), *Challenges for a service system in transition: Ensuring quality community experiences for persons with developmental disabilities* (pp. 3–22). Baltimore: Paul H. Brookes Publishing Co.

Litvak, S., Zukas, H., & Brown, S. (1991, Spring). A brief economy of personal assistance services. *Spinal Cord Injury Life, 3*–5.

Litvak, S., Zukas, H., & Heumann, J. (1991). *Attending to America: Personal assistance for supportive living.* Oakland, CA: World Institute on Disability.

Luckasson, R., Coulter, D.L., Polloway, E.A., Reiss, S., Schalock, R.L., Snell, M.E., Spitalnik, D.M., & Stark, J.A. (1992). *Mental retardation: Definition, classification and systems of supports.* Washington, DC: American Association on Mental Retardation.

Mace, R., Hardie, G., & Place, J. (1991). *Accessible environments: Toward universal design.* Raleigh, NC: Center for Accessible Housing.

Mancuso, L. (1990). Reasonable accommodations for workers with psychiatric disabilities. *Psychosocial Rehabilitation Journal, 14*(2), 3–19.

Marshall, C., Johnson, M., Martin, W., & Saravanhabhaven, R. (1992). The rehabilitation needs of American Indians with disabilities in an urban setting. *Journal of Rehabilitation, 58*(2), 13–21.

Mickulecky, T. (Ed.). (1974). *Human services integration.* Washington, DC: American Society for Public Administration.

Moreillon, J. (1992). Young people's perceptions of health and health care. *Journal of Adolescent Health, 13,* 420–430.

Mount, B., & Zwernik, K. (1988). *It's never too early, it's never too late: A booklet about personal futures planning.* St. Paul, MN: DD Case Management Project, Metropolitan Council.

National Center for Youth with Disabilities. (1993). *Teenagers at risk: A national perspective of state level services for adolescents with chronic illness and disability.* Minneapolis, MN: Author.

National Conference of State Legislators. (1988). *Mental health financing and programming.* Denver, CO: Author.

Nosek, M.A. (1989). *Personal assistance services in Japan: Effect of productivity and daily living among Japanese with severe physical disabilities.* Houston, TX: Baylor College of Medicine.

O'Brien, J. (1987). A guide to life-style planning: Using *The Activities Catalog* to integrate services and natural support systems. In B. Wilcox & G.T. Bellamy, *A comprehensive guide to* The Activities Catalog: *An alternative curriculum for youth and adults with severe disabilities* (pp. 175–189). Baltimore: Paul H. Brookes Publishing Co.

Ostroff, E., & Racino, J. (1991). *There's no place like home: Creating opportunities for housing that people want and control.* Seattle, WA: The Association for Persons with Severe Handicaps, Housing Subcommittee.

Peter, D. (1991). We began to listen. In S.J. Taylor, R. Bogdan, & J.A. Racino (Eds.), *Life in the community: Case studies of organizations supporting people with disabilities* (pp. 129–138). Baltimore: Paul H. Brookes Publishing Co.

Racino, J.A. (1991, September). *Personal assistance services for people with mental retardation.* Paper presented at the International Personal Assistance Symposium, Oakland, California.

Racino, J.A. (1992). Living in the community: Independence, support, and transition. In F. Rusch, L. Destefano, J. Chadsey-Rusch, L.A. Phelps, & E. Szymanski (Eds.), *Transition from school to adult life* (pp. 131–148). Sycamore, IL: Sycamore Publishing Co.

Racino, J.A. (1993a). *A qualitative study of self-advocacy and guardianship in New Hampshire.* Syracuse, NY: Community and Policy Studies.

Racino, J.A. (1993b, December). *Living in the community: Toward supportive policies in housing and community services* (Report prepared for the New York State Department of Health). Syracuse, NY: Community and Policy Studies.

Racino, J. (1994). Natural supports in school, at work and the community for people with severe disabilities [Book review]. *American Journal of Mental Retardation, 99,* 221–224.

Racino, J.A. (1995a). Personal assistance and personal support services for, by, and with adults, children, and youth with disabilities. *Journal of Vocational Rehabilitation, 5,* 205–211.

Racino, J.A. (1995b). *Personal assistance services for, by, and with youth with disabilities.* Syracuse, NY: Community and Policy Studies.

Racino, J.A. (1995c). *Personal assistance services for people with mental retardation and physical disabilities* (Report prepared for the World Institute on Disability, Oakland, California). Syracuse, NY: Community and Policy Studies.

Racino, J., & Knoll, J. (1986, September). Life in the community: Developing non-facility-based services. *TASH Newsletter, 6.*

Racino, J.A., & O'Connor, S. (1994). "A home of our own": Homes, neighborhoods, and personal connections. In M.F. Hayden & B.H. Abery (Eds.), *Challenges for a service system in transition: Ensuring quality community experiences for persons with developmental disabilities* (pp. 381–403). Baltimore: Paul H. Brookes Publishing Co.

Racino, J.A., Walker, P., O'Connor, S., & Taylor, S.J. (Eds.). (1993). *Housing, support, and community: Choices and strategies for adults with disabilities.* Baltimore: Paul H. Brookes Publishing Co.

Racino, J.A., with Whittico, P. (in press). Creating a community network for change: Self-advocacy and community employment. In P. Wehman & J. Kregel (Eds.), *Employment and careers for people with disabilities: A consumer-driven approach.* Baltimore: Paul H. Brookes Publishing Co.

Research and Training Center on Accessible Housing. (1993). *Application to NIDRR for a national housing and support coalition.* Raleigh: North Carolina State University.

Research and Training Center on Community Integration for Persons with Mental Retardation. (1990). *Principles for Research and Training Center on Community Integration* (Proposal to NIDRR). Syracuse, NY: Syracuse University.

Roberts, E., & O'Brien, J. (1993). Foreword. In J.A. Racino, P. Walker, S. O'Connor, & S.J. Taylor (Eds.), *Housing, support, and community: Choices and strat-*

egies for adults with disabilities (pp. xi–xii). Baltimore: Paul H. Brookes Publishing Co.

Rubin, S., & Millard, R. (1991). Ethical principles and American public policy and disability. *Journal of Rehabilitation, 57*(1), 13–16.

Schleien, S.J, Rynders, J.E., & Green, F.P. (1994). Facilitating integration in recreation environments. In M.F. Hayden & B.H. Abery (Eds.), *Challenges for a service system in transition: Ensuring quality community experiences for persons with developmental disabilities* (pp. 121–145). Baltimore: Paul H. Brookes Publishing Co.

Schleifer, M. (1989). Family support: A right for all parents [Editorial]. *Exceptional Parent, 19*(4), 39.

Schleiper, M.J. (1990). "I began to hear complaints almost from the first day": Mobility and independence. *Exceptional Parent, 21*(6), 46–48.

Smith, G. (1990). *Supported living: New directions in services for people with developmental disabilities.* Alexandria, VA: National Association of State Mental Retardation Program Directors.

Smull, M., & Harrison, S.B. (1992). *Essential lifestyle planning.* Alexandria, VA: National Association of State Mental Retardation Program Directors.

Stainback, S., & Stainback, W. (Eds.). (1990). *Support networks for inclusive schooling: Interdependent integrated education.* Baltimore: Paul H. Brookes Publishing Co.

Stewart, L. (1991). Personal assistance services for people with psychiatric disabilities. In World Institute on Disability, *Personal and political perspectives on personal assistance.* Oakland, CA: World Institute on Disability.

Susser, M. (1995). The natural history of substance use as a guide to setting drug policy [Editorial]. *American Association of Public Health, 85*(1), 12–13.

Tabitha, S. (1995, February). Young people losing interest in politics. *Syracuse Herald Journal,* A12.

Taylor, S.J. (1988). Caught in the continuum: A critical analysis of the principle of the least restrictive environment. *Journal of The Association for Persons with Severe Handicaps, 13,* 45–53.

Taylor, S., & Racino, J.A. (1987, August). Common issues in family care. *TASH Newsletter.*

Taylor, S., Racino, J.A., Knoll, J., & Lutfiyya, Z. (1987). *The nonrestrictive environment: On community integration of persons with the most severe disabilities.* Syracuse, NY: Human Policy Press.

Taylor, S., Racino, J.A., & Walker, P. (1995). Inclusive community. In W. Stainback & S. Stainback (Eds.), *Controversial issues confronting special education: Divergent perspectives* (pp. 299–312). Needham, MA: Allyn & Bacon.

Test, D., Keul, P., & Howell, J. (1993). Community resource trainers: Meeting the challenge of providing quality supported employment follow-along services. *Journal of Rehabilitation, 59*(2), 40–44.

Ulmer, D., Webster, S., & McManus, N. (1991). *Cultivating competence: Models of support for families headed by parents with cognitive limitations.* Madison, WI: Waisman Center on Mental Retardation and Human Development.

U.S. Department of Health and Human Services. (1991). *Services integration: A twenty year retrospective.* Washington, DC: Author.

Vandercook, T., York, J., & Forest, M. (1989). The McGill Action Planning System (MAPS): A strategy for building vision. *Journal of The Association for Persons with Severe Handicaps, 14*(4), 218–226.

Wehman, P., Revell, G., Kregel, J., Kreutzer, J., Callahan, M., & Banks, D. (1991). Supported employment: An alternative model for vocational rehabilitation of persons with neurologic, psychiatric, and physical disabilities. *Archives of Physical Medicine, 72,* 101–105.

Appendix: Resource List

American Academy of Pediatrics
141 Northwest Point Boulevard
P.O. Box 927
Elk Grove Village, Illinois 60009-0927
(708) 228-5005

American Association on Mental Retardation (AAMR)
444 North Capitol Street, N.W.,
Suite 846
Washington, D.C. 20001
(202) 387-1968
(202) 387-2193 (Fax)

American Association of University Affiliated Programs for Persons with Developmental Disabilities
8430 Fenton Street, Suite 410
Silver Spring, Maryland 20910
(301) 588-8252
(301) 588-2842 (Fax)

American Civil Liberties Union (ACLU) Children's Rights Project
132 West 43rd Street
New York, New York 10036
(212) 944-9800
(212) 302-7035
(212) 921-7916 (Fax)

American Speech-Language-Hearing Association (ASHA)
1801 Rockville Pike
Rockville, Maryland 20852
(301) 897-5700 (Voice/TDD)
(301) 571-0457 (Fax)

Association of Birth Defect Children
827 Irma Street
Orlando, Florida 32803
800-313-ABDC
(407) 629-1466 (Phone and Fax)
(407) 245-7035

Association for Children with Down Syndrome
2616 Martin Avenue
Bellmore, New York 11710
(516) 221-4700
(516) 221-4311 (Fax)

Association on Higher Education and Disability (AHEAD)
P.O. Box 21192
Columbus, Ohio 43221
(614) 488-4972 (Voice/TTY)
(614) 488-1174 (Fax)

Boy Scouts of America
1325 Walnut Hill Lane
Irving, Texas 75062
(214) 580-2000

Canadian Association for Community Living
4700 Keele Street
Kinsmen Building
North York, Ontario, M3J 1P3
CANADA
(416) 661-9611
(416) 661-2023 (TDD)
(416) 661-5701 (Fax)

Canadian Down Syndrome Society
12837 76th Avenue, Suite 206
Surrey, British Columbia, V3W 2V3
CANADA
(604) 599-6009
(604) 599-6165 (Fax)

Canadian Rehabilitation Council for the Disabled
45 Sheppard Avenue East, Suite 801
Willowdale, Ontario, M2N 5W9
CANADA
(416) 250-7490
(416) 250-7490 (TDD)
(416) 229-1371 (Fax)

Christian Council on Persons with Disabilities
7120 West Dove Court
Milwaukee, Wisconsin 53223
(414) 357-6672 (Phone and Fax)

Clearinghouse on Disability Information
Office of Special Education and Rehabilitative Services (OSERS)
U.S. Department of Education
Switzer Building, Room 3132
Washington, D.C. 20202-2524
(202) 708-5366

CMR/Edward I. and Fannie L. Baker International Resource Center for Down Syndrome
1621 Euclid Avenue, Suite 514
Cleveland, Ohio 44115
(216) 621-5858
(216) 621-0221 (Fax)

Coalition on Sexuality and Disability, Inc.
122 East 23rd Street
New York, New York 10010
(212) 242-3900 (answering service; staff will return calls)

DIRECT LINK for the disABLED, Inc.
Post Office Box 1036
Solvang, California 93464
(805) 688-1603 (Voice/TDD)
(805) 686-5285 (Fax)

Council for Exceptional Children (CEC)
1920 Association Drive
Reston, Virginia 22091-1589
(703) 620-3660
(703) 264-9494 (Fax)

Disabilities Rights Education and Defense Fund (DREDF)
2212 Sixth Street
Berkeley, California 94710
(510) 644-2555 (Voice/TDD)
(510) 841-8645 (Fax)

Exceptional Parent
209 Harvard Street, Suite 303
Brookline, Massachusetts 02146
(617) 730-5800
(617) 730-8742 (Fax)
(617) 730-9856 (TDD)

Families of Children Under Stress (FOCUS)
3813 Briargreen Court
Doraville, Georgia 30340
(404) 934-7529

Federation for Children with Special Needs
95 Berkely Street, Suite 104
Boston, Massachusetts 02116
800-331-0688 (in Massachusetts only—Voice/TTY)
(617) 482-2915 (Voice/TTY)
(617) 695-2939 (Fax)

Fundación John Langdon Down A.C.
Selva 4
Insurgentes Cuicuilco
Delegación Coyoacán
04530 México D.F.
MEXICO
+52 (525) 666-85-80
+52 (525) 606-38-09 (Fax)

Girl Scouts of the U.S.A.
830 Third Avenue
New York, New York 10022
(212) 940-7500

Heart to Heart
1227 President Street, Suite 1B
Brooklyn, New York 11225
(718) 778-0525
(718) 774-5723 (Fax)

HEATH Resource Center, National Clearinghouse on Postsecondary Education for Individuals with Disabilities
One Dupont Circle, Suite 800
Washington, D.C. 20036-1193
800-54H-EATH
(202) 939-9320
(202) 833-4760 (Fax)

Independent Living Aids, Inc.
27 East Mall
Plainview, New York 11803
(516) 752-8080
(516) 752-3135 (Fax)

Institute for Child Behavior Research
4182 Adams Avenue
San Diego, California 92116

Job Accommodation Network (JAN)
West Virginia University
918 Chestnut Ridge Road, Suite 1
Post Office Box 6080
Morgantown, West Virginia 26506-6080
800-526-7234
800-ADA-WORK
800-526-2262 (Canada)
(304) 293-5407 (Fax)

Joseph P. Kennedy, Jr., Foundation
1350 New York Avenue, N.W.
Suite 500
Washington, D.C. 20005-4709
(202) 393-1250
(202) 737-1937 (Fax)

Keshet-Jewish Parents of Children with Special Needs
3525 West Peterson, Suite T-17
Chicago, Illinois 60659
(312) 588-0551
(312) 588-5825 (Fax)

March of Dimes Birth Defect Foundation
1275 Mamaroneck Avenue
White Plains, New York 10605
(914) 428-7100
(914) 428-8203 (Fax)

National Association of Developmental Disabilities Councils
1234 Massachusetts Avenue, N.W., Suite 103
Washington, D.C. 20005
(202) 347-1234
(202) 347-4023 (Fax)

National Association of Private Schools for Exceptional Children
1522 K Street, N.W., Suite 1032
Washington, D.C. 20005
(202) 408-3338
(202) 408-3340 (Fax)

National Association of Protection and Advocacy Systems
900 Second Street, N.E., Suite 221
Washington, D.C. 20002
(202) 408-9514
(202) 408-9520 (Fax)
(202) 408-9521 (TDD)

National Birth Defects Center
40 Second Avenue
Waltham, Massachusetts 02154
(617) 466-9555
(617) 487-2361 (Fax)

National Catholic Office for Persons with Disabilities
Post Office Box 29113
Washington, D.C. 20017
(202) 529-2933 (Voice/TDD)
(202) 529-4678 (Fax)

National Center for Education in Maternal and Child Health
38th and R Streets, N.W.
Washington, D.C. 20057
(202) 625-8400

National Center for Youth with Disabilities
University of Minnesota
Box 721
420 Delaware Street, S.E.
Minneapolis, Minnesota 55455-0392
(612) 626-2825
(612) 626-2134 (Fax)
(612) 624-3939 (TDD)

National Council on Independent Living
2111 Wilson Boulevard, Suite 405
Arlington, Virginia 22201
(703) 525-3406
(518) 274-1979
(703) 525-3409 (Fax)

National Down Syndrome Congress (NDSC)
1605 Chantilly Drive, Suite 250
Atlanta, Georgia 30324
800-232-6372
(404) 633-1555
(404) 633-2817 (Fax)

National Down Syndrome Society
666 Broadway, Suite 810
New York, New York 10012
800-221-4602
(212) 460-9330
(212) 979-2873 (Fax)

National Foundation of Dentistry for the Handicapped
1800 Glen Arm Place, Suite 500
Denver, Colorado 80202
(303) 298-9650
(303) 298-9649 (Fax)

National Foundation for Jewish Genetic Diseases
250 Park Avenue, Suite 1000
New York, New York 10177
(212) 371-1030

National Handicapped Sports
National Headquarters
451 Hungerford Drive, Suite 100
Rockville, Maryland 20850
(301) 393-7505
(301) 217-0963 (TDD)
(301) 217-0968 (Fax)

National Information Center for Children and Youth with Disabilities (NICHCY)
Post Office Box 1492
Washington, D.C. 20013
800-695-0285 (Voice/TDD)
(202) 884-8200
(202) 884-8441 (Fax)

National Information Center for Educational Media (NICEM)
P.O. Box 40130
Albuquerque, New Mexico 87196
(505) 265-3591
(505) 256-1080 (Fax)

National Information System and Clearinghouse Center for Developmental Disabilities
University of South Carolina
Benson Building
Columbia, South Carolina 29208
800-922-9234
800-922-1107 (in SC only)
800-777-6058 (Fax)

National Organization on Disability
910 16th Street, N.W., Suite 600
Washington, D.C. 20006
800-248-ABLE
(202) 293-5960
(301) 229-1187 (in Maryland only)
(301) 293-7999 (Fax)
(301) 293-5968 (TDD)

National Parent Network on Disabilities (NPND)
1600 Prince Street, Suite 115
Alexandria, Virginia 22314
(703) 684-NPND
(703) 684-6763 (Voice/TDD)
(703) 836-1232 (Fax)

National Rehabilitation Clearinghouse
816 West 6th Street
Oklahoma State University
Stillwater, Oklahoma 74078
(405) 624-7650
(405) 624-0695 (Fax)

National Rehabilitation Information Center
8455 Colesville Road
Silver Spring, Maryland 20910
800-346-2742
800-227-0216 (Voice/TDD)
(301) 588-9285 (Able Data)
(301) 587-1967 (Fax)

Parent Educational Advocacy Training Center
10340 Democracy Lane
Fairfax, Virginia 22030
(703) 691-7826 (Voice/TTY)
(703) 691-8148 (Fax)

President's Committee on Employment of People with Disabilities
1331 F Street, N.W.
Washington, D.C. 20004-1107
(202) 376-6200
(202) 376-6205 (TDD)
(202) 376-6219 (Fax)

President's Committee on Mental Retardation (PCMR)
330 Independence Avenue
Cohen Building, Room 5325
Washington, D.C. 20201
(202) 619-0634
(202) 205-9519

Sibling Information Network
The A.J. Pappanikou Center on Special Rehabilitation
62 Washington Street
Middletown, Connecticut 06457-2844
(860) 344-7500
(860) 344-7590 (TDD)
(860) 344-7595 (Fax)

Siblings for Significant Change
United Charities Building
105 East 22nd Street, Room 710
New York, New York 10010
(212) 420-0776
(212) 677-0696 (Fax)

Social Security Administration (SSA)
6401 Security Boulevard
Baltimore, Maryland 21235
(410) 965-7700

Special Olympics International
1325 G Street, N.W., Suite 500
Washington, D.C. 20005-4709
(202) 628-3630
(202) 824-0200 (Fax)

Special Recreation, Inc.
362 Koser Avenue
Iowa City, Iowa 52246-3038
(319) 337-7578
(319) 353-6808

**Team of Advocates for Special Kids
(TASK)**
100 West Cerritos Avenue
Anaheim, California 92805
(714) 533-TASK
(714) 533-2533 (Fax)

**Technical Assistance for Special
Populations Program (TASPP)**
National Center for Research in
Vocational Education
University of Illinois Site
345 Education Building
1310 South Sixth Street
Champaign, Illinois 61820
(217) 333-0807
(217) 244-5632 (Fax)

**The Arc (formerly Association for
Retarded Citizens of the United
States)**
500 East Border Street, Suite 300
Arlington, Texas 76010
800-433-5255
(817) 261-6003
(817) 277-0553 (TDD)
(817) 277-3491 (Fax)

**The Association for Persons with
Severe Handicaps (TASH)**
29 West Susquehanna Avenue
Suite 210
Baltimore, Maryland 21204
(410) 828-8274
(410) 828-6706 (Fax)

Index